Therapy of
Moderate-to-Severe Psoriasis

The National Psoriasis Foundation gratefully acknowledges the following corporations for their generous support in helping to make this project possible. The Psoriasis Foundation was solely responsible for all development and content.

Bristol-Myers Squibb Dermatology
Centocor
Genentech
Roche
Schering Corporation

Therapy of Moderate-to-Severe Psoriasis

Second Edition, Revised and Expanded

edited by

Gerald D. Weinstein
University of California, Irvine
College of Medicine
Irvine, California, U.S.A.

Alice B. Gottlieb
University of Medicine and Dentistry of
New Jersey–Robert Wood Johnson Medical School
New Brunswick, New Jersey, U.S.A.

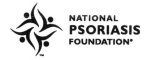

NATIONAL
PSORIASIS
FOUNDATION®

MARCEL DEKKER, INC.   NEW YORK · BASEL

The first edition was published by the National Psoriasis Foundation, 1993.

Library of Congress Cataloging-in-Publication Data
A catalog record for this book is available from the Library of Congress.

ISBN: 0-8247-4116-1

This book is printed on acid-free paper.

Headquarters
Marcel Dekker, Inc.
270 Madison Avenue, New York, NY 10016
tel: 212-696-9000; fax: 212-685-4540

Eastern Hemisphere Distribution
Marcel Dekker AG
Hutgasse 4, Postfach 812, CH-4001 Basel, Switzerland
tel: 41-61-260-6300; fax: 41-61-260-6333

World Wide Web
http://www.dekker.com

The publisher offers discounts on this book when ordered in bulk quantities. For more information, write to Special Sales/Professional Marketing at the headquarters address above.

Current printing (last digit):
10 9 8 7 6 5 4 3 2

PRINTED IN THE UNITED STATES OF AMERICA

Preface

Over the years, psoriasis has challenged physicians to achieve better control of this disease. Patients, however, must cope with its chronicity, appearance, psychological burden, expense, time-consuming treatments, and problematic therapeutic responses. Many patients—and even some physicians—have concluded that little can be done for psoriasis, but this attitude ignores the many treatment advances developed in recent years. Now, at the beginning of the 21st century, we are entering an era of many new drugs related to the immunological basis of psoriasis.

The goal of this book is to provide guidelines on state-of-the-art clinical management of moderate-to-severe psoriasis utilizing the experience of a group of experts well known in each area. There is also a chapter highlighting recent advances in our understanding of the clinical manifestations, epidemiology, and pathogenesis of the disorder. Several chapters discuss immunological aspects of psoriasis and the new group of immunomodulators or "biologics." The treatments covered include several types of ultraviolet B (UVB) phototherapy, photochemotherapy (psoralen/ultraviolet A; PUVA), methotrexate, retinoids, cyclosporine, and the first biologics likely to become available. Because pediatric patients and patients with psoriatic arthritis present special treatment problems, we have also included chapters on these patient populations. We hope that the reader will learn some new approaches to therapy or perhaps add some new wrinkles to old treatments that may improve the comfort of their patients.

We thank the distinguished clinicians who contributed to this book and especially the National Psoriasis Foundation (NPF) for sponsoring this undertaking. The NPF is the major lay advocacy group for psoriasis patients in the United States and provides outstanding services in patient education and research support. We urge all of you to join the NPF and to encourage your patients to join and reap the benefits of this organization.

Gerald D. Weinstein
Alice B. Gottlieb

Introduction

The National Psoriasis Foundation is pleased to present *Therapy of Moderate-to-Severe Psoriasis: Second Edition, Revised and Expanded,* a powerful tool that can assist you in providing the best care for your psoriasis patients. Leading experts in psoriasis and psoriatic arthritis have recently updated the chapters from the first edition and offer a concise, useful overview of the most commonly prescribed therapies for these diseases. New to this edition are chapters on the immunobiology of psoriasis and several of the new biological therapies planned for psoriasis.

Treating psoriasis can be frustrating, for both the physician and the patient. The National Psoriasis Foundation believes that caring, knowledgeable medical staff, combined with membership in the Foundation, are a winning combination to help people successfully manage their psoriasis and psoriatic arthritis. The following patient guidelines complement the clinical information found in this book.

I. WHY UNDERSTANDING THE PATIENT PERSPECTIVE IS SO IMPORTANT

Patients often have unrealistic expectations about how psoriasis treatment therapies should work, due to a lack of knowledge and widely conflicting information.

No treatment is universally effective.

The amount of time physicians have to spend with each patient is shrinking.

Alone, each of these things is frustrating, but the combination creates a situation in which treating psoriasis successfully and instilling hope in patients seems impossible. The National Psoriasis Foundation is committed to making it easier for patients to live with psoriasis and psoriatic arthritis by providing award-winning educational materials, support services, and advocacy. We give patients what they need to cope with the physical and emotional challenges of their disease. And for physicians, we offer the most comprehensive, cutting-edge diagnosis and disease treatment information available.

II. BEYOND THE TREATMENTS—TIPS FOR PATIENT SUCCESS

Since 1968, the National Psoriasis Foundation has served more than a million people with psoriasis and psoriatic arthritis. We've heard thousands of stories of success as well as of disappointment. We know what patients are seeking when it comes to treatment, and we know what makes for a successful outcome in a patient's eyes. Based on our extensive experience working with patients, and our involvement in research about their behavior, we offer the following tips.

A. Set Realistic Expectations

Addressing and clarifying patient expectations up front can have a dramatic impact on how patients view both their disease and you, the physician. Read these examples and ask yourself if they sound familiar.

A newly diagnosed patient walks into your office thinking you will dispense a cream that will make his "rash" go away permanently.

A patient tells you that the treatment you prescribed during her last visit doesn't work—she used it for one week (not the month you prescribed) before giving up because of slow or inadequate results and now wants something that "works."

A patient has been to 10 dermatologists in 20 years for his psoriasis, without ever finding an effective treatment that works—he thinks he's tried everything but "everything" has actually been only an impressive array of topical steroids.

We have heard these stories, and so have you. Many patients don't know the simple facts about their disease and have unrealistic expectations about what their physician can and can't do for them. Communicating the following key points can mean the difference between a compliant and optimistic patient and a frustrated and dissatisfied one.

Explain that psoriasis is chronic—something they will likely have (on and off) for life, requiring lifelong management.

Communicate that many treatment options are available and explain that you will work with them to find one that works best for them.

Reinforce that although not every treatment is effective, compliance can mean the difference between no results and very good results, including clearance.

B. Understand the Psychosocial Impact and Treat with Compassion

Psoriasis creates a significant stigma for many patients. The emotional impact of the disease can range from embarrassment to extreme shame. Understanding how psoriasis affects patients emotionally is paramount to the success of the physician–patient relationship.

The number-one complaint from psoriasis patients about their dermatologist is not that the doctor didn't "fix" their disease. Instead, patients feel most frustrated that their doctor didn't listen or didn't seem to care. Whether you are the first doctor they have seen for their psoriasis or the 20th, you can make a significant and valuable impact on how psoriasis patients view themselves, their disease, and you, the physician.

Here are a few simple things that demonstrate to your psoriasis patients that you care.

Acknowledge and validate the patients' feelings.

Touch their skin—patients often tell us their physician never touched their psoriasis or even looked at their skin.

Don't imply that their disease is insignificant.

Direct them to the National Psoriasis Foundation for additional support.

C. Partner with the National Psoriasis Foundation

The Foundation is the leading organization dedicated to improving the quality of life of people who have psoriasis and psoriatic arthritis. We can help make your job easier in a variety of ways.

1. Patient Education

> www.psoriasis.org (The National Psoriasis Foundation's Website).
> (800) 723-9166, toll-free support for patients and medical professionals.
> Easy-to-understand patient education on a variety of psoriasis-specific topics.

2. Emotional Support and Referrals

> Patient education and support specialists to speak with patients and lead them to the appropriate resources: (800) 723-9166.
> Programs that connect psoriasis patients—there is no better support than connecting with someone who knows exactly what you are going through.

3. Insurance Advocacy

> The Foundation educates insurance companies about psoriasis and the need for adequate and prompt reimbursement for appropriate therapies.
> The Foundation creates individual appeals letters and illustrated educational materials designed to educate insurance companies.

4. Programs for Medical Professionals

> Annual meeting for chief residents to train dermatologists about psoriasis early in their careers.
> Training sessions on effective phototherapy techniques.
> Insightful information from medical experts in the *Psoriasis Forum*, a newsletter for National Psoriasis Foundation professional members.

D. Stay Educated

The National Psoriasis Foundation wants to be your partner in patient care. We hope that you find this manual helpful. We will continue to support you as we head into an exciting time of new hope and possibility for the psoriasis and psoriatic arthritis community.

For information about professional membership please contact the National Psoriasis Foundation at (800) 723-9166, or visit www.psoriasis.org

Thank you for partnering with us to improve the quality of life of people with psoriasis and psoriatic arthritis.

Contents

Contributors

Grace Bandow, M.D. Clinical Research Fellow, Department of Dermatology, University of California, San Francisco, San Francisco, California, U.S.A.

Madhu Battu, B.A. University of Michigan Medical School, Ann Arbor, Michigan, U.S.A.

Kristina P. Callis, M.D. Clinical Research Fellow, Department of Dermatology, University of Utah Health Sciences Center, Salt Lake City, Utah, U.S.A.

Charles N. Ellis, M.D. Professor and Associate Chair, Department of Dermatology, University of Michigan Medical School, Ann Arbor, Michigan, U.S.A.

Steven R. Feldman, M.D., Ph.D. Professor of Dermatology, Pathology, and Public Health Sciences, Wake Forest University School of Medicine, Winston-Salem, North Carolina, U.S.A.

Dafna D. Gladman, M.D., F.R.C.P.C. Professor of Medicine, University of Toronto, and Senior Scientist, Toronto Western Research Institute, and Centre for Prognosis Studies in the Rheumatic Diseases, University Health Network, Toronto Western Hospital, Toronto, Ontario, Canada

Alice B. Gottlieb, M.D., Ph.D. W. H. Conzen Chair in Clinical Pharmacology, Professor of Medicine, and Director, Clinical Research Center, University of Medicine and Dentistry of New Jersey–Robert Wood Johnson Medical School, New Brunswick, New Jersey, U.S.A.

John Koo, M.D. Professor and Vice Chair, Department of Dermatology, University of California, San Francisco, San Francisco, California, U.S.A.

Tanya Kormeili, M.D. Clinical Research Specialists, Santa Monica, and Division of Dermatology, UCLA School of Medicine, Los Angeles, California, U.S.A.

Gerald G. Krueger, M.D. Professor, Cumming Presidential Endowed Chair, Department of Dermatology, University of Utah Health Sciences Center, Salt Lake City, Utah, U.S.A.

Mark Lebwohl, M.D. Professor and Chairman, Department of Dermatology, Mount Sinai School of Medicine, New York, New York, U.S.A.

Craig L. Leonardi, M.D. Clinical Associate Professor, Department of Dermatology, St. Louis University School of Medicine, St. Louis, Missouri, U.S.A.

Peggy Lin, M.D. Department of Pediatrics, Children's Memorial Hospital and Northwestern University Feinberg School of Medicine, Chicago, Illinois, U.S.A.

Nicholas J. Lowe, M.D., F.R.C.P. Clinical Research Specialists, Santa Monica, and Clinical Professor, Division of Dermatology, UCLA School of Medicine, Los Angeles, California, U.S.A.

M. Alan Menter, M.D. Chief, Division of Dermatology, Baylor University Medical Center, Dallas, Texas, U.S.A.

Warwick L. Morison, M.D., F.R.C.P. Professor of Dermatology, Johns Hopkins Medical School, Baltimore, Maryland, U.S.A.

Amy S. Paller, M.D. Chair, Division of Dermatology, Children's Memorial Hospital and Professor of Pediatrics and Dermatology, Northwestern University Feinberg School of Medicine, Chicago, Illinois, U.S.A.

Rickie Patnaik, M.D. Clinical Research Specialists, Santa Monica, and Division of Dermatology, UCLA School of Medicine, Los Angeles, California, U.S.A.

Dalia Rizk, M.D. Clinical Research Specialists, Santa Monica, and Division of Dermatology, UCLA School of Medicine, Los Angeles, California, U.S.A.

Gerald D. Weinstein, M.D. Professor and Chairman, Department of Dermatology, University of California, Irvine, College of Medicine, Irvine, California, U.S.A.

Paul S. Yamauchi, M.D., Ph.D. Clinical Research Specialists, Santa Monica, and Division of Dermatology, UCLA School of Medicine, Los Angeles, California, U.S.A.

Therapy of
Moderate-to-Severe Psoriasis

1

An Overview of Psoriasis

Gerald D. Weinstein
University of California, Irvine, College of Medicine, Irvine, California, U.S.A.

M. Alan Menter
Baylor University Medical Center, Dallas, Texas, U.S.A.

I. INTRODUCTION

Psoriasis has traditionally been considered an inflammatory skin disorder of unknown etiology producing red scaly patches of mere cosmetic nuisance to patients. However, with recent knowledge gleaned from the immunopathogenesis and genetics of psoriasis together with what may be termed the biological revolution in therapy, all of which will be discussed in later chapters, psoriasis now has to be considered a dynamic, genetic, immunological, systemic disorder manifesting on the body surface as well as in the joints in a significant proportion of patients. Patients and dermatologists alike thus need to shift their focus from considering psoriasis as a mere skin disease likely to be controlled with topical therapy to a condition no different from other immune-mediated disorders such as Crohn's disease, rheumatoid arthritis, and lupus erythematosus, all of which have a vast range of clinical manifestations. Just as the full spectrum of these disorders of the immune system need to be carefully considered, so too does psoriasis need a careful clinical evaluation, taking into account the extent of disease, the form of the disease, and quality of life issues for each individual patient as well as the potential for coexistent psoriatic joint disease. All of this, particularly on an initial patient visit, will not be accomplished in a 5–10 min patient encounter. It will require time and dedication from the physician and his or her support staff to improve patient compliance as well as the disappointment factor currently prevalent in the psoriatic population. Never has psoriasis been so much at the forefront; the buzz among researchers, clinicians, and indeed patients with the advent of new therapies, is palpable. It behooves us as dermatologists to rise to the challenge, refocus our energies and thought processes to the treatment of this most prevalent of all immune-mediated diseases, and take center stage along with our rheumatology and gastro-enterology colleagues in biotechnology, target-based therapeutics. Certainly, we will continue to utilize the full therapeutic armamentarium currently available to us, as will be discussed later in this chapter. The explosion of this new knowledge, and with it new therapeutics, will enable patients and physicians alike to tailor therapy to individual forms of psoriasis as well as to individual patient needs.

II. CLINICAL MANIFESTATIONS

Psoriasis is defined by the Committee on Guidelines of Care and the Task Force on Psoriasis of the American Academy of Dermatology as follows: "A chronic skin disease that is classically characterized by thickened, red areas of skin covered with silvery scales" (1). The extent of skin involvement can range from discrete, localized areas to generalized body involvement. The joints, nails, and mucous membranes may also be affected with the disease. "Psoriasis has a tremendous range of phenotypic variability," with a range of clinical manifestations from mild disease with a few isolated discoid plaques to multiple different morphological variants together with more serious forms of the disease involving major portions of the body surface, and, finally, coexistent psoriatic joint disease. Psoriasis may be symptomatic throughout one's lifetime, may progress with age, or may wax and wane in severity. The disease may be readily apparent to others and cause functional impairment, disfigurement, and emotional distress out of all proportion to the actual extent of clinical disease. When severe, in the judgment of the patient, the effects of psoriasis can have a deleterious impact on work performance, social performance and acceptability, sexual function, and mental health. The diagnosis of psoriasis is normally relatively easy to make, although conditions such as cutaneous T-cell lymphoma (CTCL), mycosis fungoides, eczema, tinea infections, and secondary syphilis may occasionally cause confusion and should be considered in the differential diagnosis, particularly when patients' conditions fail to respond to traditional antipsoriatic therapy. A full medical, family, and personal history is likewise important (Table 1). The classic morphological variants are noted in Table 2.

While psoriasis normally remains true to form during one's lifetime with discoid plaques predominating, the whole range of morphological

Table 1 Important Factors in Patient's History

Medical history
  Chronic scaling of the ears
  Coexistent or previously diagnosed immune-mediated diseases
  Long-standing "dandruff"
  Atopy
  Pruritus ani or vulvae
  Associated joint problems
Family history
  Atopy
  Psoriasis
  Rheumatological disorders
Precipitating factors
  Antecedent infections, particularly streptococcal
  Stress (physical, emotional, or metabolic)
Medications (see Table 7)

Source: From Menter A, Barker J, Fonelli WN. Psoriasis in practice.
Lancet 1991; 338: 231–234.

subtypes may present in an individual patient either simultaneously or progressively with increasing age. Thus patients with palmar–plantar psoriasis may have no other clinical evidence of psoriasis, may have coexistent flexural psoriasis, or may have classic discoid plaque psoriasis involving a few anatomical sites or major portions of the body surface area. In addition, erythrodermic psoriasis also classically shows severe palmar–plantar involvement. It is likely that as we unravel the genetics of psoriasis (see below), this

Table 2 Morphological Variants of Psoriasis

Discoid
Elephantine
Erythrodermic
Flexural
Guttate
Palmar-plantar
Pustular
  Localized
  Generalized

Source: From Menter A, Barker J, Fonelli WN.
Psoriasis in practice. Lancet 1991; 338: 231–234.

Table 3 Classification of Psoriasis

Mild psoriasis	Disease does not alter the patient's quality of life
	Patients can minimize the impact of disease and may not require treatment.
	Treatments have no known serious risks (e.g., class 5 topical steroids)
	Generally less than 5% of body surface area is involved with disease.
Moderate psoriasis	Disease does alter the patient's quality of life.
	The patient expects therapy will improve quality of life.
	Therapies used for moderate disease have minimal risks, (i.e., although these therapies may be inconvenient, expensive, time-consuming, and less than totally effective, they are not recognized as having the potential for altering short- or long-term health).
	Generally between 2% and 20% of body surface area is involved with disease.
Severe psoriasis	Disease alters the patient's quality of life.
	Disease does not have a satisfactory response to treatments that have minimal risks.
	Patients are willing to accept life-altering side effects to achieve less disease or no disease.
	Generally more than 10% of body surface area is involved with disease.
	Other factors
	Patient's attitude about disease
	Location of disease (e.g., face, hands, fingernails, feet, genitals)
	Symptoms (e.g., pain, tightness, bleeding, or severe itching)
	Arthralgias/Arthritis

Source: Adapted from Ref. 2.

clinical range will have a genotypic basis. The recognition that psoriasis is a condition of wide clinical variability, just like lupus erythematosus, will make evident that what we call psoriasis is in reality an umbrella term for more than one disease with a similar histopathological picture of a hyperplastic epithelium, and an inflammatory cell infiltrate in both the epidermis and the dermis consisting predominantly of T lymphocytes. Before considering the various clinical forms and manifestations of psoriasis more specifically, it is worthwhile to review definitions of mild, moderate, and severe psoriasis.

Psoriasis has traditionally been classified purely on the basis of body surface area: mild corresponds to less than 5% body surface area, moderate psoriasis equals 5–15% body surface area, and severe psoriasis over 15–20% body surface area. Krueger et al. (2) attempted to revise these definitions to include not only body surface area involvement, but also quality of life issues as well as the patient's perception and his or her ability to withstand as well as deal with side effects relating to their individual treatments (see Table 3).

III. THE GENETICS OF PSORIASIS

A. Psoriasis Relating to Age of Onset

Traditionally, two distinct forms of psoriasis have been noted: Type I disease with early onset (before age of 40), likely genetic in origin: and Type II late-onset (over 40 years of age), less likely to be genetic. In a recent clinical and epidemiological study from Spain (3), 1774 patients were studied. In this population, the disease started at a wide range of ages, with a mean age of onset of 29.1 years, with a slight female preponderance for earlier age of onset. In accordance with other studies, over 60% of patients experienced their psoriasis before the age of 30. As in similar prior studies, this large cohort of patients confirmed the association of a positive family history (in up to 40% of patients) with early-onset psoriasis showing an increasing family history of disease. From a morphological point of view, the only significant relationship between the age of onset and clinical forms of the disease related to guttate psoriasis (more frequently seen in patients with early-onset psoriasis) and palmar–plantar pustular psoriasis (more prevalent in late-onset psoriasis). In addition, patients with the early-onset form tended to have more extensive disease and a more severe clinical course.

In a large series of patients followed at the University of Kiel, Germany, a bimodal age of onset of psoriasis was noted with one peak occurring in young patients (mean age 16–22 years), and a second peak occurring in older patients (mean age 57–60 years) (4), which are similar findings to the Spanish study. The features of psoriasis in these two patient groups, Type I and Type II disease, are summarized in Table 4.

Thus in the Kiel population, Type I psoriasis had a strong association with a human leukocyte antigen (HLA)-Cw6 genotype with 85% having this gene compared to 15% of Type II psoriatics. Overall, about 70% of psoriatics were classified as having Type I disease, with the clinical course of Type I psoriasis tending towards more severe involvement.

The genetic influence on psoriasis is best illustrated in twin studies comparing the development of this disorder in monozygotic and dizygotic twin pairs (5). In dizygotic (not genetically identical) twins, psoriasis was

Table 4 Characteristics of Type I and Type II Psoriasis

Characteristics	Type I	Type II
Age at onset	Peak around age 20	Peak around age 60
Family history	Common	Rare
HLA association	Cw6 definite, B13 and B17 probable	Rare
Clinical course	Tends towards more generalized refractory or severe disease	Milder

Source: Adapted from Ref. 4.

found in both individuals in about one-fourth of the pairs, whereas in monozygotic (genetically identical twins), psoriasis was found in both individuals in about two-thirds of the pairs. The significantly higher prevalence of psoriasis in identical twins strongly suggests a genetic component to its development. However, since in only one-third of identical twin pairs only one individual developed psoriasis, there is also an epigenetic influence on its expression. The genetic transmission of psoriasis has been evaluated in some families in which this trait occurs in a higher percentage of individuals (6). Its transmission in some of these families suggests that a dominant gene is responsible, but that, as in the twin studies, acquiring the gene does not always produce the condition (variable genetic penetrance). In large population studies, a clear grouping of psoriasis in families has been confirmed, but the transmission has not followed simple autosomal dominant or recessive patterns. It has thus been proposed that its inheritance in the broad population is multifactorial, combining both a genetic component and an environment influence.

B. Recent Research

Let us now consider the most recent research relating to the genetics of psoriasis. It has been known for years that there is a significant association between HLA and psoriasis, specifically, class I antigens HLA-B57, B13, Cw6, and Cw7, with HLA-Cw6 appearing to confer the highest risk. The first susceptibility locus at the distal end of chromosome 17 was described in 1994 in a publication in Science (7). This came about as a result of research at the National Psoriasis Tissue Bank based in Dallas at Baylor University Medical Center, sponsored by the National Psoriasis Foundation. In 1997, the Michigan-Kiel Group confirmed this susceptibility locus (8). In this study of 224 sib-pairs, Nair and colleagues found linkages in the HLA region as well as additional loci on chromosome 16q and chromosome 20p. Of interest was the overlap in the 16q region with a previously described locus for Crohn's disease: psoriasis appears more commonly in patients with Crohn's disease. Furthermore, an Italian group has shown a locus on chromosome 1: i.e., 1q21 (9). Drs. A. Bowcock (the discoverer of the original 17q locus) and Bhalerao in 1999 also confirmed this Italian finding (10). Other susceptibility loci have also been found on chromosomes 3 and 4 with no confirmation of these findings to date yet published for these two loci. The various psoriasis loci have been designated:

Psors1 = 6p
Psors2 = 17q
Psors3 = 4q
Psors4 = 1q
Psors5 = 3q

The majority of interest and work in this field of psoriasis genetics has been confined to Psors1 on chromosome 6p21.3, which is considered the most important locus for psoriasis susceptibility in the majority of populations studied. Fortunately in 1999, the full sequence and gene map of the human MHC was described (11). In a study from the United Kingdom published in *Lancet* in 1999 (12), the polymorphic S gene ("S for skin") that lies 160 kb telomeric of HLA-C showed significant evidence for gene linkage and disease association, thus supporting evidence that the S gene plays a major role in psoriasis susceptibility. This S gene encodes the corneodesmosin protein, which plays a role in epidermal differentiation as well as the adhesion of the stratum corneum. It was the authors' conclusion that the S gene was a more attractive potential candidate gene than HLA-C itself. Subsequently, other genes in this region including the HCR gene have been considered to play a role in the pathogenesis of psoriasis. Despite intensive investigation within and around this HLA-Cw6 region, the definitive candidate gene in this area has hitherto not been identified. More recent evidence suggests that the S gene (also called the CDSN gene) may not appear to account for disease suscept-ibility any better than HLA-Cw6 itself, as underscored by a recent paper in 2000 from the Michigan-Kiel group (13). In this paper, Nair and co-workers defined the psoriasis susceptibility gene as a 60 kb region between HLA-C and HCR, suggesting that this region is the region most likely to carry the disease allele at the 6p 21 locus.

Thus, in conclusion, to quote A. D. Burden in his 2000 review (14),

> Classical HLA loci are not themselves psoriasis genes, but by virtue of their position, are in strong linkage disequilibrium with a non-HLA

susceptibility locus. In addition, it is quite likely that different ethnic groups may have produced different disease-associated haplotypes which possibly could explain both the different HLA associations as well as the decreased incidence in the Chinese population as compared to the Caucasian population (15).

In summary, the identification of the specific gene/s for psoriasis has been narrowed, with multiple loci almost certainly implicated. Once a specific candidate gene on chromosome 6p21.3 (Psors1) is identified, potential interactions (epistasis) between this gene and other psoriatic loci previously discovered (Psors2–Psors5) appear likely to be confirmed. The collaboration between molecular geneticists around the world, under the sponsorship of the National Psoriasis Foundation, certainly is bearing fruit and the potential exists for the exact molecular defect underlying psoriasis susceptibility being discovered in the not too distant future.

IV. PATHOPHYSIOLOGY OF PSORIASIS

A. Epidermal Hyperproliferation

The histopathology of the psoriatic epidermis was always noted to have many mitoses. In 1963, Van Scott determined that there was a marked increase in mitoses per surface of psoriasis in comparison to the normal epidermis. He developed the concept called the hyperplasia of psoriasis (16). This information was then expanded in a series of studies using radioactive isotopic techniques to examine both static and dynamic aspects of psoriatic epidermal hyperproliferation. The data showed that the transit time of psoriatic basal cells moving upward to the beginning of the stratum corneum took only 2 days in comparison to the normal epidermis, which had a slower upward movement of about 12 days through a much thinner epidermis (17). Further studies using tritiated thymidine injected in vivo into psoriatic skin determined a cell cycle of approximately 37 h compared to about 300 h in normal skin (18). While finding that psoriatic cells were hyperproliferative, it did not reveal the mechanism(s) by which the skin would change its pattern of proliferation and conversion into the phenotype of psoriasis. However, it did suggest at least one reason why a drug such as methotrexate might be active in the treatment of this disease. Additional studies indicate that lymphocytes are more sensitive to methotrexate than epidermal cells, suggesting that methotrexate may affect at least two different cellular components of psoriatic tissue (19).

B. Immunology of Psoriasis

Since the mid-1980s, evidence has appeared that there might be an immunological component to the pathogenesis of psoriasis. This concept was
expanded by the serendipitous observation that patients receiving an immunosuppressive drug, cyclosporine, who also had psoriasis, found that their
skin disease was clearing. This is not unlike a similar serendipitous observation in 1951 that the folic acid antagonist, aminopterin (later replaced by
methotrexate) produced clearing of psoriasis. The immunological milieu of
psoriatic skin includes the presence of many T lymphocytes, particularly
CD4 + (helper) and CD8 + (suppressor/cytotoxic) cells. Related to these and
other cells, many cytokines were and are still being discovered that influence
the inflammatory aspects of psoriasis and trigger, directly or indirectly, the
hyperproliferation of psoriatic keratinocytes.

The science of immunology as it pertains to many diseases is now being
utilized to develop new therapeutic approaches to diseases including psoriasis, rheumatoid arthritis, psoriatic arthritis, multiple sclerosis, Crohn's
disease, and others. From research on the immunopathogenesis of psoriasis,
these findings are creating an extensive pipeline of new drugs described in this
book (20,21) (see Chapter 11).

V. CLINICAL MANIFESTATIONS

A. Scalp Psoriasis

The majority of patients with psoriasis will show evidence of scalp involvement. Despite the full range of therapeutic modalities now available, including topicals, light treatments, and systemic therapies including the new
biological agents, scalp psoriasis remains one of the most difficult areas to
control. Psoriasis is classically a highly symmetrical disease, but lesions on the
scalp are frequently asymmetrical, almost certainly related to the inevitable
koebnerization of scalp psoriasis due to the patient's picking, scratching, and
harsh shampooing. This leads to lichenified plaques with involvement usually
on the posterior scalp or above either ear (i.e., areas of easy accessibility).
When scalp psoriasis predominates with or without associated facial involvement, overlap with seborrheic dermatitis may produce the clinical variant
known as sebopsoriasis.

B. Guttate Psoriasis

This form is well known to most dermatologists, often presenting in young
adults or children with a prior history of a streptococcal throat infection.

Numerous other trigger factors, such as viral infections, medications, major stress episodes, and rapid discontinuation of systemic therapy (steroids, methotrexate, or cyclosporine) may also produce this inflammatory, papular form of psoriasis. In addition, patients with previous stable plaque psoriasis may experience, at intervals, guttate flares, either related to the aforementioned trigger factors or spontaneously. It is fortunate that pure guttate psoriasis is one of the forms of psoriasis most amenable to treatment with phototherapy and, if necessary with culture-proven streptococcal infection, concomitant antibiotics. Parents of children presenting with guttate psoriasis as a first indication of the condition should be counseled about the likelihood of more classic discoid-type psoriasis supervening in young adult life as well as the need to interact with their pediatrician for future interventions with subsequent upper respiratory infections, particularly streptococcal ones.

C. Discoid Plaque Psoriasis

This most common form of the disease usually presents as symmetrical plaques ranging in size from small coin-sized plaques to larger plaques that may coalesce to form large geographic areas (Fig. 1). As discussed in the definitions of mild, moderate and severe disease, it is essential to do a full-body evaluation of the patient's plaque involvement to ascertain whether topical therapy, for instance, is likely to be both of value as well as appropriate for each individual's needs and potential long-term compliance.

D. Erythrodermic Psoriasis

This inflammatory severe form of psoriasis, fortunately affecting only a minority of patients, is frequently precipitated by trigger factors such as infections, inappropriate systemic steroid usage, or burns incurred during phototherapy. Other trigger factors may relate to abrupt discontinuation of systemic therapy, particularly methotrexate and cyclosporine. It is important to differentiate other forms of erythroderma, particularly in patients with no known prior history of stable chronic plaque psoriasis. Thus, eczema of all forms, particularly atopic in nature, Sézary form of cutaneous T-cell lymphoma, pityriasis rubra pilaris, and drug-related causes may need to be differentiated. Despite the continued decrease in hospitalization of psoriasis patients, erythrodermic psoriasis is the one form of the disease that frequently necessitates inpatient therapy. In our experience, it is critical to rule out systemic sepsis prior to initiating specific antipsoriatic therapy since a certain proportion of patients will have staphylococcal sepsis. In fact, a

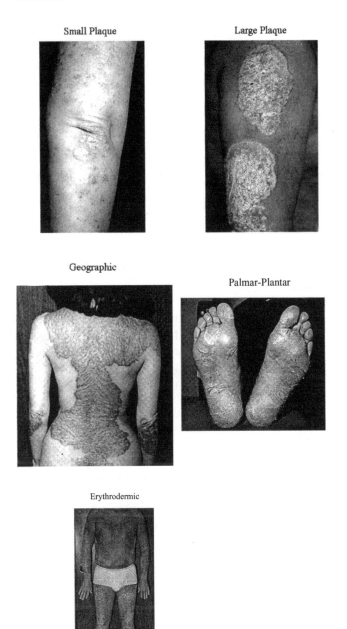

Small Plaque

Large Plaque

Geographic

Palmar-Plantar

Erythrodermic

Figure 1 Morphological variants of psoriasis: Is this one disease? (Refer to the color insert.)

recent referral to our clinic in Dallas was a young patient with prior stable plaque psoriasis well controlled on cyclosporin who experienced sudden worsening and increased inflammation. The dosage of cyclosporin was increased by his referring dermatologist to 5 mg/kg/day, despite which his psoriasis continued to worsen. Coagulase-positive *Staphylococcus* was cultured in his blood, on initiation of appropriate systemic antibiotics, his psoriasis responded dramatically with no further need for antipsoriatic therapy. Likewise, it is important to observe these patients for evidence of cardiac and renal failure, particularly in elderly patients in whom these organ systems may already be compromised. A certain proportion of these patients do respond to hospitalization and treatment with wet compresses, dilute topical steroids with or without occlusion, and supportive therapy, such as fluid balance control (22).

E.   Flexural Psoriasis

This form of psoriasis, like scalp psoriasis, is frequently resistant to traditional forms of therapy. In obese patients, areas such as breast folds and groin folds may frequently be complicated with secondary candidiasis necessitating specific anti-*Candida* therapy. In addition to standard antipsoriatic therapy, such as dilute topical steroids, the newer nonsteroidal topicals tacrolimus and pimecrolimus both appear to be effective in this location compared to their rather poor effect in other cutaneous sites except for the face.

F.   Palmar–Plantar Psoriasis

This is classically divided into the hyperkeratotic form and the pustular form. In many instances there is an overlap between these two polar types with fissuring, erythema, crusting, and pustules coexisting in individual patients, with or without evidence of cutaneous disease on other anatomical sites. Intensive topical therapy is frequently difficult. A significant proportion of patients have disease that is not well controlled on purely topical therapy leading to problems in quality of life, particularly in day-to-day activities, including ambulation, and manual activities. Many patients with this form of psoriasis will require systemic therapy and/or phototherapy.

G.   Psoriatic Arthritis

Why is it important that the dermatologist recognize this condition? First, psoriatic arthritis is far more common than has previously been considered (23). It has always been considered to affect only about 10% of patients with psoriasis, yet it is well known that over 35% of patients with psoriasis will complain of joint tenderness without necessarily having confirmed psoriatic arthritis. According to a recent National Psoriasis Foundation survey, up to 20% of patients may indeed have psoriatic arthritis. Psoriatic arthritis is often considered a relatively benign arthropathy associated with cutaneous psoriasis. However, it can frequently be debilitating and disabling, and, like rheumatoid arthritis, is frequently progressive leading to disability and eventual need for surgical intervention. Five clinical patterns of psoriatic arthritis have been recognized that can coexist with overlapping clinical expressions (Table 5).

Patients with distal interphalangeal (DIP) disease are likely to have psoriatic nail changes, and thus it is imperative that at all clinic visits the dermatologist inquire whether the patient has morning stiffness and/or joint pain or swelling elsewhere (Table 6).

While we do not ask all dermatologists to delineate the type or degree of psoriatic arthritis, because we are frequently the portal of entry for psoriatic patients, diagnosis by us and/or referral to our rheumatological colleagues may prevent further disability and progression of the disease. This is especially important with the array of medications, particularly the new biological agents, currently available.

Table 5 Classification of Psoriatic Arthritis: Types and Incidence

Type	Key clinical features	Incidence (%)
Asymmetrical polyarthritis or oligoarthritis	Morning stiffness, distal (DIP) and proximal interphalangeal (PIP) involvement, nail disease, ≤4 joints involved	> 47
Symmetrical polyarthritis	Simultaneous development of psoriasis and arthritis	25
Ankylosing spondylitis	Progressive low back pain, morning stiffness, sacroiliac and axial joint involvement	23
Distal interphalangeal joint disease	Nail and joint involvement (DIP) predominate	Rare
Arthritis mutilans	Destructive form of arthritis, telescoping, joint lysis, typically in phalanges and metacarpals	Rare

Source: Courtesy of Amgen Corporation.

Table 6 What is the Role of the Dermatologist in Identifying Psoriatic Arthritis?

No one expects dermatologists to be rheumatologists
However, dermatologists should be aware of, and vigilant for the arthritic
   component of psoriasis and refer as needed

Dermatologists should:

Examine for	*Ask about*
PIP and DIP involvement	Morning stiffness
Tender and/or swollen joints	Persistent joint pain or other arthritic symptoms
Nail involvement	Fluctuations of joint pain with exacerbations of psoriasis
	Family history of psoriatic arthritis

Source: Courtesy of Amgen Corporation.

VI. ITCHING IN PSORIASIS

Most major texts state that itching of psoriasis, while present in a fairly
significant proportion, is frequently mild in nature. Prevalence is frequently
higher in patients with more severe disease. In this regard, a study of 200
psoriasis patients found that 92% had pruritus at some time (24). In a study
of patients from a psoriasis outpatient clinic with significant plaque involvement, pruritus was a feature in 84% of 108 patients, being daily in 77% of
patients, weekly in 18% of patients, and less frequently in 5%. All body
sites were affected, with the back, legs, and arms the most commonly
involved. The face and neck were less commonly involved (25). Important
in this study was the fact that the pruritus in the majority of patients was
unresponsive to treatment with traditional antipruritics. Phototherapy also
did not significantly relieve the itch. Thus itching is a symptom, like many
other symptoms of psoriasis, that has a negative impact on the quality of
life in the majority of patients with psoriasis. This will be discussed in more
detail subsequently.

VII. FACTORS AFFECTING REMISSIONS AND FLARES

Since psoriasis is a chronic condition that often waxes and wanes in severity, it
is clearly desirable to identify factors that can worsen disease activity or
prolong the duration of therapy-induced remission. Much more is known
about circumstances under which psoriasis worsens than about favorable
conditions or treatments that will significantly extend a period of remission or

low-level disease activity. Presently many psoriatic patients are continued on standard therapeutic agents following clinical clearing of their disease in order to suppress recurrences (maintenance therapy). Other than maintenance therapy, there are no specific treatments for extending remission periods, except through efforts made to avoid skin injury or drugs for other therapies that will lead to worsening of psoriasis. Warm weather, summertime, and rest and relaxation in beach-type vacation environments may provide significant periods of improvement without accompanying medical treatments. The relaxation component may be the most significant part of the improvement in a stress-prone patient. Factors that have been shown to exacerbate psoriasis are summarized in Table 7.

Expression of active, lesional psoriasis is linked to mitotic and biochemical activation of both keratinocytes and immunological cells within a localized area of skin. Because both sets of cells are functionally activated by common cytokines, it is not surprising that psoriasis can be triggered by a variety of different stimuli that activate either epidermal keratinocytes or lymphocytes locally in skin. Any form of injury to the epidermis that triggers resting keratinocytes into a wound repair pathway can also trigger psoriasis in susceptible (Koebner-responsive) patients. Thus tape stripping, superficial or deep abrasions, lacerations, thermal burns, sunburns, or other physical injury can locally trigger psoriasis (26). In normal individuals, each of these forms of injury would lead to a transient period of altered epidermal activity (termed regenerative epidermal maturation) or an alternative pathway of keratinocyte differentiation that would repair the injury. In this regard, the difference between Koebner-responsive psoriatics and nonresponsive individuals is probably the ability to turn off or downregulate a physiologically relevant cell growth pathway. Another physiological cell-activation process that can occur locally in skin is delayed-type hypersensitivity local T-cell activation via antigen presentation by epidermal Langerhans cells. The most common expression of this pathway in skin is contact allergy to an external substance, but local immunity can also be triggered by focal skin infections, vaccinations, or reactions to systemic medications. Each of these conditions that activates cellular immunity has also been shown to cause a flare of psoriasis in some susceptible individuals. Flares of guttate psoriasis, especially in adolescents, are often attributed to antecedent pharyngeal infections with group A streptococci. Although the skin is not directly infected with this organism, systemic immunological activation may lead to increased T-cell activation in skin as the initiating reaction in a guttate flare. It should also be emphasized that widespread systemic immune dysfunction induced by human immunovirus (HIV) sometimes leads to a form of psoriasis that, paradoxically, worsens with decreasing T-cell counts (27).

Table 7   Factors that Can Induce or Exacerbate Psoriasis in Susceptible Individuals

---

Physical trauma to skin
  Superficial abrasion
  Blister
  Laceration/incision
  Thermal burn
Phototoxic reactions
  Solar
  Ultraviolet B
  PUVA-induced
Activation of local cellular immunity
  Contact allergens
  Immunizations in skin
  Infections in skin (bacterial or viral)
Systemic immunological activation or alteration
  Hypersensitivity to drug or other antigen
  Group A streptococcal infections
  HIV infection
Systemic drugs (probable action through pharmacological properties of the agent)
  Corticosteroids
  Interferons
  Lithium
  Antimalarials (chloroquine, hydroxychloroquine, quinacrine, quinidine)
  Beta-blockers (adrenergic receptor antagonists: many different agents both selective and nonselective)
  Nonsteroidal anti-inflammatory drugs
  Angiotensin-converting enzyme inhibitors
  Gemfibrozil and a number of other drugs in case reports
Emotional stress

Psoriasis can be exacerbated or induced in some susceptible individuals by a number of systemic drugs (28, 29). Drugs that have been reported to worsen psoriasis include lithium, β-adrenergic receptor blockers, antimalarials, nonsteroidal anti-inflammatory drugs, angiotensin-converting enzyme inhibitors, gemfibrozil, and corticosteroids (Table 7). In individuals with demonstrated or suspected worsening of psoriasis due to one of these agents, it is desirable to discontinue the suspected drug or to try an unrelated alternative if the patient's medical condition permits and other therapeutic options are available. Although systemic corticosteroids are occasionally used to treat psoriasis, the response in this regard is limited by significant exacerbation of baseline disease activity (termed rebound or flaring), including induction of pustular flares, following their discontinuation. Unless a concurrent medical condition dictates the need for systemic corticosteroids, their use in the treatment for psoriasis should be avoided because of their tendency to worsen psoriasis after withdrawal. In a study of 103 patients with generalized pustular psoriasis, over 30% had previously received treatment with oral steroids (30). Such exacerbations of psoriasis have also have been seen after extensive use of topical corticosteroids, particularly when they are applied under occlusion. Rebound and flaring of psoriasis following discontinuation of systemic corticosteroids are probably not obligate consequences of systemic immunological suppression, since psoriasis recurs without rebound or pustular flares less frequently following discontinuation of cyclosporine therapy.

VIII. STRATEGY OF THERAPY

The strategy of therapy starts with an educational process that informs the patient as to the nature of psoriasis and the therapeutic capabilities available today for the type and extent of disease in the particular patient. The initial visit with a patient will usually include consideration of topics that pertain to the current disease manifestations, exacerbating factors, familial hereditary concerns, and psychological factors (Table 8). The discussion soon reaches the major goal, which is to improve the patient's quality of life without producing undue harm medically, fiscally, or emotionally. The physician is challenged with presenting to the patient a realistic but, it is hoped, optimistic big picture of therapy, keeping in mind the chronicity of this disease. Extended therapy with any treatment leads to the potential for resistance and/or toxicity.

Table 8 Doctor–Patient Discussion of Psoriasis

Lesions/symptoms/diagnosis
Hereditary aspects
Systemic manifestations: arthritis
Exacerbating and favorable factors
Response to past treatments
Range of therapeutic options
Chronic long-term disease
Psychological ramifications
Optimism for tomorrow, new therapies in the pipeline

The therapeutic approaches to psoriasis today include topical or local medications, phototherapeutic modalities, and systemic drugs. The simplest and safest treatments are topical agents used primarily in patients with limited amounts of skin involvement. There is no precise definition of limited (or mild) disease. Our definition is that the location and amount of body surface area (BSA) affected can be practically and effectively treated with topical medications.

Quality of life comes into this consideration: smaller areas but those in critical areas (such as for employment or social appearance) may override consideration of a simple body surface area calculation (2). Topical therapy of BSA greater than 20% requires large quantities of medications with commensurate higher costs, time for applications, and inconvenience depending on the drug. Currently available topical therapy does not usually produce long-term clinical improvement. Patients with minimal disease undergo continual trials of different medications and accumulate a medicine chest filled with topical preparations. At some point, however, those frustrated patients with more disease (i.e., 10% or more BSA), or those unresponsive to topical therapy) become candidates for more aggressive forms of therapy, such as phototherapy and/or systemic drugs. In these patients, now defined as having moderate-to-severe disease, more effective therapies are, fortunately, available.

In 1993 a survey of American Academy of Dermatology members revealed that there were approximately 2.4 million visits annually to dermatologists by psoriatic patients, with each dermatologist seeing an average of 28 patients with psoriasis per month (31). Using a working definition of mild psoriasis as a patient being treated with topical therapy, 77% were estimated to have mild (limited) disease. The remainder of the patients received photo/systemic treatment and were considered to have moderate-to-severe disease. Other criteria frequently used to define moderate-to-severe disease are listed in Table 9.

In patients receiving topical therapy, corticosteroids are the choice of 85% of physicians. The remaining patients receive either topical calcipo-

Table 9 Working Definitions of Moderate-to-Severe Psoriasis

Greater than 20% of body surface area involved
Psoriasis not responsive to topical therapy
Extensive disease not economically feasible to treat topically
Psychologically stressful disease
Gainful employment prevented
Pustular or erythrodermic psoriasis

triene, topical tazarotene, or combinations of each with corticosteroids. See Chaps. 2 and 8. Within the steroid selection category, class I–II (potent-superpotent) steroids were chosen by 62% of the dermatologists and 37% selected the mid-potency compounds. Potent steroids generally produce good to excellent results, but the major problem is that these results do not persist for long periods of time. The survey information indicates that by 3 months after maximal improvement with steroids, relapse of disease is seen in about 50% of patients, even with continuing use of medication. The well-known phenomenon of tachyphylaxis somehow prevents the continuing responsiveness of psoriasis to topical steroids. Older therapies—tars and an-thralin—are much less effective than the potent steroids and are used less today. In summary, while the potent topical steroids may be reasonably effective for the treatment of psoriasis, their value is limited by lack of long-term remission and maintenance. The frequency with which patients carry bags of different topical medications into their physician's office testifies to this frustrating dilemma.

The moderate-to-severe psoriatic patient presents a much more inter-esting, satisfying, and valuable therapeutic challenge. There is probably no other extensive (noninfectious) dermatological disease that has available such an armamentarium of effective therapeutic approaches. There are at least se-ven forms of psoriasis therapy (Table 10) for which much information has been acquired. These treatments are the subject of this book.

It is interesting to consider the advances in therapy of psoriasis that have occurred in the last half-century. These advances represent approximately half of all the new medications that have been developed for our most common dermatological diseases to the present (Table 11).

In the treatment of moderate to severe psoriasis, there are some interesting concepts worth noting. The moderate/severe patient population comprises 20–25% of all the psoriatics seen in the average practice (31).

Table 10 Therapeutic Approaches to Moderate-to-Severe Psoriasis

---

Phototherapy:UVB with or without tar
Photochemotherapy
Methotrexate
Acitretin
Cyclosporine
Isotretinoin (pustular psoriasis)
Immunomodulatory drugs (biologicals)

Table 11 Major Dermatology Drug Discoveries

Pre 1950	**Tar/UVB**; penicillin, antibiotic era begins
1950s	**Corticosteroid** era begins, **methotrexate**, griseofulvin, antifungals, antihistamines
1960s	5-fluorouracil, topical retinoids
1970s	Retinoids (isotretinoin), **PUVA,** acyclovir
1980s	**Retinoids (etretinate, acitretin)**
1990s	**Cyclosporine, topical calcipotriene, topical tazarotene**
2000s	Tacrolimus, **"immunomodulatory drugs"**

Bold names indicate psoriasis therapies.
The bold therapies used for psoriasis represent half of the therapeutic medical advances in dermatology.

Estimates of which therapies dermatologists use are presented in Table 12. It is readily apparent that ultraviolet B (UVB) phototherapy with or without tar is the most frequently utilized modality. This is followed in frequency by psoralen combined with ultraviolet A phototherapy (PUVA) and methotrexate. The oral retinoid, etretinate, now acitretin, is used to a significantly lesser extent. Since cyclosporine was approved at about the time of the survey, its usage is probably significantly higher now than found in the survey. Several other treatments are used for occasional patients. The data also indicate that a small percentage of physicians continue to use systemic steroids in about one-third of their patients. The concern with this treatment is the number of patients presenting with pustular psoriasis associated with recent or continuing use of systemic steroids.

Table 12 Selection of Photo/Systemic Treatments for Moderate-to-Severe Psoriasis

Therapy	% Dermatologists using this form of treatment	Mean % of patients receiving this therapy
Goeckerman; UVB ± tar	82	62
PUVA	56	25
Methotrexate	56	22
Etretinate	43	9
Cyclosporine	3	2
Sulfasalazine	18	15
Systemic steroids	11	35
Other (referral out)	8	44

Source: From Ref. 31.

In treating patients with a chronic disease such as psoriasis, treatment effectiveness, duration of effectiveness, and safety are integral components of a treatment plan. As indicated earlier, topical steroids may have good short-term effects but long-term lesion clearance is far from satisfactory.

The surveyed dermatologists were asked for their perception of the effectiveness of topical therapy for mild psoriasis in comparison to the effectiveness of photo/systemic treatments for more extensive psoriasis. The criteria for judgment included both quality and duration of improvement. Each of the photo/systemic treatments was perceived to work *better* than topical steroids (Fig. 2). In a recent report, an analysis of multiple studies on the effectiveness of these therapies was performed (32). This report quantitates the clearance rates of available treatments (Fig. 3). One can conclude that the available topical forms of therapy are not yet as effective for psoriasis, lesion for lesion, as the photo/systemic modalities. Subsequent chapters in this book will describe in detail the quality and duration of improvement achieved by these treatments.

With moderate-to-severe psoriasis the assumption must be made that this disease will generally remain active in some form for much of the patient's

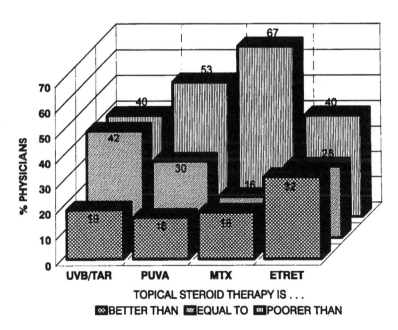

Figure 2   Comparison of efficacy of topical steroid therapy for mild psoriasis with photo/systemic therapy for widespread disease in the opinion of physicians surveyed. (From Ref. 31.)

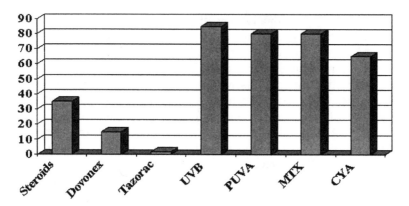

Figure 3 Clearance rate is not a realistic expectation of psoriasis treatment. (Courtesy of S. Feldman.)

future. Therapeutic planning must consider that the currently available treatments will be used for many years. Thus they must be used in a manner that will minimize long-term toxicity so that they can be safely used intermittently for possibly the remainder of the patient's life. For two of our major treatments, UVB with tar and methotrexate, we have clinical experience for over 70 and 50 years, respectively. Long-term experience with PUVA and the oral retinoids, etretinate and acitretin, is still being accumulated, while cyclosporine experience with psoriasis is about 10 years old. Unfortunately, all the current therapies are accompanied by toxicity to a greater or lesser extent. At some point during treatment, the therapeutic index for each therapy suggests that the risks may begin to outweigh the benefits. These risk factors appear to accumulate with continuing therapy, as seen, for example, in the liver changes accompanying large cumulative dosages of methotrexate or skin cancers following many PUVA treatments.

The development of long-term toxicity in patients receiving large amounts of individual treatments has led to the concept of periodically *rotating* the different available therapies (33). In this way, a patient would not remain on a specific medication for a long enough time to reach early levels of predictable toxicity, but instead would be switched to an alternative treatment. If one were to rotate these treatments at 1–3 year intervals (depending on the intensity of usage), it would theoretically take several years to return to the original drug or phototherapy (Fig. 4). By that time, after a several-year rest period off that treatment, some of the cumulative toxic effects in the body might have diminished. With such an approach one can hope to extend the useful and safe duration of therapy for many years. As

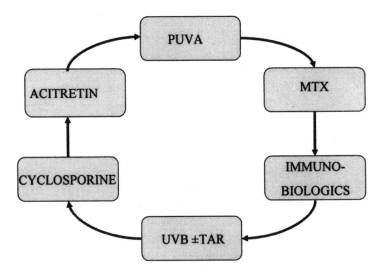

Figure 4 Multiple approaches to rotating available therapies for moderate-to-severe psoriasis. (Adapted from Ref. 33.)

new forms of therapy become available, which now includes cyclosporine and the newly available biologicals, the rotational circle then becomes larger and longer. (See Chap. 8).

Today, more than ever, the economics of therapy of a long-term disease psoriasis must be considered. Recent reports detail the annual costs of therapies for moderate-to-severe psoriasis (34). Outpatient forms of therapy range in cost from $1,400 to $6,600 (Table 13). Inpatient therapy, which is generally a modified form of the Goeckerman regimen, is substantially more expensive and is now used infrequently because of current health economic

Table 13 Mean Annual Costs of Psoriasis Care

Treatment	Total ($)	Lab Work	Drug
Outpatient Goeckerman (day-care setting)	3,914	0	0
PUVA	2,604	138	473
Outpatient UVB (3 times/wk)	1,966	0	0
Methotrexate	1,381	470	458
Etretinate	1,995	465	1,267
Cyclosporine	6,648	1,021	4,119

Source: From Ref. 34.

changes relating to hospitalization and length of stay issues. The overall costs of treating psoriasis may exceed $3 billion in the United States on an annual basis as of 1993, a figure that identifies psoriasis as a major health-care problem. Psoriasis, especially in those patients with moderate-to-severe disease, should not be viewed as a minor cosmetic problem.

IX. COUNSELING AND EDUCATION

As dermatologists we are faced with the very difficult and sensitive responsibility of discussing a chronically discomforting, cosmetically disfiguring disease. The physically discomforting problems of itching, dryness, irritation, fissuring, and a host of other symptoms are the more immediate difficulties that therapy is asked to overcome. The issue of cosmesis may be more distressing than anything else, leading to psychological difficulties because of an altered self-image. With new patients, particularly young adults who are socially distressed, it has always been of value to spend at least a short time discussing the emotional aspects of the disease. It often allows the patient to vent many pent-up feelings and frustrations to which the sympathetic physician can respond and offer encouragement. The availability of local support groups for psoriasis, and particularly the materials of the National Psoriasis Foundation, becomes very helpful. The patient needs optimism and education. Both of these needs can be discussed in terms of the considerable amount of research being done on psoriasis. The research has led to the development of several new therapies in the past 25 years, including PUVA, oral retinoids, cyclosporine, and the potential of the new immunomodulators or biologicals. As dermatologists accumulate more experience with each of the therapeutic modalities, additional patients with borderline severe disease may be included in the treatment groups for some of the drugs described in this book. With the basic mystery of psoriasis continuing to unravel and with more emphasis on immunological mechanisms, we are seeing new therapies that will attempt to interdict immunological pathways affecting the skin.

X. PSYCHOLOGICAL INTERVENTION

The physician's role is, and always has been, very much that of educator and psychotherapist. To know how to induce peace of mind in the patient and to enhance his or her faith in the healing powers of the health-care provider requires psychological knowledge and skills, not merely charisma (36, 37). The practitioner's sensitivity to changes in body image and to fears of social rejection, and a willingness to listen to and understand the familial, social, and sexual impact of the disorder aids the recovery of the whole person. Within this supportive context, encouragement is more readily received.

The relationship between stress and psoriasis has been investigated by Baughman and Sobel, (38) and by Arnetz et al. (39) among others. Cognitive interpretation (how stressful life events are perceived by each individual) may be a crucial factor in what constitutes what we call stress (40). Cognitive interpretation, as an intervening variable, mediating between stressful life events and somatic reactivity, may explain why some patients with psoriasis believe their disorder is caused or exacerbated by stress while others do not. Thus, patients in Baughman and Sobel's sample are described as stress reactors and nonstress reactors. In contrast, the Arnetz et al. study suggests that, during stressor exposure, the psoriatic group reported significantly higher strain levels "accompanied by higher levels of urinary adrenaline and lower levels of plasma cortisol."

The continuing "stress and psoriasis" controversy makes research into treatment programs that combine state-of-the-art dermatological therapy with psychological intervention worth investigating. Yet self-control strategies and/or psychotherapy are not generally incorporated into treatment. Relaxation training and psoriasis-specific guided imagery as adjuvant treatment to dermatological therapy have been investigated (41). Twenty-five subjects with severe psoriasis were randomly assigned to one of three treatment groups: PUVA only; PUVA plus a series of individual psychotherapy sessions; or PUVA plus a self-control strategy; psoriasis-specific relaxation training/guided imagery. Each patient in the two psychological intervention treatment conditions met individually with a psychologist each week for 7 weeks. The dependent measures were qualitative evaluation of psoriatic lesional severity, and quantitation of percentage of psoriatic body involvement. At the 3 month follow-up, PUVA plus *either* of the adjuvant psychological intervention treatment conditions produced significant differences ($p < 0.05$) in both qualitative and quantitative dermatological measurements, indicating better psoriatic status compared with PUVA treatment alone. Both the adjuvant psychological treatment groups showed 80–89% psoriatic improvement in qualitative and quantitative measures compared with pretreatment values, while the PUVA-only treatment conditions showed 58–60% improvement. The results suggest a useful place for adjuvant psychological intervention in the management of severe psoriasis. There is a strong need for further research in this area.

REFERENCES

1. Drake LA, Ceilley RI, Cornelison RL, Dinehart SM, Dorner W, Goltz RW, Graham GF, Hordinsky MK, Lewis CW, Pariser DM, et al. Guidelines of care for psoriasis. J Am Acad Dermatol 1993; 28:632–637.
2. Krueger GG, Feldman SR, Camisa C, Duvic M, Elder JT, Gottlieb AB, Koo J, Krueger JG, Lebwohl M, Lowe N, Menter A, Morison WL, Prystowsky JH, Shupack JL, Taylor JR, Weinstein GD, Barton TL, Rolstad T, Day RM. Two considerations for patients with psoriasis and their clinicians: what defines mild, moderate, and severe psoriasis? What constitutes a clinically significant improvement when treating psoriasis? J Am Acad Dermatol 2000; 43:281–285.
3. Ferrandiz C, Pujol RM, Garcia-Patos V, Bordas X, Smandia, JA. Psoriasis of early and late onset: a clinical and epidemiologic study from Spain. J Am Acad Dermatol 2002; 46:867–873.
4. Henseler T, Christophers E. Psoriasis of early and late onset: characteristics of two types of psoriasis vulgaris. J Am Acad Dermatol 1985; 13:450–456.
5. Farber EM, Nall ML, Epidemiology: Natural history and genetics. In: Roenigk HHJ, Maibach HI, eds. Psoriasis, 2nd ed. New York: Marcel Dekker, 1991:209–253.
6. Farber EM, Nall ML, Genetics of psoriasis: twin study. In: Farber EM, Cox AJ, eds. Psoriasis—Proceedings of the International Symposium. Stanford, CA: Stanford University Press, 1971:7–13.
7. Tomfohrde J, Silverman A, Barnes R, Fernandez-Vina MA, Young M, Lory D, Morris L, Wuepper KD, Stastny P, Menter A, Bowcock A. Gene for familial psoriasis susceptibility mapped to the distal end of chromosome 17q. Science 1994; 264:1141–1145.
8. Nair RP, Henseler T, Jenisch S, Stuart P, Bichakjiam CK, Lenk W, Westpahl, Guo SW, Christophers E, Voorhees JJ, Elder JT. Evidence for two psoriasis susceptibility loci (HLA and 17q) in two novel candidate regions (16q and 20p) by genome-wide scan. Hum Mol Genet 1997; 6:1349–1356.
9. Capon F, Novelli G, Semperini S, Clementi M, Nudo M, Vultaggio P, Mazzanti C, Gobello T, Botta A, Fabrizi G, Dallapiccola B. Searching for psoriasis susceptibility genes in italy: genome scan and evidence for a new locus to chromosome 1q. J Invest Dermatol 1999; 112:32–35.
10. Bhalerao J, Bowcock A. The genetics of psoriasis: a complex disorder of the skin and immune system. Hum Mol Genet 1999; 7:1537–1545.
11. Beck S, Geraghty D, Inoko H. Complete sequence and gene map of a human major histocompatibility complex. Macher 1999; 401:921–923.
12. Allen MH, Veal C, Faassen A, Powis SH, Vaughan RW, Trembath RC, Barker JN. A non-HLA gene within the MHC in psoriasis. Lancet 1999; 353:1589–1590.
13. Nair RP, Stuart P, Henseler T, Jenisch S, Chia NV, Westphal E, Schork NJ, Kim J, Lim HW, Christophers E, Voorhees JJ, Elder JT. Localization of psoriasis susceptibility locus. PSORS 1 to a 60 kilobase interval telomeric 2 HLA-C. Am J Hum Genet 2000; 66:1833–1844.

14. Burden AD. Identifying a gene for psoriasis on chromosome 6 (Psors1). Br J Dermatol 2000; 143:238–241.

15. Lin XR. Psoriasis in China. J Dermatol 1993; 20:746–755.

16. Van Scott EJ, Ekel TM. Kinetics of hyperplasia in psoriasis. Arch Dermatol 88:373–381.

17. Weinstein GD, Van Scott EJ. Turnover time of human normal and psoriatic epidermis by autoradiographic analysis. J Invest Dermatol 1966; 45:561–567.

18. Weinstein GD, McCullough JM, Ross PA. Cell kinetic basis for the pathophysiology of psoriasis. J Invest Dermatol 1985; 85:579–583.

19. Jeffes EWB III, McCullough JL, Pittelkow MR, McCormick A, Almanzor J, Lieu G, Dang M, Voss J, Schlotzhauer A, Weinstein GD. Methotrexate therapy of psoriasis: differential sensitivity of proliferating lymphoid and epithelial cells to the cytotoxic and growth-inhibitory effects of methotrexate. J Invest Derm 1995; 104:183–188.

20. Nickoloff BJ. The immunologic and genetic basis of psoriasis. Arch. Dermatol 1999; 135:1104–1110.

21. Gottlieb AB. Psoriasis: immunopathology and immunomodulation. Derm Clinics 2001; 19:649–657.

22. Boyd AS, Menter A. Erythrodermic psoriasis. Precipitating factors, course, and prognosis in 50 patients. J Am Acad Dermatol 1989; 985–991.

23. Gladman DD, Farewell VT, Nadeau C. Clinical indications of progression in psoriatic arthritis: multivariate relative risk model. J Rheumatol 1995; 22:675–679.

24. Newbold PCH. Pruritus in Psoriasis. In: Farber EM, Cox AJ, eds. Proceedings of the Second International Symposium. New York: Yorke Medical Books, 1977: 334–336.

25. Yosip OV, Itca G, Goon A, Wee J. The Prevalence and Clinical Characteristics of Pruritus Among Patients with extensive Psoriasis. Br J Dermatol 2000; 143:969–973.

26. Eyre RW, Krueger GG, Response to injury of skin involved and uninvolved with psoriasis, and its relation to disease activity: Koebner and 'reverse' Koebner reactions. Br J Dermatol 1982 Feb; 106:153–159.

27. Kaplan MH, Sadick N, McNutt NS, Dermatologic findings and manifestations of acquired immunodeficiency syndrome (AIDS). J Am Acad Dermatol 1987; 16:485–506.

28. Able EA, DiCicco LM, Orenberg EK, Fraki JE, Farber EM. Drugs in exacerbation of psoriasis. J Am Acad Dermatol 1986; 1007–1022.

29. Gilleaudeau P, Vallat VP, Carter DM. Arniotensim converting enzyme inhibitor as possible exacerbating drugs in psoriasis. J Am Acad Dermatol 1993; 28:490–492.

30. Baker H, Ryan T. Generalized pustular psoriasis: a clinical and epidemiological study of 103 cases. Br J Dermatol 1968; 80:771–773.

31. Liem W, McCullough JL, Weinstein GD. Effectiveness of topical therapy for psoriasis: results of a national survey. Cutis 1993; 55:306–310.

32. Al-Shevarden S, Feldman S. Clearance is not a realistic expectation of psoriasis treatment. J Am Acad Dermatol 42:796–802.
33. Weinstein GD, White GM. An approach to the treatment of moderate to severe psoriasis with rotational therapy. J Am Acad Dermatol 1993; 28:454–459.
34. Sander HM, Morris LF, Phillips CM, Harrison PE, Menter A. The annual cost of psoriasis. J Am Acad Dermatol 1993; 28:422–425.
35. Lee GC, Weinstein GD. Comparative cost effectiveness of different treatments for psoriasis. In: Rajagopalan R, Sherertz EF, Aderson RT, eds. Care and Management of Skin Diseases: Life Quality and Economic Impact, New York: Marcel Dekker, Inc. 21:269–298.
36. Section contributed by Marcia Z. Weinstein, Ph.D.
37. Engel GL. The need for a new medical model: a challenge for biomedicine. Science 1977; 196:4286.
38. Baugham R, Sobel R. Psoriasis, stress, and strain. Arch Dermatol 1971; 103:599–605.
39. Arnetz BB, Fjellner B, Eneroth P, Kallner A. Stress and psoriasis: psychoendocrine and metabolic reactions in psoriatic patients during standardized stressor exposure. Psychosom Med 1985; 47:528–541.
40. Lazarus RS. Psychological Stress and the Coping Process. New York: McGraw Hill, 1966.
41. Weinstein MZ. Psoriasis-specific relaxation training/guided imagery as adjuvant treatment for intractable psoriasis. Doctoral dissertation, Nova University, 1988.

2

Topical Agents in the Treatment of Moderate-to-Severe Psoriasis

Kristina P. Callis and Gerald G. Krueger
University of Utah Health Sciences Center, Salt Lake City, Utah, U.S.A.

I. INTRODUCTION

The topical treatment of psoriasis is firstline and mainstream in the United States. Topical agents are generally considered to be easy to administer, cost-effective, safe, and acceptable to patients. They are typically prescribed as the initial treatment when plaque psoriasis affects less than 20% of the body surface. However, for patients with moderate to severe disease, topical agents may not be appropriate or acceptable. Application to a large body surface area is time-consuming, expensive, and puts the patient at increased risk for systemic adverse effects. Cutaneous side effects may be intolerable over a large area. Topical agents can be messy and may look or feel unacceptable to the patient. Using quality-of-life parameters, response to treatment has been used to define severity; by this definition severe psoriasis does not have a satisfactory response to treatments that have minimal risks (1). Thus moderate-to-severe psoriasis may, by definition, be moderate to severe because it does not respond to topical agents.

Despite their limitations, topical therapies have a useful role in the treatment of moderate-to-severe psoriasis. Select patients may be able to clear their psoriasis and sustain the response with the use of topical agents. Realistically, however, most patients with moderate-to-severe psoriasis will not be able to enjoy clearance or long-term remission with topical agents alone. In these cases topical agents are more appropriately used by adding them to systemic or light-based therapies where they can augment effect, reduce cumulative dosages of systemic or light-based therapies, or treat recalcitrant areas. Following clearance with systemic therapies, topical agents may provide a bridge until systemic agents need to be reintroduced. Occasionally, patients with moderate-to-severe psoriasis will be unable or unwilling to use systemic agents, even when systemic agents may be more appropriate. Side effect profiles, laboratory monitoring, and costs related to systemic or phototherapy may be unacceptable to some patients. In these settings the physician is obliged to develop the most appropriate and efficacious topical regimen (Table 1).

This volume is not directed at treating mild psoriasis, thus the aim of this chapter is to assist in answering the following questions that arise when topical therapies are used to treat moderate-to-severe disease:

1. What are the most effective topical therapies for the treatment of psoriasis?
2. How should they be used?
3. What toxicities can be expected?
4. Which topical agents can be combined with others?
5. What are the most effective topical combinations?
6. Is there any advantage to combining topical therapy with systemic or phototherapy?

II. CORTICOSTEROIDS

Topical corticosteroids are the cornerstone of most topical psoriasis treatment regimens. Used as single agents, superpotent corticosteroids have the most potential to temporarily clear or nearly clear psoriatic plaques more effectively than other topical therapies. However, side effects such as atrophy and tachyphylaxis limit their quantity, duration, and location of use. This

Table 1 Indications for Use of Topical Therapies in Moderate-to-Severe Psoriasis

Initial treatment after determining severity, patient's desires (comfort only to complete clearing), ability and willingness to apply medication, and prior response to topical therapies
Maintenance therapy after clearance with topical and/or systemic agents
Combination therapy with oral agents or phototherapy for augmentation of effect, dose-sparing, or treatment of recalcitrant areas
Palliative therapy (i.e., patient comfort while awaiting onset of systemic therapy)
Initial, maintenance, or palliative therapy in patients unable or unwilling to use systemic agents

section will present strategies advocated to maximize efficacy and compliance while minimizing risks.

A. Pharmacology and Mechanism of Action

Corticosteroids act on psoriasis via anti-inflammatory, immunosuppressive, and antiproliferative properties. At the molecular level, corticosteroids act on gene transcription by forming complexes with receptors and binding to DNA to modulate transcription. Corticosteroids exert their anti-inflammatory actions by inhibiting the movement and function of leukocytes, reduction of dermal edema, and vascular permeability. T lymphocytes are particularly sensitive to the effects of corticosteroids. Corticosteroids cause reduced total circulating lymphocyte count and cytokine production. In the epidermis and dermis, corticosteroids inhibit the proliferation of keratinocytes and fibroblasts (2–5).

Topical corticosteroids are ranked in the Stoughton-Cornell classification, originally based on an assay of the corticosteroid's ability to cause vasoconstriction (6). The efficacy of most topical corticosteroids is generally well correlated with the potency (7–9). Potency of a corticosteroid is associated with its chemical modification, such as presence of an acetate moiety, its vehicle formulation, hydration status of the skin, and occlusion. Penetration is also enhanced in certain sites of application such as the eyelids and face (10).

B. Efficacy

The efficacy of superpotent (class I) corticosteroid ointments in the treatment of plaque type psoriasis is well established (11–14). Katz et al. showed that clobetasol-17-propionate and betamethasone dipropionate produced clearance or marked improvement in 75% and 80% of patients, respectively, treated for 3 weeks (15). In another study, the onset of therapeutic effect of halobetasol propionate 0.05% was demonstrated to occur within 5 days of starting treatment, and resulted in clearance or marked improvement in 88% of patients over a 4 week period, compared to 64% of patients treated with betamethasone valerate (12). The use of class II corticosteroids is less impressive: only 10% of patients achieve clearance with an average of 47% of patients achieving 75% improvement, (12, 16–18).

Other formulations of corticosteroids have proven efficacious and useful in treating psoriasis. Flurandrenolide tape (Cordran tape) applied once daily has been shown to produce > 75% improvement in 64% of patients over 4 weeks and found to be superior to diflorasone diacetate ointment applied twice daily over 4 weeks (14). This vehicle is particularly useful in the treatment of more lichenified plaques. Corticosteroids available as lotions, solutions, and foams are most effective for the treatment of scalp psoriasis. In one study, clobetasol scalp solution resulted in > 50% clearance in 81% of patients compared to placebo, with 26% of patients achieving complete clearance (19). More recently, betamethasone valerate (Luxiq) and clobetasol propionate (Olux) have become available in a foam vehicle. Betamethasone valerate foam cleared or nearly cleared scalp psoriasis in 72% of patients and was preferred by patients over the lotion vehicle (20). Clobetasol foam resulted in clearance or near-clearance of scalp psoriasis in 74% of patients in one study (21) and has also been shown to be efficacious in treatment body plaques (22).

C. Cutaneous Side Effects

The adverse effects of topical corticosteroids are well known and limit the frequency and continuity of treatment (Table 2). Cutaneous adverse events are the most common and usually occur when corticosteroids are used with excessive frequency or duration, or on steroid-sensitive sites such as the face or intertriginous areas. The same antiproliferative and antimitotic actions of topical corticosteroids that make them effective in psoriasis also contribute to

Table 2 Adverse Effects of Topical Corticosteroids

Cutaneous	Systemic
Irritation	HPA axis suppression
Burning	Cushing syndrome
Pruritus	Glaucoma
Atrophy of the skin	
Striae	
Telangectasia	
Acneiform eruption	
Rosacea	
Perioral dermatitis	
Folliculitis	
Infection (bacterial, fungal)	
Contact dermatitis	
Hypopigmentation	
Purpura/ecchymoses	
Folliculitis	
Rebound of psoriasis	
Tachyphylaxis	

their atrophogenic potential. Early signs of atrophy include visualization of the superficial vascular plexus (23). With further atrophy of the epidermis and dermis the skin becomes thin and fragile and is easily lacerated and bruised. Further loss of dermal elements leads to vascular dilatation with telangectasia formation and tearing of dermal connective tissue, causing irreversible, purplish striae. Acneiform eruptions may occur, particularly if high-potency agents are used on the face. Irritation may occur as a result of epidermal atrophy or intolerance to components of vehicle. Allergic contact dermatitis is rare, but has been reported (24). Rebound, or the abrupt worsening of psoriasis or the development of pustular psoriasis after discontinuation of topical steroids, has been observed, particularly when agents are applied under occlusion (25–27).

D. Systemic Side Effects

Although this is rarely clinically evident, topical corticosteroids can cause the same systemic side effects as systemically administered steroids. Hypothalamic–pituitary–adrenal (HPA) axis suppression can be demonstrated on laboratory testing after only 1–2 weeks of using moderate to superpotent corticosteroids, but is rarely clinically significant (28). Exacerbation of hyperglycemia, hyperglycuria, and hypertension may be seen. Iatrogenic Cushing syndrome (29) and osteonecrosis of the femoral head (30), both rare side effects of systemic corticosteroid use, have been reported from long-term topical steroid application. By virtue of their body surface involvement, patients with moderate to severe psoriasis require increased vigilance for systemic effects of corticosteroids.

E. Guidelines for Administration of Topical Corticosteroids in Moderate-to-Severe Psoriasis

1. Select the Appropriate Strength and Vehicle for the Body Surface

Superpotent corticosteroids are the most suitable choice for initial treatment of scalp and body surfaces excluding the face, axilla, groin, and genitals. Less than superpotent steroids are less likely to result in clearance but may be used if relief of symptoms is the treatment goal. Superpotent corticosteroids in an ointment vehicle are the most efficacious and appropriate choice for body plaques. However, patients frequently dislike the greasy nature of ointments. To improve compliance, a cream vehicle can be prescribed for morning dosing, for example, prior to dressing for work. Solutions and foams are the most acceptable formulations for scalp treatment.

2. Limit Frequency and Duration

If it is used as a single agent, continuous twice-daily application of a super potent corticosteroid should be, in accordance with Food and Drug Administration (FDA) approved package insert, limited to a 2-week course. How often these courses can be repeated safely and the length of the intervals between courses has never been clearly established. It is the authors' opinion that twice-daily application to nonintertriginous areas for 2 months will result in visible atrophy. When used once daily, onset of atrophy is delayed, but does occur, as early as 2–3 months. The scalp is more resistant to atrophy but it does occur; frequently telangiectasia precedes atrophy. Application on one or two consecutive days out of each week, known as pulse therapy, provides adequate maintenance in some patients However, maintenance therapy in combination with calcipotriene or tazarotene is more efficacious (see sections on these agents below).

3. Prescribe the Appropriate Quantity for the Frequency of Application and the Area to be Treated

Limiting quantities and refills, requiring frequent follow up and close observation, educating the patient, and combining corticosteroids with other non-steroid therapy will help maximize effectiveness of therapy and minimize side effects.

4. Monitor for Lack of Response: Tachyphylaxis and Compliance

One of the most frustrating aspects of treating psoriasis with topical corticosteroids is that over time their effectiveness wanes. This is frequently attributed to the phenomenon of tachyphylaxis, defined as the diminished or lack of response to an agent after repeated applications, which has been observed with corticosteroid application on normal skin (31, 32). However, in a study of 32 patients who applied betamethasone dipropionate twice daily for 12 weeks, tachyphylaxis was not observed (33). The authors suggested that lack of therapeutic efficacy and poor compliance may be responsible for what is perceived as tachyphylaxis. Carefully reviewing the patient's actual application practice is therefore imperative when evaluating lack of response. If tachyphylaxis is suspected, a break from corticosteroids is warranted. The time needed to recover from what is termed the tachyphylactic state is unknown. Likewise, there is no information that would indicate that, once tachyphylaxis develops, switching to a different steroid in the same class is of benefit. It is our prejudice that recovery from tachyphylaxis occurs in about 3 months and the topical corticosteroid will

Table 3 Selection of Topical Corticosteroids

Area of body	Strength	Examples of compounds/vehicles
Trunk and extremities	Class I	Clobetasol propionate ointment or cream 0.05%
		Halobetasol propionate ointment or cream 0.05%
		Betamethasone dipropionate ointment 0.05%
		Diflorasone diacetate ointment 0.05%
Scalp	Class I	Clobetasol propionate solution 0.05%
		Clobetasol propionate foam 0.05%
	Class IV	Betamethasone valerate foam or lotion 0.12%
Face, body folds, axilla, groin, genitals	Class V–VI	Hydrocortisone butyrate cream 0.1%
		Tridesilon cream 0.05%
Lichenified body plaques	Class I	Flurandrenolide tape

once again provide benefit. Once tachyphylaxis has occurred, it is likely to recur. If it develops with a lower-potency corticosteroid, switching to a more potent agent will likely restore, at least temporarily, the response. (See Table 3.)

III. CALCIPOTRIENE/CALCIPOTRIOL (DOVONEX, DAIVONEX)

Calcipotriene (known as calcipotriol outside the United States) is a vitamin D_3 analog that was developed after patients with psoriasis experienced improvement when treated with oral and topical calcitriol (1,25-dihydroxy vitamin D_3). It is the most commonly prescribed therapy for psoriasis in the United States, in part attributable to its paucity of side effects, aesthetic acceptability, and therapeutic advantages over anthralin and tar. Calcipotriene is available as a 0.0025% and 0.005% ointment and cream, and as a solution for scalp use. Although as monotherapy it is less effective than superpotent topical corticosteroids, it can be combined with topical steroids to provide better efficacy than either agent alone. It can also be combined with systemic agents such as cyclosporine and acitretin and with phototherapy to provide more rapid clearance of disease with potential dose-sparing effects.

A. Pharmacology and Mechanism of Action

Calcipotriene is the structural analog of calcitriol (1,25-dihydroxy vitamin D_3). Calcitrol and calcipotriene exhibit similar keratinocyte receptor binding and affinity but calcipotriene is 100 times less potent in its effects on calcium metabolism. Although its mechanism of action on psoriasis is not completely understood, the beneficial effects of calcipotriene on psoriasis are based on gene-regulatory events. Calcipotriene has been shown to promote terminal differentiation and inhibition of proliferation of keratinocytes (34). The metabolite of vitamin D3, 1,25 $(OH)_2$ D_3, may modulate the proliferation of T lymphocytes (35, 36).

Calcipotriene is a relatively unstable molecule and is inactivated by an acid pH. It is therefore not compatible in combination with some therapies. In vitro it was found to be compatible with halobetasol propionate 0.05% ointment and cream, tazarotene gel, and Estargel (37, 38). Some degradation was found in combination with hydrocortisone-17-valerate 0.2% ointment and ammonium lactate 12% lotion. Mixing with salicylic acid 6% caused rapid degradation of calcipotriene. Ultraviolet B (UVB) may inactivate calcipotriene; therefore, when used in combination with UVB therapy, it should be applied after exposure.

B. Efficacy

As a single agent calcipotriene is comparable to the efficacy of a class II corticosteroid ointment such as fluocinonide 0.05% (18, 39–41). However, several regimens that combine calcipotriene with class I corticosteroids have been shown to provide greater efficacy than either agent alone. Lebwohl et al. showed that subjects who applied calcipotriene ointment in the morning and halobetasol ointment in the evening for 2 weeks responded significantly better than those who applied halobetasol ointment twice daily or calcipotriene twice daily (42). A similar 2 week treatment of morning calcipotriene and evening halobetasol followed by a maintenance regimen of calcipotriene twice daily on weekdays with halobetasol twice daily on weekends subsequently provided a 6 month remission in 76% of patients, compared to only 40% of patients who used weekend halobetasol and weekday vehicle (43).

Another regimen compared augmented betamethasone applied once daily for 4 weeks to betamethasone applied daily on weeks 1 and 3, and calcipotriene applied twice daily on weeks 2 and 4. The alternating calcipotriene/betamethasone regimen resulted in clearance or marked improvement in 96% of patients, compared to 40% with the single-agent regimen (44).

In a 6 week study of 39 patients with palmoplantar psoriasis, twice-weekly overnight calcipotriol under occlusion was found to be equivalent to twice-daily calcipotriol nonocclusive therapy. No significant adverse events were reported (45).

C. Administration

It is the authors' opinion that topical calcipotriene, as a single agent administered twice daily, is not used by the great majority of patients for months on end. This is because the onset of action is slow and the response is usually less than the patient feels they should get based on the current cost. Most who use it successfully do so in combination with other agents. Experience has led us to two currently favored ways of using calcipotriene. The first is a program in which superpotent corticosteroids are applied twice daily for 2 weeks, followed by a week of twice-daily calcipotriene. Thereafter each of these is used twice daily on alternating weeks. In the second, superpotent corticosteroids are applied twice daily for 2 weeks, which is followed by calcipotriene twice daily on weekdays and superpotent corticosteroids on weekends. Vehicle choice is optimally ointment-based, but for compliance reasons more cosmetically acceptable vehicles can be used at least when applied prior to dressing for work. (See Table 4.)

D. Combination with Systemic Agents

Addition of calcipotriene to some systemic agents has been shown in small clinical trials to provide increased efficacy with a lower dosage of the

Table 4 Use of Calcipotriene in Moderate-to-Severe Psoriasis

Prescribe as part of a combination regimen with topical corticosteroids or tazarotene.
Limit application to 100 g per week (this will treat a body surface area of 15% twice daily).
Apply twice daily to body plaques.
Apply once or twice daily to face, axilla, groin, body folds, and genitals.
If facial irritation occurs, reduce frequency of application or discontinue use. Instruct patient to wash hands after application to other areas to avoid inadvertent contact of medication with face.
Apply with petrolatum jelly to reduce irritation.
Discontinue treatment if lesional or perilesional irritation persists.

systemic agent. Adding calcipotriene to cyclosporine has been shown to be beneficial and dose sparing (46,47). In the study by Goodman et al., calcipotriene applied concomitantly with low-dosage oral cyclosporine (2 mg/kg/day) resulted in > 90% improvement in 50% of patients compared to 11.8% of patients treated with cyclosporine and vehicle. Calcipotriene and systemic retinoids can also be combined with the similar dose-sparing and efficacy benefits. In one study the addition of calcipotriene to acitretin therapy resulted in clearance or marked improvement in 67% of patients compared to 41% of patients receiving acitretin and vehicle (48). Formal studies of the combination of methotrexate and calcipotriene have not been published. However, in a survey of dermatologists who actively treat psoriasis, responders indicated that 21/22 patients have achieved > 75% improvement after 8 weeks of combination therapy (49). To date, no additional safety concerns have been raised in studies of combination therapy with calcipotriene.

E. Combination with Phototherapy

Topical calcipotriene has been combined with UVB to improve efficacy and reduce cumulative exposure. Although one study of 53 patients did not show increased efficacy when calcipotriene was applied twice daily in conjunction with narrowband UVB, a more recent study of broadband UVB twice weekly with calcipotriene cream applied twice daily was shown to be equivalent in efficacy to UVB three times weekly with vehicle, significantly decreasing cumulative UVB exposure (50).

F. Cutaneous Side Effects

The only significant cutaneous side effect associated with calcipotriene therapy is skin irritation. This usually presents as lesional or perilesional burning, stinging, erythema, or scaling. Facial irritation is common, either due to intentional application or transfer of the medication from the hands after application elsewhere. Reducing the frequency of application or diluting calcipotriene with petrolatum has been advocated to reduce irritation (51). Hardening does occur, (i.e., the irritative effect lessens with time).

G. Systemic Side Effects

Long-term studies of calcipotriene have demonstrated few significant effects on calcium metabolism. Hypercalcemia has been reported in patients who have applied excessive quantities over large surface areas over a significant amount of time (52, 53). Subjects with renal impairment have developed hypercalcemia when 170–180 g are applied each week. Hypercalcuria, although clinically insignificant, has been observed in subjects applying 100 g/week for 4 weeks. No effect on bone metabolism has been observed (54).

IV. TAZAROTENE (TAZORAC)

Tazarotene is a topical retinoid that was approved for use in the United States in 1997. It is available as a 0.1% and 0.05% gel and cream. Although this agent is effective as monotherapy, many patients experience significant local irritation that limits its use. Using it in combination with topical corticosteroids increases efficacy and diminishes irritation, and can be used as part of a long-term combination maintenance regimen. Tazarotene can also be added to UVB therapy for more rapid improvement, increased efficacy, and cumulative UV dosage reduction.

A. Pharmacology and Mechanism of Action

Tazarotene is a vitamin A derivative that selectively binds to the γ and β retinoic acid receptors (RAR). In vivo it is rapidly converted to its biologically active metabolite, tazarotenic acid (55). Its mechanism of action in psoriasis may include reduction of number of lymphocytes in the dermis, decreased expression of inflammatory markers such as intracellular adhesion molecule 1 (ICAM-1), and modification of abnormal keratinocyte differentiation and proliferation (56).

B. Efficacy

Under clinical trial conditions tazarotene 0.1% gel applied as a single agent once daily resulted in 70% of patients having reached the clinical endpoint of treatment success, with 41% maintaining significant improvement 12 weeks after stopping use of the drug (57). More rapid improvement, improved efficacy, and decreased irritation have been shown in clinical trials combining tazarotene with intermediate and superpotent corticosteroids (58–60) A reported additional benefit to concomitant application of retinoids and corticosteroids is the prevention of atrophy (61). A recent review article by Lebwohl notes unpublished data showing that tazarotene has similar potential to reduce corticosteroid-related atrophy (62).

Tazarotene also appears to be stable in vitro when combined with a variety of topical corticosteroids and calcipotriene, and does not appear to affect adversely the stability of the other compounds (38). A recent left–right comparison study has shown that a 2 week course of tazarotene gel 0.1%

applied once daily combined with calcipotriene twice daily was comparable to clobetasol dipropionate 0.05% ointment applied twice daily (63).

C. Administration

Patients using tazarotene as monotherapy should apply the medication once daily, taking care to avoid surrounding unaffected skin. Patients should be warned of the likelihood of irritation, particularly if the agent is used on the face and neck. Intertriginous regions and genitals should be avoided. If significant irritation occurs, the patient may benefit from what is termed a short contact regimen (64). The patient is instructed to apply the medication for a shortened period of time (5–60 mins) then to wash the medication off. This can be followed by application of an emollient. Utilizing tazarotene every other day or changing to the 0.05% concentration or cream formulation may also help to reduce irritation but may also be less effective.

Tazarotene may be most efficacious and best tolerated (therefore improving compliance) when applied in combination with topical cortico-steroids. Initial treatment with once-daily application of tazarotene coupled with once-daily application of a super-potent corticosteroid, with subsequent tapering of the frequency of each agent (Table 5), is an effective regimen to prolong response.

D. Photocombination: UVB and Tazarotene

Tazarotene has been successfully combined with both broadband (65, 66) and narrowband UVB (67) for more effective and rapid clearing of psoriasis compared with either treatment alone. In a study of 54 patients, tazarotene

Table 5   Use of Tazarotene in Moderate-to-Severe Psoriasis

Apply once daily.
If irritation develops, try "short contact" therapy:
Apply tazarotene to plaques for a short period of time. We suggest that the first time be 10 min, but therapeutic effect is claimed with as little as 1 min.
Gradually increase application time by 1–5 minutes as tolerated.
Wash medication off after prescribed time period and apply an emollient.
In combination with superpotent corticosteroid:
Apply corticosteroid after short contact with tazarotene or apply tazarotene in the morning and the corticosteroid each evening.
Wean superpotent corticosteroid after 2 weeks to avoid atrophy.
In combination with UVB:
Apply after UV exposure.
If added to an already existing UVB regimen, reduce UV dosage by 1/3.

applied immediately after UVB phototherapy three times weekly achieved initial treatment success in half the time with significantly reduced cumulative UVB exposure and no unusual photosensitivity (66). Tazarotene applied nightly combined with narrowband UVB 5 times per week was likewise shown to be more effective than narrowband UVB alone (67). No unusual photosensitivity has been reported in these studies. Irritation from tazarotene also appears to be reduced when combined with UV therapy. Although no trials have been reported using tazarotene immediately prior to UVB exposure, the compound is stable with UV exposure (68). To date, no trials have assessed efficacy or safety of tazarotene use prior to UVB exposure. Therefore, if used in combination with UVB, tazarotene should be applied after light treatment. Since tazarotene has been shown to reduced epidermal thickness, concerns have been expressed regarding the increased risk of burning. It has been suggested that the UV dosage be reduced by one-third if tazarotene is added during phototherapy (68). (See Table 6.)

E. Side Effects

The most frequently reported side effect at lesional and perilesional application sites is irritation, including itching, burning, stinging, and erythema.

Table 6 Combination Topical Regimens for Resistant Lesions and Maintenance Treatment After Improvement with Systemic or Ultraviolet Therapy for Moderate-to-Severe Psoriasis

---

Initial treatment (2 weeks)
    Super-potent corticosteroid twice daily (BID)
    Calcipotriene (am) + superpotent corticosteroid (pm)
    Tazarotene (am) + superpotent corticosteroid (pm)
    Tazarotene and calcipotriene (am) + calcipotriene (pm)
Maintenance
    Calcipotriene BID weekdays + superpotent corticosteroid BID weekends
    Calcipotriene BID × 1 week alternating with superpotent corticosteroid
        BID × 1 week
    Short-contact[a] tazarotene then calcipotriene (pm) + calcipotriene (am) × 1 week,
        alternating with short-contact tazarotene then superpotent corticosteroid
        (pm) + corticosteroid (am)

Patients should be evaluated within 4–6 weeks after initiating treatment to monitor for efficacy, side effects, compliance, and patient satisfaction.
These combinations can be used for patients with moderate to severe psoriasis who cannot use or are fearful of systemic or UV treatment.
[a] 5–30 min application, then wash off prior to application of second agent.

Although the medication is not phototoxic or photoallergenic, the FDA-approved package insert cautions against sunlight and sunlamp exposure. When combined with UVB, thinning of the stratum corneum has been demonstrated, predisposing patients to burn more easily (68). Tazarotene is potentially teratogenic (pregnancy category X): women of childbearing potential should have a pregnancy test prior to use and use adequate contraception during therapy.

V. ANTHRALIN

Anthralin, or dithranol, has never been widely used in the United States. Historically, anthralin has been employed in the treatment of moderate to severe psoriasis in the hospital or daycare setting in combination with ultraviolet therapy, but its use has been superceded by more effective and convenient systemic therapies. Due to its lower efficacy than calcipotriene and undesirable side effect profile, its role in moderate to severe psoriasis is reserved for well-motivated patients whose disease has demonstrated intolerance to other agents.

A. Pharmacology and Mechanism of Action

Anthralin is the synthetic equivalent of chrysarobin, the active component in Goa powder used since the mid-19th century. Synthetic anthralin has been used since the 1930s when it was successfully substituted for coal tar by Ingram in the Goeckerman regimen. Its exact mechanism of action in psoriasis is unknown. Possible mechanisms include inhibition of DNA synthesis and proliferation (69), generation of free radicals, alteration in the epidermal growth factor receptor pathway, and alterations in mitochondrial respiratory function. Dithranol may suppress the interferon-gamma-induced up-regulation of cytokeratin 17 as a putative psoriasis autoantigen in vitro (70).

As of press time, the only commercially available anthralin was Psoriatec (1% anthralin cream), which recently replaced Micanol, formulated in a temperature-sensitive vehicle that released active medication when applied to skin (71). This controlled-release technology may reduce staining of fabrics and hair as long as cool water is used for washing. Anthralin can be compounded by an experienced pharmacist for the desired strength and vehicle.

B. Efficacy

As a single agent, anthralin appears most effective when given as short contact therapy. Studies have demonstrated clearance in approximately 30% of patients treated an average of 5 weeks (72–74). However, twice-daily application of calcipotriol was shown to be superior to short contact anthralin cream with better patient acceptability (41). Anthralin has been shown to enhance efficacy of many agents when used in combination; however, the disadvantages frequently outweigh the benefits. It is therefore seldom used in clinical practice in the United States.

C. Administration

For motivated patients whose disease has failed to respond to other topical and systemic modalities, short contact anthralin programs can be developed (Table 7).

Table 7 Directions for Application of Anthralin

Application
    Apply to body plaques for prescribed time period once daily
    Avoid face, axilla, intertriginous sites, genitals, and eyes
    Use a bland emollient, such as petrolatum jelly, on noninvolved contiguous skin
        surrounding plaques to prevent contact and irritation
Removal
    After allotted time, remove anthralin completely
    Medication should be completely washed off so that the skin is dry
        and completely without medication
    Use baby wipes, or baby, mineral, or vegetable oil on an old cloth or towel
    Shower or bathe with neutral pH soap
    Apply an emollient (i.e., Eucerin, Cetaphil, or Aquaphor)
Observation
    Patient should observe area over the next 48 h for erythema.
    Discontinue treatment if significant erythema or irritation occurs
Stain prevention
    Apply medication with disposable latex gloves
    Completely wash and dry area of application prior to dressing
    Use an old or disposable cloth or towel for removal and drying
    Cleanse tub or shower fixture immediately
    If staining occurs to a noncolored surface, remove with household bleach

Patients selected for this treatment should be motivated and able to follow detailed instructions. Patients should carefully adhere to total duration of application prescribed by the dermatologist; duration should begin at 10–30 min. Basic application instructions are supplied in this table.

D. Side Effects

The cutaneous side effects of anthralin include erythema, edema, and staining. Erythema usually occurs within 6 h and peaks in 48–72 hours. Allergic contact dermatitis has been reported rarely. Oxidation of anthralin causes staining of the skin, hair (particularly blonde), and clothing or other household fabrics.

VI. OTHER TOPICAL AGENTS: TACROLIMUS, SALICYLIC ACID, EMOLLIENTS

A. Tacrolimus (Protopic)

Tacrolimus ointment is the topical formulation of FK 506, an immuno-modulatory agent first used as an oral drug in patients undergoing organ transplantation. The topical ointment (available in 0.03% and 0.1% concentrations) is very effective in the treatment of atopic dermatitis and is being investigated in the treatment of psoriasis. Although initial trials failed to demonstrate efficacy in plaque-type psoriasis, there have been reports that it is effective for psoriasis on the face (75). It is the author's experience, as well as that of colleagues, that tacrolimus ointment is effective for facial plaques and inverse psoriasis. Application of a low- to midpotency steroid such as tridesilon cream or hydrocortisone butyrate with tacrolimus ointment reduces the pruritus and burning seen with initial treatment with tacrolimus. Studies are planned to evaluate other formulations in the treatment of psoriasis.

B. Salicylic Acid

Salicylic acid has been used in the treatment of psoriasis for years. It likely acts on the stratum corneum by disrupting desmosomes and may reduce thickness and scaling. It is available as a 6% gel but is most commonly found in shampoos or compounded with other psoriasis therapies. Salicylic acid enhances penetration and efficacy of corticosteroids (76). The combination of 5% salicylic acid and 0.1% mometasone furoate ointment has been shown more effective than either agent alone (77), but to date there are no commercially available combinations of salicylic acid and high-potency corticosteroids in the United States.

C. Emollients

Emollients are commonly used and highly recommended as concomitant therapy in the treatment of psoriasis. Use of emollients usually increases comfort by relieving dryness, scaling, and pruritus. The authors recommend frequent application of a cream or ointment (such as Cetaphil, Eucerin, Aquaphor and petrolatum).

VII. TREATMENT OF MODERATE-TO-SEVERE SCALP PSORIASIS WITH TOPICAL THERAPIES

All of the agents discussed in this chapter can be utilized on the scalp when prescribed in an acceptable vehicle. However, as previously discussed, patients with moderate to severe psoriasis isolated to the scalp often have tried and failed to respond to topical agents. It is the authors' opinion that moderate to severe psoriasis, even if isolated to the scalp, can (and some would argue should) be treated with systemic agents once topical therapies have been proven ineffective for the individual patient. The challenge to the treating dermatologist is determining treatment failure. It is our assessment that the most common reason for patients declaring that topical treatments do not work for scalp psoriasis is because they have not been compliant and or have had unreal expectations. Our approach in these patients is to determine if topical therapy has a chance of reaching their expectations. For this we prescribe the vigorous program outlined in Table 8: a combination regimen of superpotent corticosteroids, calcipotriene, and/or tazarotene and occlusion.

Table 8 Aggressive Therapy for Moderate-to-Severe Scalp Psoriasis

Evening
   1. Superpotent corticosteroid (solution or foam vehicle)
   2. Calcipotriene solution
   3. Tazarotene 0.1% gel
   4. Cover with plastic wrap and conform to scalp with thigh section of ladies nylon stocking
   Leave in place for 8–12 h
Morning
   1. Shampoo with tar-based shampoo (with or without keratolytics)
   2. Superpotent corticosteroid (solution or foam vehicle)
   3. Calcipotriene solution

Patients are asked to adhere to this regimen for 2 months. If the patient is compliant but his or disease is not 75% improved, systemic therapy should be considered.

To assess improvement, patient should be asked the following question at baseline, at follow-up, and at the end of the 2 month trial: "If '1' is equivalent to having no psoriasis, and '10' is equivalent to psoriasis being the worst ever, what is it today?" A score of 3 or less is considered a success.

Patients are asked to adhere to this regimen for 2 months. We announce to the patient that we have high expectations: if they are compliant and do not gain 75% improvement in 2 months, we will have to turn to systemic therapy or to adjust topical approaches to achieve less than clearance, (i.e., comfort measures). We find that a follow-up in the first 2–4 weeks is useful for answering questions and to emphasize the need for an assessment of response by the patient (see Table 8).

REFERENCES

1. Krueger GG, Feldman SR, Camisa C, et al. Two considerations for patients with psoriasis and their clinicians: what defines mild, moderate, and severe psoriasis? What constitutes a clinically significant improvement when treating psoriasis? J Am Acad Dermatol 2000; 43(2 Pt 1): 281–285.
2. Boumpas DT, Chrousos GP, Wilder RL, Cupps TR, Balow JE. Glucocorticoid therapy for immune-mediated diseases: basic and clinical correlates. Ann Intern Med 1993; 119(12): 1198–1208.
3. Barnes PJ, Adcock I. Anti-inflammatory actions of steroids: molecular mechanisms. Trends Pharmacol Sci 1993; 14(12): 436–441.
4. Gower WR, Jr. Mechanism of glucocorticoid action. J Fla Med Assoc 1993; 80(10): 697–700.
5. Kragballe K. Topical corticosteroids: mechanisms of action. Acta Derm Venereol Suppl (Stockh) 1989; 151: 7–10; 47–52.
6. Cornell RC, Stoughton RB. Correlation of the vasoconstriction assay and clinical activity in psoriasis. Arch Dermatol 1985; 121(1): 63–67.
7. Cornell RC. Clinical trials of topical corticosteroids in psoriasis: correlations with the vasoconstrictor assay. Int J Dermatol 1992; 31 Suppl 1: 38–40.
8. Gibson JR, Kirsch JM, Darley CR, Harvey SG, Burke CA, Hanson ME. An assessment of the relationship between vasoconstrictor assay findings, clinical efficacy and skin thinning effects of a variety of undiluted and diluted corticosteroid preparations. Br J Dermatol 1984; 111 Suppl 27: 204–12.
9. Barry BW, Fyrand O, Woodford R, Ulshagen K, Hogstad G. Control of the bioavailability of a topical steroid; comparison of desonide creams 0.05% and 0.1% by vasoconstrictor studies and clinical trials. Clin Exp Dermatol 1987; 12(6): 406–9.
10. Feldmann RJ, Maibach HI. Regional variation in percutaneous penetration of 14C cortisol in man. J Invest Dermatol 1967; 48(2): 181–3.
11. Goldberg B, Hartdegen R, Presbury D, Smith EH, Yawalkar S. A double-blind, multicenter comparison of 0.05% halobetasol propionate ointment and 0.05% clobetasol propionate ointment in patients with chronic, localized plaque psoriasis. J Am Acad Dermatol 1991; 25(6 Pt 2): 1145–8.
12. Blum G, Yawalkar S. A comparative, multicenter, double blind trial of 0.05% halobetasol propionate ointment and 0.1% betamethasone valerate ointment in

the treatment of patients with chronic, localized plaque psoriasis. J Am Acad Dermatol 1991; 25(6 Pt 2): 1153–6.

13. Katz HI, Gross E, Buxman M, Prawer SE, Schwartzel EH, Gibson JR. A double-blind, vehicle-controlled paired comparison of halobetasol propionate cream on patients with plaque psoriasis. J Am Acad Dermatol 1991; 25(6 Pt 2): 1175–8.

14. Krueger GG, O'Reilly MA, Weidner M, Dromgoole SH, Killey FP. Comparative efficacy of once-daily flurandrenolide tape versus twice-daily diflorasone diacetate ointment in the treatment of psoriasis. J Am Acad Dermatol 1998; 38(2 Pt 1): 186–90.

15. Katz HI, Hien NT, Prawer SE, Mastbaum LI, Mooney JJ, Samson CR. Superpotent topical steroid treatment of psoriasis vulgaris—clinical efficacy and adrenal function. J Am Acad Dermatol 1987; 16(4): 804–11.

16. Tristani-Firouzi P, Krueger GG. Efficacy and safety of treatment modalities for psoriasis. Cutis 1998; 61(2 Suppl): 11–21.

17. Molin L, Cutler TP, Helander I, Nyfors B, Downess N. Comparative efficacy of calcipotriol (MC903) cream and betamethasone 17-valerate cream in the treatment of chronic plaque psoriasis. A randomized, double-blind, parallel group multicentre study. Calcipotriol Study Group. Br J Dermatol 1997; 136(1): 89–93.

18. Bruce S, Epinette WW, Funicella T, et al. Comparative study of calcipotriene (MC 903) ointment and fluocinonide ointment in the treatment of psoriasis. J Am Acad Dermatol 1994; 31(5 Pt 1): 755–9.

19. Olsen EA, Cram DL, Ellis CN, et al. A double-blind, vehicle-controlled study of clobetasol propionate 0.05% (Temovate) scalp application in the treatment of moderate to severe scalp psoriasis. J Am Acad Dermatol 1991; 24(3): 443–7.

20. Franz TJ, Parsell DA, Halualani RM, Hannigan JF, Kalbach JP, Harkonen WS. Betamethasone valerate foam 0.12%: a novel vehicle with enhanced delivery and efficacy. Int J Dermatol 1999; 38(8): 628–32.

21. Melian EB, Spencer CM, Jarvis B. Clobetasol propionate foam, 0.05%. Am J Clin Dermatol 2001; 2(2): 89–92; 93.

22. Lebwohl M, Sherer D, Washenik K, et al. A randomized, double-blind, placebo-controlled study of clobetasol propionate 0.05% foam in the treatment of nonscalp psoriasis. Int J Dermatol 2002; 41(5): 269–274.

23. Katz HI, Prawer SE, Mooney JJ, Samson CR. Preatrophy: covert sign of thinned skin. J Am Acad Dermatol 1989; 20(5 Pt 1): 731–5.

24. Alani MD, Alani SD. Allergic contact dermatitis to corticosteroids. Ann Allergy 1972; 30(4): 181–5.

25. Mommers JM, van Erp PE, van De Kerkhof PC. Clobetasol under hydrocolloid occlusion in psoriasis results in a complete block of proliferation and in a rebound of lesions following discontinuation. Dermatology 1999; 199(4): 323–7.

26. Volden G, Successful treatment of chronic skin diseases with clobetasol propionate and a hydrocolloid occlusive dressing. Acta Derm Venereol 1992; 72(1): 69–71.

27. van de Kerkhof PC, Chang A, van der Walle HB, van Vlijmen-Willems I, Boezeman JB, Huigen-Tijdink R. Weekly treatment of psoriasis with a hydrocolloid dressing in combination with triamcinolone acetonide. A controlled comparative study. Acta Derm Venereol 1994; 74(2): 143–6.

28. Levin C, Maibach HI. Topical corticosteroid-induced adrenocortical insufficiency: clinical implications. Am J Clin Dermatol 2002; 3(3): 141–7.

29. Nathan AW, Rose GL. Fatal iatrogenic Cushing's syndrome. Lancet 1979; 1(8109): 207.

30. Kubo T, Kojima A, Yamazoe S, Ueshima K, Yamamoto T, Hirasawa Y. Osteonecrosis of the femoral head that developed after long-term topical steroid application. J Orthop Sci 2001; 6(1): 92–4.

31. du Vivier A, Stoughton RB. Tachyphylaxis to the action of topically applied corticosteroids. Arch Dermatol 1975; 111(5): 581–3.

32. du Vivier A. Tachyphylaxis to topically applied steroids. Arch Dermatol 1976; 112(9):1245–8.

33. Miller JJ, Roling D, Margolis D, Guzzo C. Failure to demonstrate therapeutic tachyphylaxis to topically applied steroids in patients with psoriasis. J Am Acad Dermatol 1999; 41(4): 546–9.

34. Smith EL, Walworth NC, Holick MF. Effect of 1 alpha,25-dihydroxyvitamin D3 on the morphologic and biochemical differentiation of cultured human epidermal keratinocytes grown in serum-free conditions. J Invest Dermatol 1986; 86(6): 709–14.

35. Tsoukas CD, Provvedini DM, Manolagas SC. 1,25-dihydroxyvitamin D3: a novel immunoregulatory hormone. Science 1984; 224(4656): 1438–40.

36. Lemire JM, Adams JS, Kermani-Arab V, Bakke AC, Sakai R, Jordan SC. 1,25-Dihydroxyvitamin D3 suppresses human T helper/inducer lymphocyte activity in vitro. J Immunol 1985; 134(5): 3032–5.

37. Patel B, Siskin S, Krazmien R, Lebwohl M. Compatibility of calcipotriene with other topical medications. J Am Acad Dermatol 1998; 38(6 Pt 1): 1010–1.

38. Hecker D, Worsley J, Yueh G, Lebwohl M. In vitro compatibility of tazarotene with other topical treatments of psoriasis. J Am Acad Dermatol 2000; 42(6): 1008–11.

39. Kragballe K. Calcipotriol for psoriasis. Lancet 1991; 337(8751): 1229–30.

40. Cunliffe WJ, Berth-Jones J, Claudy A, et al. Comparative study of calcipotriol (MC 903) ointment and betamethasone 17-valerate ointment in patients with psoriasis vulgaris. J Am Acad Dermatol 1992; 26(5 Pt 1): 736–43.

41. Berth-Jones J, Chu AC, Dodd WA, et al. A multicentre, parallel-group comparison of calcipotriol ointment and short-contact dithranol therapy in chronic plaque psoriasis. Br J Dermatol 1992; 127(3): 266–71.

42. Lebwohl M, Siskin SB, Epinette W, et al. A multicenter trial of calcipotriene ointment and halobetasol ointment compared with either agent alone for the treatment of psoriasis. J Am Acad Dermatol 1996; 35(2 Pt 1): 268–9.

43. Lebwohl M, Yoles A, Lombardi K, Lou W. Calcipotriene ointment and

halobetasol ointment in the long-term treatment of psoriasis: effects on the duration of improvement. J Am Acad Dermatol 1998; 39(3): 447–50.

44. Singh S, Reddy DC, Pandey SS. Topical therapy for psoriasis with the use of augmented betamethasone and calcipotriene on alternate weeks. J Am Acad Dermatol 2000; 43(1 Pt 1): 61–5.

45. Duweb GA, Abuzariba O, Rahim M, al-Taweel M, al-Alem S, Abdulla SA. Occlusive versus nonocclusive calcipotriol ointment treatment for palmoplantar psoriasis. Int J Tissue React 2001; 23(2): 59–62.

46. Grossman RM, Thivolet J, Claudy A, et al. A novel therapeutic approach to psoriasis with combination calcipotriol ointment and very low-dose cyclosporine: results of a multicenter placebo-controlled study. J Am Acad Dermatol 1994; 31(1): 68–74.

47. Kokelj F, Torsello P, Plozzer C. Calcipotriol improves the efficacy of cyclosporine in the treatment of psoriasis vulgaris. J Eur Acad Dermatol Venereol 1998; 10(2): 143–6.

48. van de Kerkhof PC, Cambazard F, Hutchinson PE, et al. The effect of addition of calcipotriol ointment (50 micrograms/g) to acitretin therapy in psoriasis. Br J Dermatol 1998; 138(1): 84–9.

49. Katz HI. Combined topical calcipotriene ointment 0.005% and various systemic therapies in the treatment of plaque-type psoriasis vulgaris: review of the literature and results of a survey sent to 100 dermatologists. J Am Acad Dermatol 1997; 37(3 Pt 2): S62–8.

50. Ramsay CA, Schwartz BE, Lowson D, Papp K, Boldue A, Gilbert M. Calcipotriol cream combined with twice weekly broad-band UVB phototherapy: a safe, effective and UVB-sparing antipsoriatric combination treatment. The Canadian Calcipotriol and UVB Study Group. Dermatology 2000; 200(1): 17–24.

51. Koo J. Diluting Dovonex. Psoriasis Forum 1995; 1: 6.

52. Georgiou S, Tsambaos D. Hypercalcaemia and hypercalciuria after topical treatment of psoriasis with excessive amounts of calcipotriol. Acta Derm Venereol 1999; 79(1): 86.

53. Dwyer C, Chapman RS. Calcipotriol and hypercalcaemia. Lancet 1991; 338(8769): 764–5.

54. Mortensen L, Kragballe K, Wegmann E, Schifter S, Risteli J, Charles P. Treatment of psoriasis vulgaris with topical calcipotriol has no short-term effect on calcium or bone metabolism. A randomized, double-blind, placebo-controlled study. Acta Derm Venereol 1993; 73(4): 300–4.

55. Chandraratna RA. Tazarotene–first of a new generation of receptor-selective retinoids. Br J Dermatol 1996; 135 Suppl 49: 18–25.

56. Duvic M, Asano AT, Hager C, Mays S. The pathogenesis of psoriasis and the mechanism of action of tazarotene. J Am Acad Dermatol 1998; 39(4 Pt 2): S129–33.

57. Krueger GG, Drake LA, Elias PM, et al. The safety and efficacy of tazarotene gel, a topical acetylenic retinoid, in the treatment of psoriasis. Arch Dermatol 1998; 134(1): 57–60.

58. Koo JY, Martin D. Investigator-masked comparison of tazarotene gel q.d. plus mometasone furoate cream q.d. vs. mometasone furoate cream b.i.d. in the treatment of plaque psoriasis. Int J Dermatol 2001; 40(3): 210–2.

59. Lebwohl M, Ast E, Callen JP, et al. Once-daily tazarotene gel versus twice-daily fluocinonide cream in the treatment of plaque psoriasis. J Am Acad Dermatol 1998; 38(5 Pt 1): 705–11.

60. Lebwohl M, Lombardi K, Tan MH. Duration of improvement in psoriasis after treatment with tazarotene 0.1% gel plus clobetasol propionate 0.05% ointment: comparison of maintenance treatments. Int J Dermatol 2001; 40(1): 64–6.

61. Lesnik RH, Mezick JA, Capetola R, Kligman LH. Topical all-trans-retinoic acid prevents corticosteroid-induced skin atrophy without abrogating the anti-inflammatory effect. J Am Acad Dermatol 1989; 21(2 Pt 1): 186–90.

62. Lebwohl M, Ali S. Treatment of psoriasis. Part 1. Topical therapy and phototherapy. J Am Acad Dermatol 2001; 45(4): 487–98; 499–502.

63. Bowman PH, Maloney JE, Koo JY. Combination of calcipotriene (Dovonex) ointment and tazarotene (Tazorac) gel versus clobetasol ointment in the treatment of plaque psoriasis: a pilot study. J Am Acad Dermatol 2002; 46(6): 907–13.

64. Persaud A, Bershad S, Lamba S, Lebwohl M. Short-contact tazarotene therapy for psoriasis. Poster presentation, American Academy of Dermatology, Nashville, TN, 2000.

65. Lowe NJ. Optimizing therapy: tazarotene in combination with phototherapy. Br J Dermatol 1999; 140 Suppl 54: 8–11.

66. Koo JY, Lowe NJ, Lew-Kaya DA, et al. Tazarotene plus UVB phototherapy in the treatment of psoriasis. J Am Acad Dermatol 2000; 43(5 Pt 1): 821–8.

67. Behrens S, Grundmann-Kollamnn M, Schiener R, Peter RU, Kerscher M. Combination phototherapy of psoriasis with narrow-band UVB irradiation and topical tazarotene gel. J Am Acad Dermatol 2000; 42(3): 493–5.

68. Hecker D, Worsley J, Yueh G, Kuroda K, Lebwohl M. Interactions between tazarotene and ultraviolet light. J Am Acad Dermatol 1999; 41(6): 927–30.

69. Klem EB. Effects of antipsoriasis drugs and metabolic inhibitors on the growth of epidermal cells in culture. J Invest Dermatol 1978; 70(1): 27–32.

70. Bonnekoh B, Bockelmann R, Ambach A, Gollnick H. Dithranol and dimethylfumarate suppress the interferon-gamma-induced up-regulation of cytokeratin 17 as a putative psoriasis autoantigen in vitro. Skin Pharmacol Appl Skin Physiol 2001; 14(4): 217–25.

71. Volden G, Bjornberg A, Tegner E, et al. Short-contact treatment at home with Micanol. Acta Derm Venereol Suppl (Stockh) 1992; 172: 20–2.

72. Goransson A. Comparison of dithranol and butantrone in short contact therapy of psoriasis. Acta Derm Venereol 1987; 67(2): 149–53.

73. Schaefer H, Farber EM, Goldberg L, Schalla W. Limited application period for dithranol in psoriasis. Preliminary report on penetration and clinical efficacy. Br J Dermatol 1980; 102(5): 571–73.

74. Statham BN, Ryatt KS, Rowell NR. Short-contact dithranol therapy–a comparison with the Ingram regime. Br J Dermatol 1984; 110(6): 703–8.

75. Yamamoto T, Nishioka K. Topical tacrolimus is effective for facial lesions of psoriasis. Acta Derm Venereol 2000; 80(6): 451.

76. Krochmal L, Wang JC, Patel B, Rodgers J. Topical corticosteroid compounding: effects on physicochemical stability and skin penetration rate. J Am Acad Dermatol 1989; 21(5 Pt 1): 979–84.

77. Koo J, Cuffie CA, Tanner DJ, et al. Mometasone furoate 0.1%-salicylic acid 5% ointment versus mometasone furoate 0.1% ointment in the treatment of moderate-to-severe psoriasis: a multicenter study. Clin Ther 1998; 20(2): 283–91.

3

The Art and Practice of UVB Phototherapy for the Treatment of Psoriasis

John Koo and Grace Bandow
University of California, San Francisco, San Francisco, California, U.S.A.

Steven R. Feldman
Wake Forest University School of Medicine, Winston-Salem, North Carolina, U.S.A.

Ultraviolet light B (UVB) is one of the oldest therapeutic modalities for the treatment of psoriasis. Because of its long track record of both safety and efficacy, UVB phototherapy continues to enjoy widespread use in spite of the development of many newer modalities for treating psoriasis, including psoralen and ultraviolet A (PUVA) therapy and various systemic agents. Certain forms of UVB phototherapy, such as the traditional Goeckerman regimen, induce a prolonged remission according to available published data; indeed, Goeckerman treatment is often used as the gold standard against which newer modalities are compared in terms of remission times (1).

This chapter will discuss the entire spectrum of UVB phototherapy. UVB regimens range from simple treatments in a UVB phototherapy box, with or without concurrent use of commercially available tar preparations, to a much more elaborate and aggressive modality in which the intensity of UVB radiation used varies not only among patients, but also according to different anatomical regions within the same patient. Combining UVB phototherapy with various topical and systemic agents can also enhance UVB phototherapy. Even though some of these techniques are discussed in the context of the psoriasis day treatment program, it is important to note that these techniques can be carried out for selected recalcitrant psoriatic lesions in a regular office setting. These techniques will be discussed one by one, starting with the simplest regimen followed by more effective, but also more involved, uses of this modality. We will also discuss new developments in phototherapy including narrowband UVB, UVB laser, and other forms of localized phototherapy.

I. BASIC OUTPATIENT UVB PHOTOTHERAPY

The simplest method of administering UVB phototherapy involves treatment in a UVB box, with or without the use of commercially available tar preparations. Since even the simplest use of UVB phototherapy requires some commitment, time, and effort from patients, outpatient UVB phototherapy is usually reserved for patients whose disease does not adequately respond to topical medications such as steroids, calcipotriol, tazarotene, tar, or anthralin. It is also indicated for those patients who initially respond to topical agents but who develop tachyphylaxis over time, or for patients with such extensive involvement that topical therapy is nearly impossible. For patients with generalized psoriasis, UVB phototherapy is a reasonable first choice among the various available options because of its proven safety profile.

A.   Contraindications

UVB phototherapy is contraindicated in patients who react badly to light, either because of medication they are taking or because of an underlying photosensitive disease. Numerous medications can potentially photosensitize patients, including thiazide diuretics and certain antibiotics such as tetracycline or doxycycline. However, such medications do not always induce photosensitivity. In fact, if phototherapy is strongly indicated, it is frequently possible to go ahead and conduct phototherapy after exposing a selected test area of the skin to UVB light without a reaction. Another option is scheduling phototherapy so that the maximum time elapses between administration of the photosensitizing medication and UVB therapy. This ensures minimum blood level of the photosensitizing medication at the time of light exposure, thereby minimizing the risk of a phototoxic reaction.

UVB phototherapy is contraindicated in patients with photosensitizing diseases such as systemic lupus erythematosus or polymorphous light eruption, unless the phototherapy is specifically utilized to harden the skin as a therapeutic strategy in patients with such conditions. Although much of the published literature regarding this hardening process refers to PUVA, UVB can be used for this purpose (2, 3). A discussion of each photosensitizing medication and disease is beyond the scope of this monograph, but detailed references regarding these conditions can be readily found in standard text-books (4).

Some in vitro data suggest that UVB exposure may enhance activation of human immunovirus (HIV) infection. (5–8) However, in practice, UVB therapy is utilized to treat not only HIV-infected patients with psoriasis but also cases of HIV pruritus and folliculitis, including eosinophilic folliculitis. After almost two decades of use, practitioners have not noticed widespread occurrence of adverse reactions to this therapy in HIV-infected patients. UVB phototherapy is still considered safer, by most practitioners, than other therapeutic alternatives, including PUVA, methotrexate, and cyclo-sporine, especially in light of a recent publication describing the lack of changes in immune function among HIV-positive patients undergoing UVB phototherapy (9).

B. Dosage and Administration

There are two ways to determine the initial dose of UVB radiation for any given patient. The first method involves formal minimal erythema dose (MED) testing, in which small, defined areas of skin are sequentially exposed to different intensities of UVB radiation (Figs. 1, 2). The MED is defined as the amount of UVB that produces barely perceptible erythema in non-involved skin 12–18 h after exposure. Once the MED for a particular patient has been determined, the initial exposure may range anywhere from 50% to 100% of the MED, depending on the desired aggressiveness of the dosing schedule, ranging from suberythemogenic to erythemogenic. In an erythemo-genic schedule, an attempt is made to maintain barely perceptible erythema following each UVB treatment session (10–15). To compensate for tanning and other forms of tolerance, subsequent dosages of UVB radiation may be increased by 15%–25% of the previously applied dosage, if necessary, to maintain mild, nontender erythema in the noninvolved skin.

The erythemogenic schedule is ideal in theory since UVB phototherapy tends to produce maximal results when used at or near a patient's MED (16–19). In practice, the erythemogenic dosage schedule is not practical for many patients either because they experience uncomfortable burning sensations at MED, or because practitioners do not want to risk burning patients by attempting to maintain MED. The alternative is the suberythemogenic schedule and tar as outlined by Frost in 1978 (20). In this schedule, the initial dosage of UVB radiation is 50% of the MED, and the subsequent dose of UVB is increased as shown in Table 1 only if the patient stops showing steady improvement clinically. The rationale behind using a less aggressive, suberythemogenic schedule is to minimize the cumulative dosage of UVB radiation and also to minimize the risk of inducing UVB burns.

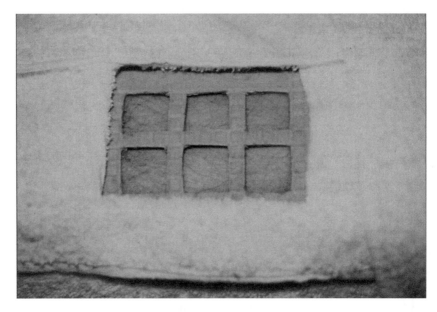

Figure 1 In conducting formal MED testing, a different amount of UVB radiation is applied sequentially to each opening in the template, which is made of an opaque material such as a thick piece of cardboard. The increment of UVB exposure used is usually 15 or 30 s when a UVB box with fluorescent lights is utilized. (Refer to the color insert.)

However, patients also tend to respond more slowly when a less aggressive schedule is utilized. As discussed in the section on tar, this shortcoming can be largely overcome by using tar preparations concurrently.

In a busy phototherapy practice, with a high volume of patients, formal MED testing may be cumbersome since it is labor-intensive and potentially disruptive to the natural flow of patients undergoing phototherapy. In our clinic, instead of MED testing a defined guideline is used to determine the starting dosage for UVB therapy based on patients' skin types (Table 2). As illustrated in Table 2, within these guidelines a wide range of UVB dosages is suggested both for starting and increasing the dosage of UVB radiation. Using this table as a general guideline, our phototherapy nurses use their judgement in determining a particular starting dosage, an incremental dosage, and the timing of dosage adjustment. The underlying principle is to increase UVB gradually until the MED is reached and then try to maintain the UVB dose *just below* the MED. This approach eliminates the need for formal MED testing in most patients. It is also simpler and more efficient than methods using incremental dosages calculated as a certain percentage of the previous

Figure 2 The result of MED testing on the body. (Refer to the color insert.)

dosage. However, the author does not recommend this approach unless the nursing staff is highly experienced in phototherapy and in making this type of judgment.

C. Efficacy

To induce steady improvement of existing psoriatic lesions, outpatient UVB phototherapy should be performed three to five times per week. If UVB phototherapy is conducted less than three times per week, the rate of clinical

Table 1 Determining UVB Dosage Increment

Previous Treatment Dose (mj)	Increment (mj)
0–12	1.5
12–30	3.0
30–60	6.0
> 60	12.0

Source: Modified from Lowe NJ, ed. Practical Psoriasis Therapy. 2nd ed. St. Louis, Mo: Mosby-Year Book Inc, 1993:102.

Table 2 Protocol for UVB Therapy at UCSF
Phototherapy Unit

Skin Type	Start and Increases (mJ)
I	10–20
II	20–30
III	30–40
IV & V (Asian, Spanish, Italian)	40–50
VI (Black)	50–100

improvement diminishes significantly; it is unusual to see significant improvement in clinical status if UVB is conducted less than twice per week. It generally takes 20 UVB treatment sessions to induce significant improvement or clearance in an average patient with scattered plaque-type psoriasis. In the author's experience, the success rate for basic UVB phototherapy ranges from 50% to 80%, depending on the definition of success. With basic UVB phototherapy, most patients show significant improvement or clearance of trunk lesions. In other words, if one makes an allowance for residual lesions on the extremities such as on the elbows, knees, and shins, approximately 80% of the patients can be considered to be successfully treated. However, if one defines success as significant improvement or clearing on both the trunk and the extremities, the rate of success with basic UVB therapy decreases to about 50% of patients treated.

D. Comparison with Other Therapies

A distinct advantage of UVB phototherapy is that it has essentially no systemic side effects compared to systemic agents. In order to minimize both the acute and long-term systemic side effects of systemic agents such as methotrexate, acitretin, or cyclosporine, ideally, a therapeutic trial with phototherapy should be performed before resorting to use of systemic agents.

In comparison with PUVA phototherapy, UVB phototherapy tends to be less effective. However, patients are spared the possibility of annoying side effects such as nausea, headaches, and dizziness that sometimes come with systemic PUVA therapy (see Chap. 4). In addition, long-term UVB phototherapy appears to result in much less photodamage. In fact, most of the epidemiological studies in which patients on long-term UVB therapies were followed for up to two decades in the United States and Europe failed to show any increase in skin cancer rates when compared to the general population (21–23). This is surprising since many of these patients were also treated with various tar preparations and both UVB and tar are potentially carcinogenic.

Decreased efficacy rates of UVB phototherapy compared to PUVA can be overcome in many patients, but requires more labor-intensive and specialized applications of UVB as described below, and/or conducting UVB phototherapy on a more frequent basis. If the physician does not have the equipment or skilled phototherapy nurses for more specialized UVB procedures, or if the patient has logistical constraints to doing phototherapy more than twice per week, PUVA phototherapy would be a more effective mode of treatment.

II. AGGRESSIVE UVB THERAPY

There are many different ways to enhance UVB phototherapy. Generally, the strategies for enhancement fall into three different categories: optimizing UVB exposure, combining UVB phototherapy with topical agents, and combining UVB phototherapy with systemic agents. These three strategies are not mutually exclusive. For a physician faced with a truly recalcitrant case, it is often possible to prevail by combining all three approaches since they generally work synergistically. By making use of these strategies, it is possible to make UVB therapy as therapeutically efficacious as PUVA therapy or systemic agents. In the following section, these three strategies will be discussed separately.

A. Optimizing UVB Exposure

For both UVB and PUVA phototherapy, adequate intensity of UV exposure is a basic requirement before any therapeutic benefit can be expected. As stated earlier, it has been determined by many studies that optimal UVB exposure lies at the MED for most patients with psoriasis (16–19). However, the task of delivering adequate UVB exposure is complicated by the fact that the MED differs in different anatomical areas (Fig. 3) (24). In most patients, the MED assumes its highest value on distal extremities such as elbows and shins; it is lowest in flexural areas such as popliteal and antecubital fossas, the face, and anterior chest, and the MED usually assumes some midpoint value for the trunk. In fact, the MED for so-called difficult to treat areas such as the elbows and shins typically runs two to three times that of the trunk. This is thought to be one explanation for the fact that many patients experience only a partial response to UVB box therapy: they improve adequately on their trunk but relatively poorly on their distal extremities.

Rather than declaring these patients UVB-resistant cases, a logical approach is to give extra exposure to those areas that require higher intensity of UVB for optimal therapeutic effect. The simplest way to accomplish this is

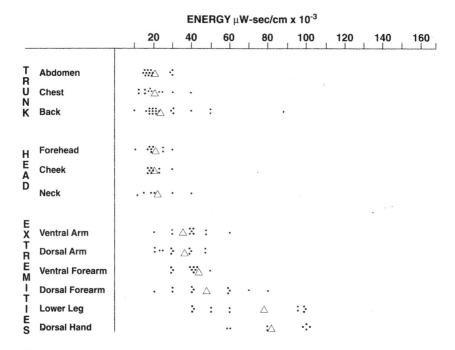

Figure 3 As shown here, the MED differs in different parts of the body. (From Ref. 24.)

to practice two-step UVB box phototherapy. The patient goes into a UVB box for overall exposure, comes out of the box to cover areas with a low MED such as the face (the face should be covered from the start if there are no psoriatic lesions), trunk, and flexural areas, and then goes back into the UVB box for a second, additional exposure to the extremities. One drawback of this method is that the intensity of UVB radiation drops off sharply at both the top and bottom of UVB boxes (Fig. 4) (25). Ironically, patients end up getting less UVB exposure in precisely the areas that need it most. Because of this, even the two-step approach may not be adequate for optimal UVB exposure to areas such as the shins. A better approach is using equipment such as hot quartz lamps, or Dermalight, that are designed to give intense exposure to localized areas (Figs. 5, 6). These metal–halide units give off several times the intensity of UVB radiation of traditional fluorescent lamp boxes, and they do not have the fall-off effect characteristic of fluorescent lamps. In short, by exposing different anatomical areas to different intensities of UVB radiation, one can frequently clear lesions that are otherwise resistant to regular UVB box therapy.

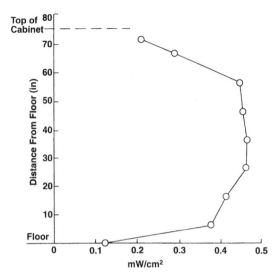

Figure 4 The intensity of UVB output drops off dramatically at the top and bottom sections of a typical phototherapy box lined with fluorescent lights. (Adapted from Ref. 25.)

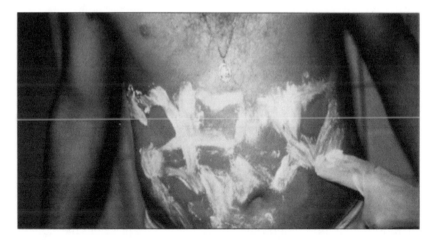

Figure 5 Since noninvolved skin burns much more easily than psoriatic plaques, zinc oxide paste is used to protect the noninvolved skin in between the psoriatic plaques before the patient is treated with a high-intensity UVB source such as a hot quartz lamp.

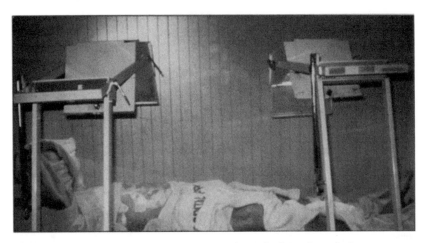

Figure 6   One advantage of a hot quartz lamp is that, since patients are treated lying down, it is relatively easy to cover the noninvolved areas with towels to avoid unnecessary exposure to UVB.

B.   Enhancing UVB Phototherapy with Topical Agents

1.   Keratolytics

Thick, micaceous psoriatic scales scatter light, and any light that is not absorbed into the skin is wasted. Using keratolytic agents to remove as much scale as possible diminishes this problem and enhances the therapeutic effect of phototherapy. This measure is especially important in UVB phototherapy, since UVB rays cannot penetrate the skin as deeply as UVA rays. Keralyt Gel is a topical salicylic acid preparation most often used for this purpose. For thicker and more resistant lesions, pharmacists can compound higher concentrations of salicylic acid in liquor carbonis detergents (LCD) or crude coal tar for use under occlusion for maximal keratolytic effect. At UCSF Medical Center, 10% crude coal tar (black tar, Koppers Company, Pittsburgh, PA) with up to 10% salicylic acid (Spectrum Chemical Manufacturing, Gardena, CA) in petrolatum is often used for extremely hyperkeratotic lesions on the palms, soles, elbows, and shins under plastic wrap, gloves, or shower cap occlusion. Shower caps work well for occluding the soles when held in place with a sock. If the patient cannot tolerate salicylic acid, topical lactic acid preparations up to prescription strength can be used in place of salicylic acid. Ideally, psoriatic lesions should be kept relatively free of scaling during UVB phototherapy. In a minority of cases where the above measures are still not adequate, low-dosage acitretin can be used to minimize hyperkeratosis and induration. Lastly, in addition to removing the scales, UVB penetration can be enhanced by applying mineral oil or petrolatum to change the skin surface's refractive index. This is accomplished by instructing the patient to apply mineral oil to the psoriatic lesions sometime before he or she goes into the UVB box.

2. Tar

There are many commercially available tar preparations, including creams, shampoos, and soaks. Tar in higher concentrations can also be compounded by most pharmacists to enhance its therapeutic effect. If the pharmacist has the right equipment, LCD can be compounded up to 20% concentration in Aquaphor, and the original black tar can be compounded up to 10% concentration in petrolatum. It is generally accepted by dermatologists who run day treatment programs that black tar holds a significant therapeutic advantage over LCD or other refined tar products. Several studies suggest that when the MED is reached in UVB therapy, tar may not add much additional benefit for most patients with psoriasis (16–19). As mentioned previously, in practice, it is frequently not feasible to attain minimal erythema since patients often complain of burning, stinging, and other uncomfortable symptoms. On the other hand, when the intensity of the UVB therapy is titrated to a *sub*erythemogenic level, tar preparations have been well demonstrated to provide additional therapeutic benefit (12). In practice, if patients are willing, *sub*erythemogenic doses of UVB are used together with tar preparations.

At our Center, patients admitted for all-day, daily Goeckerman therapy have previously failed to respond to outpatient regimens using 20% LCD in Aquaphor and intense UVB exposure, yet their skin routinely clears with the use of true black tar supplemented with UVB phototherapy. While this may represent greater efficacy of black tar over other tar preparations, it may also reflect the difficulty with compliance with tar products in the home setting.

In the day treatment setting, 10% crude coal tar with up to 10% salicylic acid in petrolatum is typically the strongest regimen used. This preparation is very difficult to use at home because of its messiness. Yet if patients are highly motivated, it is possible to prescribe for home application to localized resistant areas such as shins and elbows. Many patients with truly recalcitrant and indurated lesions find that they can apply this under plastic wrap occlusion overnight without experiencing irritation or folliculitis. For them, the use of black tar at home in conjunction with UVB therapy can offer additional therapeutic benefits for resistant lesions.

3. Anthralin

Ingram therapy consists of the combined used of anthralin and UVB phototherapy. Anthralin powder (Paddock Labs, Minneapolis, MN) is available commercially, and can be compounded up to 10% concentration. Compounded anthralin can be prepared in a cream base with salicyclic acid in concentrations of 3%, 5%, or 10%. Salicylic acid functions both as the preservative for anthralin and as a keratolytic agent. Higher concentrations of anthralin should be used only on patients who can tolerate 1% anthralin (Psoriatec, Sirius Laboratories, Sweden) without irritation. Compounded anthralin is most often used as a short contact agent and applied to the skin for at least 30–60 min once daily. Some patients with recalcitrant, indurated psoriatic plaques can tolerate even higher concentrations of anthralin under plastic wrap occlusion overnight.

The use of compounded anthralin and black tar is not mutually exclusive. In fact, some have suggested that patients would experience less irritation from anthralin if black tar were used concurrently. At our Center, the most common use of compounded anthralin in an outpatient setting is a short contact application in the evening to be washed off at bedtime and followed by tar. If the patient tolerates prolonged applications of compounded anthralin, the tar is then simply applied over the anthralin at bedtime, and they are both washed off in the morning. In this way, both anthralin and tar can be used to enhance UVB phototherapy. In patients with both large plaques and scattered small plaques, anthralin can be used on the larger lesions while tar may be used on the scattered lesions that are less amenable to the careful application of anthralin.

III. COMBINATION USE OF UVB PHOTOTHERAPY AND CALCIPOTRIENE OR TAZAROTENE

A number of calcipotriene and UVB regimens have been studied (26). Twice-weekly UVB with twice-daily calcipotriol cream proves to be just as effective as UVB three times per week with only vehicle cream applied twice daily (27). This equivalent therapeutic result was obtained with less than one-third the cumulative UVB exposure in the calcipotriol cream group compared to the vehicle cream group. This finding is important because there are many patients who are too busy to do UVB phototherapy three times per week, but could do it twice per week. For patients who pay copayments for visits, cutting down on the number of UVB visits per week is ideal. Due to rare reports of an immediate burning sensation when calcipotriol is applied around the same time as UVB phototherapy, it should not be applied within 2–3 h prior to exposure.

Tazarotene also enhances UVB phototherapy significantly, even if phototherapy is conducted aggressively three times per week (28). In a multicenter study headed by Koo et al., tazarotene 0.1% gel applied only three times per week was found to enhance aggressive UVB phototherapy regimen, significantly. A statistically significant difference was noted between active agent plus UVB phototherapy compared to UVB alone or UVB plus vehicle in the number of patients who achieved marked improvement (i.e., 75% or better). The cumulative UVB exposure for the group receiving tazarotene three times per week plus UVB phototherapy was less than one-quarter the UVB exposure required in the other two groups to reach threshold of 50% improvement in their lesional scores. No unusual photosensitivity from tazarotene was noted in the entire trial. Since tazarotene was only applied three times per week after UVB phototherapy, whether any photo-sensitivity would have occurred if tazarotene were applied daily or just prior to UVB exposure is not known.

IV. COMBINATION THERAPY WITH PUVA PHOTOTHERAPY

UVB therapy and PUVA therapy can be combined for an additive effect. This combination is especially useful for those patients who experience a flare of their psoriasis despite the use of their home UVB box. In theory, PUVA and UVB can be combined as long as each session is separated by at least 24 h to ensure that the blood level of psoralen reaches zero before the patient is exposed to UVB. This so-called washout time is critical since many UVB boxes also emit some UVA radiation leading to overexposure if treatments were conducted without adequate time between them. There are many patients whose skin clears adequately when PUVA therapy is based on the above schedule, even though these patients fail to respond adequately to PUVA or UVB alone. For patients who are using home UVB and yet experience a gradual flare, twice-weekly supplementation with PUVA frequently allows their psoriatic lesions to clear. Also, patients undergoing UVB therapy who are left with a few truly resistant lesions in areas such as elbows and shins can often clear with topical paint PUVA therapy. Oxsoralen 0.1% in solution or ointment is applied selectively to the resistant plaques followed in 30 min by exposure to UVA radiation (Fig. 7).

V. DAY TREATMENT PROGRAM

Day treatment programs can be viewed as the ultimate attempt short of hospitalization to maximize the efficacy of UVB phototherapy. This regi-men was developed mainly to minimize the cost of treatment from inpatient hospitalization, since patients with severe, generalized psoriasis often require a treatment period of 4 weeks or longer to clear their psoriasis

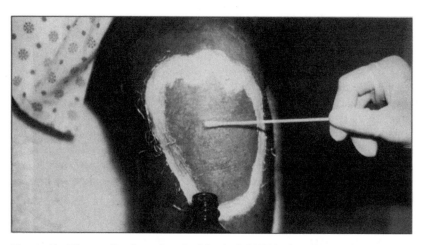

Figure 7 The application of topical "paint" PUVA therapy to selected, resistant psoriatic plaques is shown. Zinc oxide paste is sometimes used to prevent inadvertent application of 0.1% Oxsoralen solution to the noninvolved skin. (Refer to the color insert.)

completely. Traditionally, day treatment programs can be classified into two main types: Goeckerman therapy and Ingram therapy. However, with enough attention to detail, it is possible to use tar and Anthralin simultaneously, as stated earlier. Topical PUVA can also be conducted simultaneously with UVB therapy. At the UCSF Medical Center, the main treatment modality in the day treatment program is Goeckerman therapy, which combines crude coal tar with UVB phototherapy. If a patient proves to have a truly recalcitrant case of psoriasis, therapy can be escalated to combine Goeckerman, Ingram, and bath PUVA, while supplementing with oral retinoids, calcipotriol, and/or tazarotene.

Initially, patients with generalized psoriasis admitted to the day treatment program are started on 2% crude coal tar with total body UVB exposure. The concentration of crude coal tar and the exposure time for UVB is gradually increased as described previously. Localized, intense application of UVB phototherapy is initiated for resistant areas. If a patient's condition does not respond adequately to black tar and UVB phototherapy, compounded anthralin and, eventually, topical PUVA are added. Consequently, a patient with truly recalcitrant generalized psoriasis may eventually end up with a very intense regimen, as described in Table 3. This regimen is repeated daily including weekends (except for topical PUVA, which is conducted every other day) until clearance is achieved. If a patient still has recalcitrant lesions, 25 mg/day acitretin, tazarotene 0.1% cream, and calcipotriene are added.

Table 3 Maximum Day Treatment Regimen at UCSF Psoriasis Center

8:00–9:00 AM	Arrival at Center, Whole-body UVB treatment in UVB box followed by intense, localized UVB to resistant areas with hot quartz lamp or Dermalight®.
9:00 AM	Application of up to 10% concentrations of black tar and salicylic or lactic acid. Patient stays coated in tar until afternoon.
10:00–11:00 AM	Staff-conducted patient education and group discussion.
11:00–12:00 PM	Rounds with the attending physician.
12:00–1:00 PM	Lunch (catered).
2:00 PM	Compounded anthralin application to resistant areas.
3:00–3:30 AM	Wash off anthralin and tar. Second-round UVB treatment using UVB box, hot quartz lamp or Dermalight®, followed by whole-body application of 20% LCD in Aquaphor.
3:30–4:00 AM	For recalcitrant localized lesions, topical "paint" PUVA using 0.1% Oxsoralen® in Aquaphor is conducted before application of 20% LCD in Aquaphor.
Bedtime at home	One more whole-body application of 20% LCD in Aquaphor

By definition, the day treatment program is designed for resistant patients who have failed to respond to outpatient PUVA and UVB therapy. It is also well-suited for patients with generalized, recalcitrant psoriasis who cannot take systemic agents because of underlying medical problems, side effects, lack of efficacy, or a reluctance to be exposed to the risk of systemic side effects. When the day treatment program is optimized in the manner previously described, there are very few patients who still need systemic agents other than low-dosage oral retinoids. Unfortunately, due to constraints of reimbursement, despite its efficacy and safety, this type of intensive treatment is available only at a limited number of locations in the United States. It is still widely practiced in Canada, Europe, Scandinavia, and new centers are becoming operational in the Middle East.

VI. COMBINATION THERAPY WITH SYSTEMIC AGENTS

A. Retinoids

In many ways, retinoids such as acitretin are better suited for use in low dosages to enhance phototherapy than in high dosages as monotherapy (see Chap. 6 on Systemic Retinoids). When acitretin is used to enhance PUVA or UVB phototherapy, the dosage required often ranges from 25 mg every other day up to 50 mg a day. Sometimes as little as 10 mg a day may be adequate to enhance phototherapy. Patients tolerate low dosages much better than higher doses, such as 1 mg/kg/day, which is often required when etretinate is used as monotherapy in the treatment of psoriasis. Acitretin is especially useful for patients with extremely indurated and hyperkeratotic lesions in whom UVB radiation may not penetrate adequately unless the lesion is thinned by keratolytic agents (as previously described) or by retinoids. Lastly, if a female patient of childbearing age requires retinoid supplementation, isotretinoin in a similar dosage can be used to enhance phototherapy. This agent is also teratogenic but has a shorter half life.

There are two approaches when using acitretin to enhance UVB phototherapy. The first is to start the patient on acitretin approximately 2 weeks before starting phototherapy in order to prepare the skin for phototherapy. The second is to reserve low-dosage acitretin as a supplement after attempted UVB phototherapy alone proves unsatisfactory. Many patients who are motivated to commit the time and effort required for phototherapy prefer the latter approach to avoid the use of systemic agents. On the other hand, adding low-dosage etretinate to established UVB phototherapy increases the possibility of developing delayed photosensitivity. Many patients experience significant photosensitivity approximately 7–14 days following the addition of acitretin to optimized UVB phototherapy. To minimize the risk of burning, it is important to decrease the intensity of UVB therapy by up to 50% approximately 5–10 days after initiating low-dosage acitretin supplementation. If no photosensitivity develops, UVB radiation can be gradually increased to previous levels.

B. Hydroxyurea

Hydroxyurea (Hydrea) is another systemic agent that can be used to enhance UVB or PUVA phototherapy. The usual dosage for a healthy, average-sized adult is 500 mg orally twice daily. Although hydroxyurea is certainly not as effective as methotrexate, like low-dosage acitretin, it is well-suited for long-term enhancement of phototherapy in patients who experience a partial but less than adequate response to phototherapy alone. One of the main advantages of hydroxyurea is the minimal risk of hepatotoxicity associated with its long-term use. Hydroxyurea can be an alternative for a patient who is a candidate for methotrexate but refuses to consider the possibility of undergoing a liver biopsy. Also an advantage over methotrexate or acitretin, hydroxyurea used to enhance UVB phototherapy does not increase the risk of photosensitivity. However, hydroxyurea has a narrow therapeutic index and can be associated with bone marrow suppression and nephrotoxicity.

Therefore, complete blood count (CBC), liver function tests (LFT), and measurements of blood urea nitrogen (BUN) and creatinine should be periodically followed while using this agent.

Almost every patient who is on long-term treatment with hydroxyurea develops macrocytosis. Since it is usually not associated with anemia, the clinical relevance is questionable. Taking 1 mg/day folic acid minimizes the risk of macrocytic anemia. Although hydroxyurea is well described in the medical literature with respect to its use in psoriasis therapy, this drug is not approved by the Food and Drug Administration (FDA) for the treatment of psoriasis.

C. Methotrexate

Methotrexate can be used in conjuction with UVB phototherapy, however, with extreme caution due to the rare risk of acute photosensitivity (see Chap. 5 on Methotrexate) (29). There are at least three settings in which methotrexate may be combined with phototherapy or used prior to the initiation of phototherapy:

> Methotrexate is used to control widespread inflammation in a patient presenting with intense erythroderma prior to starting UVB phototherapy. This is especially useful if the patient is not a candidate for cyclosporine or is unable to participate in day treatment.
> Methotrexate is used in the short-term while initiating UVB phototherapy as an initial push to the therapeutic process.
> Methotrexate is used to enhance phototherapy when a patient's response to UVB phototherapy plateaus. In this situation, hydroxyurea or acitretin can also be used to accomplish the same result. A decision to use methotrexate depends on factors such as the patient's prior response to methotrexate, intolerance to other agents, or, in the case of acitretin, reproductive status.

Because of the above mentioned risk of acute photosensitivity induced by methotrexate, it is critical that the patient not be exposed to phototherapy for 48–72 h during and following methotrexate treatment. For example, a patient undergoing UVB phototherapy on Mondays, Wednesdays, and Fridays may start a weekly dose of methotrexate on Friday mornings right after receiving phototherapy. By the time he or she returns for UVB phototherapy on Monday, the risk of methotrexate photosensitivity is negligible. By using this combination, one can minimize the cumulative methotrexate needed to clear the psoriasis. Once psoriasis clears completely, methotrexate can be discontinued altogether and patient's disease can usually be controlled with UVB therapy alone.

Lastly, some patients are referred to outpatient UVB therapy or the day treatment program for the specific purpose of tapering off methotrexate. These are generally patients who have already received a high cumulative dosage of methotrexate. The same precautions regarding acute photosensitivity must be observed while initiating UVB phototherapy.

D. Cyclosporine

In theory, the combination of cyclosporine and phototherapy (especially PUVA therapy) can increase the risk of skin cancer in white patients. Long-term use of cyclosporine with phototherapeutic modalities is not currently recommended (30). However, there is one frequently encountered setting in which cyclosporine can be of great assistance in conducting phototherapy: patients with widespread, highly inflammatory lesions. Controlling inflammation is critical in setting the stage for initiating phototherapy. Erythrodermic patients have a great risk of developing a paradoxical reaction with either UVB or PUVA therapy: their skin becomes even more inflamed if phototherapy is initiated. Therefore, adequate control of the inflammatory state is critical before these patients can be safely started on phototherapy.

For many decades, this process of cooling down was accomplished in an inpatient setting with topical steroids, cool compresses, and soothing baths.

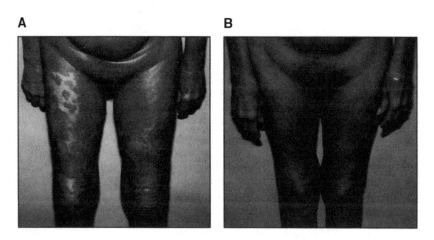

Figure 8 Erythrodermic patient with psoriasis and intense leg edema before (A) and after (B) short-term cyclosporine followed by long-term UVB phototherapy. This therapeutic regimen makes use of the powerful anti-inflammatory property of cyclosporine while minimizing the risk of systemic effects, which may be associated with long-term use of cyclosporine. (Refer to the color insert.)

More recently, limited reimbursement has led to new approaches such as short-term oral cyclosporine (3–5 mg/kg divided twice daily), which can be extremely effective in controlling erythema and inflammation (Fig. 8) (see Chap. 7 on Cyclosporine). One can conceivably use methotrexate or acitretin for controlling erythroderma; however, cyclosporine has a faster onset of action, no required test dose, and more reliably controls widespread inflammation. Once the skin is no longer beefy red, phototherapy with UVB or PUVA can be initiated and the cyclosporine dosage tapered down to 3 mg/kg/day. It can be gradually tapered altogether once phototherapy is optimized and the patient's erythroderma has resolved. Using cyclosporine for short periods of time (three months or less) decreases the risk of side effects such as nephrotoxicity. Hypertension may be encountered but is readily reversible with initiation of an antihypertensive agent or adjusting the dosage of cyclosporine. Moreover, the theoretical increased risk of malignancy can also be minimized by short-term use (31, 32).

VII. SUMMARY

UVB phototherapy is one of the safest therapeutic options available for treating widespread psoriasis. If it is not adequate, there are many creative ways to enhance treatment. Even though these methods may be more labor-intensive for health care providers and patients alike, patients who are especially wary of the systemic side effects of other treatment options often appreciate this option.

VIII. NARROW-BAND UVB

Through decades of study and clinical experience, UVB and psoralen plus UVA (PUVA) have become essential components of the treatment of psoriasis. Given the prevalence of disease and wide variability in patient profiles, researchers and physicians are constantly seeking new and different treatment options to offer their patients. Narrow-band UVB (NB-UVB) is an exciting, new modality that may be a boon not only for treatment-resistant patients or patients for whom other therapies are contraindicated, but also as a first- or second-line agent once practitioners become more familiar with it.

   Ultraviolet light lies between visible light and x-rays on the electro-magnetic spectrum. UVB ranges from 290–320 nm in wavelength. Standard UVB bulbs emit a wide range of light within this spectrum in addition to a small amount of UVA. NB-UVB light therapy uses a limited range of this spectrum. The TL-01 lamps emit a distinct and narrow band of high-intensity light ranging only from 311–313 nm, thus eliminating high-energy, shorter wavelengths responsible for burning, premature aging, and increased incidence of skin cancer. During early studies in the 1980s, authors examined various wavelengths and discovered that 313 nm allowed for the lowest effective dosage of light with the least erythema (33–35). The particular efficacy of this band of light should not be misinterpreted to mean that other UV wavelengths are not effective, only that UV in the range around 312 has the best phototherapy index. Improvement in psoriasis is also seen with a wide range of UVB and UVA wavelengths. NB-UVB has been utilized extensively throughout Europe and Australia and is now gaining popularity in the United States as evidence documenting its effectiveness continues to accumulate. Philips Company manufactures the lamps and reports that Europe has converted almost entirely to either narrow band lamps or PUVA, whereas only about 15 % of the company's narrow-band sales go to the United States. This number continues to grow as more US dermatologists learn the benefits of NB-UVB phototherapy.

A. NB-UVB Compared to BB-UVB

For the treatment of psoriasis, multiple studies have shown NB-UVB to be more effective than BB-UVB (36–40). Clearance is more rapid (38, 41), requires fewer treatments in some cases, and is preferred by more patients (40, 42). One disadvantage is that NB-UVB requires higher dosages of light to achieve minimal erythema, and thus requires longer treatment times than compared to BB-UVB (37–42). This could be difficult for disabled or elderly patients who do not tolerate long periods of standing, and busy clinics may not be able to accommodate large volumes of patients.

To compensate for higher required dosages of light, several options are available. NB-UVB boxes are sold containing 24–48 bulbs whereas standard UVB boxes typically contain 8–16 bulbs. More bulbs correspond to shorter treatment times. Several reports indicate that psoriasis does clear with less aggressive NB regimens that do not lead to erythema (33, 43–45). Therefore, treatment times may be shortened without sacrificing efficacy. Finally, as discussed above, combination therapy should be considered as a way to shorten treatment times. Each method of treatment may not clear psoriasis completely, but when used in combination may produce results better than either modality used alone. NB-UVB is no exception to this rule. Combination therapy can reduce light treatment times and light dosing requirements. Recent studies demonstrate that combining NB-UVB with tazarotene gel, anthralin, or calcipotriol can provide faster, more effective clearance with less irradiation and fewer treatments (46–48).

B. Remission Rates with NB-UVB

Few data are available comparing remission rates of NB-UVB and UVB. In one study, authors reported a stark difference in remission rates favoring NB-UVB (49). Thirty-eight percent of the NB-UVB group was still in remission 1 year after cessation of therapy. The average time to relapse was 3 months for the remaining 62%. Only 5% of UVB patients in a different study conducted by the same investigators were still in remission one year after treatment. Time to relapse was not mentioned for this group. This comparison may be flawed because the UVB group was much smaller than the NB-UVB group, the studies were conducted at different times, and the UVB therapy may have been suboptimal as evidenced by the high burning rates even with a regimen of only twice-weekly therapy.

C. NB-UVB Compared to PUVA

The advantages of NB-UVB diminish when compared to PUVA. There are several factors to consider when comparing the two therapies, including efficacy, carcinogenesis, remission rates, and ease of administration. The first investigations comparing the efficacy of PUVA and NB-UVB were done in 1990 using bilateral comparison methods in patients with widespread psoriasis (50). Although the two treatments were found to be equally effective, more patients preferred NB-UVB. Looking more closely at the data revealed that PUVA was actually more effective in clearing extremities and NB-UVB was more effective in clearing trunk psoriasis. These findings indicate that PUVA may be better for clearing lesions that are more recalcitrant to therapy, such as those usually found on the extremities. Other studies have reported similar findings (51, 52). It is interesting to note that differences may be notable only in groups of patients with high Psoriasis Area and Severity Index (PASI) scores, or those with more severe disease. Thus, for many patients, NB-UVB and PUVA are equivalent first-line treatments, but for patients with severe, hard-to-treat psoriasis, PUVA is still a better option. The largest study comparing NB-UVB to PUVA involved 100 patients, and demonstrated that given twice weekly, PUVA is more effective than narrow-band UVB with significantly fewer treatments and almost three times the remission rate at 6 months after treatment (53). PUVA is well known to induce remission rates of 4–6 months or even longer, a definite advantage over NB-UVB.

One major disadvantage of PUVA is the risk of carcinogenesis. The increased risk of squamous cell carcinoma in patients treated with UVA is well documented (69), while comparable data evaluating the safety of NB-UVB is not yet definitive. (See Safety of NB-UVB) However, NB-UVB offers some major logistic advantages over PUVA that may be important when choosing therapy for an individual patient. It is less time-consuming, easier to perform, and does not require concomitant administration of a photosensitizer that may cause nausea, cataracts, phototoxic reactions, and unwanted drug reactions. Other advantages also include safe use in pregnant women and children and no drug costs.

D. NB-UVB for the Treatment of Other Skin Diseases

Although NB-UVB is promoted as an advancement for the treatment of psoriasis, and most studies focus on this, it may prove to be beneficial for other recalcitrant skin diseases. As any dermatologist knows, management of atopic dermatitis (AD) can be challenging and often unsatisfactory. Current methods of treatment can result in severe cutaneous and systemic side effects. Over the past 10 years, several studies have shown NB-UVB to be a hopeful option for patients with AD (54–57). Seborrheic dermatitis (SD) is another persistent skin disease affecting 2–10% of the adult population. One study has shown the effectiveness of NB-UVB (58). It is also a suitable alternative for treating photodermatoses and may be especially useful for UVA-sensitive patients, and those with actinic prurigo, hydroa vacciniforme, idiopathic solar urticaria, and polymorphic light eruption (59–61). In these patients, NB-UVB produces a hardening photoprotective effect while avoiding the risk of provocation by UVA wavelengths. NB-UVB treatment has been shown to be promising for treatment of vitiligo, (62, 63) and to be safe and effective in childhood vitiligo, significantly improving patients' quality of life (64).

E. Side Effects of NB-UVB

Similar to other phototherapies, the side effects of NB-UVB include erythema and blistering, but may be more severe. Compared to PUVA, a greater proportion of patients treated with NB-UVB develop erythema, but PUVA-treated patients are more likely to miss treatments due to burning, which is a reflection of the long-lasting nature of PUVA erythema (53). Data on the incidence and severity of burning when compared to UVB are controversial. Burning episodes with NB-UVB have been reported as fewer than (40, 41), equal to (39), and more (38, 65) than with UVB. Tissue biopsies obtained from 1.0 and 2.0 MED sites reveal that the frequency of sunburn cells is similar at 1.0 MED, but 10–12 times greater in NB-UVB than BB-UVB at 2.0 MED (38). In addition, these cells are more widely distributed throughout the epidermis in NB-UVB-treated skin. These findings suggest more damaging potential of NB-UVB when 1.0 MED is exceeded. Animal studies similarly demonstrated more severe and persistent burning (66).

With NB-UVB therapy, there have also been some reports of rare blistering strictly at the site of psoriatic lesions while the surrounding normal skin remains completely unaffected (51, 67, 68). Some have speculated that due to the rapid clearance by NB-UVB, the psoriatic plaques may not gain the same photoprotection as the surrounding normal skin, thus exposing them to a burning dose midway through treatment (67). Other authors similarly concluded after histological examination that blisters result from quick reduction of acanthosis and desquamation before the development of tolerance, which results from an increase in pigmentation and stratum corneum thickness (68).

F. Safety of NB-UVB

In patients treated for many years with conventional UVB, there is little or no increased risk of skin cancer (69). Unfortunately, comparable data evaluating the safety of NB-UVB are not yet available. Murine experiments that have examined the carcinogenicity of NB-UVB offer conflicting data thus far. NB-UVB has been shown to be less (36, 37), equally (71), and more carcinogenic than BB-UVB (66, 72). Studies differ in mouse strains used, dosages of light, and treatment schedules, making comparison difficult. Studies demonstrating increased carcinogenesis also had higher rates of burning (66). This has particular relevance to the clinical setting where higher rates of burning may be a problem, and higher dosages larger doses of light are being delivered. Thus, adjusting the dosage of light may be the key to limiting carcinogenesis of NB-UVB, since lower-dosage regimens are as effective as high-dosage regimens, and require only a few more treatments (52).

G. Current Use of NB-UVB

There are two regimens currently available for treating patients with NB-UVB. The first involves determining a patient's MED (60). This requires patch testing with varying quantities of light to determine the dosage that produces a mild sunburn, or just perceptible erythema 24 h after irradiation. Once the MED has been determined, a patient can commence treatment using a percentage based protocol similar to those used in standard UVB. Typically first exposures start at 70% MED. Subsequent exposures given three times weekly are determined based on the reaction to the previous treatment. MED determination is difficult and time-consuming, and based on anecdotal reports, most clinicians do not do it. For those who do, Phillips Company makes four different lamp sizes, the smallest of which is a 7 inch twin tube for which Daavlin has designed a handheld unit, which could be used as an MED tester. Daavlin also sells MED testing kits and supplies.

Table 4   Narrow-Band Skin Type-Based Dosing Protocol,
Established by Leone Dermatology Center

Skin Type	Initial Dose (mj)	Subsequent Increase in Dose (mj)	Estimated Goal Range (mj)
I	130	15	520
II	220	25	880
III	260	40	1040
IV	330	45	1320
V	350	60	1400
VI	400	65	1600
Vitiligo	170	30	680

Source: Reprinted from Dermatol Nurs 2000; 12(6): 407–411, with permission from the publisher.

Most clinicians prefer to use a more practical dosing approach based on skin type. Skin-type treatment schedules vary widely in the reported literature, and protocols continue to evolve as clinicians gain more experience with this treatment. One schedule outlined by Leone Dermatology Center in Chicago is particularly good, in the author's opinion (73). This busy NB-UVB treatment center established a percentage-based protocol based on skin typing, using National Biologic Corporation equipment (Tables 4 and 5). Light is increased based on a patient's reaction to prior treatments. Patients

Table 5   Adjustments for Missed Treatments

Treatments Missed	% Of Last Treatment to Give
1–7 days	Increase per standard protocol
8–11 days	100% (no conditioning lost)
12–14 days	Decrease by two treatments
15–20 days	75% of last dose, but not less than base dose (25% of conditional may be lost)
21–27 days	50% of last dose but not less than base dose (50% of conditioning may be lost)
28 or more days	Start over at base dose (100% of conditioning may be lost)

Source: Reprinted from Dermatol Nurs 2000; 12(6): 407–411, with permission from the publisher.

are treated three times weekly with a goal dosage of approximately four times the initial dosage. This center estimates that the number of treatments to clear a patient is similar to conventional UVB: 30–35 treatments. Patients should expect to be treated for at least 3 months followed by maintenance therapy. In general, significant reduction in scaling may be noted after the first three to six treatments, and a significant response seen after six to nine treatments. Extra treatments to the extremities can be given as in conventional UVB. This can be initiated with the first treatment or added at any time during treatment. Maintenance tends to be every 7–10 days to prevent relapse. A practical text of broadband and narrow-band light treatment protocols for psoriasis and other skin disorders is available (74). Readers should note that different equipment can dramatically change the required protocol. These are guidelines and should be interpreted with flexibility for each patient's requirements. Adjustments should be made according to each patient's response in conjunction with physician judgement.

H. Economics of NB-UVB

Starting an NB-UVB practice or adding it to an existing one is costly, due to the requirements for equipment, replacement parts, bulbs, staff training, and increased overhead costs. Currently, reimbursement for NB-UVB is no different from UVB: a separate current procedural terminology (CPT) billing code has not yet been established. Many options are available when purchasing a NB-UVB unit. Units with 48 bulbs cost $16,000–$17,500. Units with fewer bulbs are cheaper. The best unit for a busy practice is probably that with the most bulbs so that clinics are not slowed, and patients are not forced to stand for long periods of time due to longer treatments. Combination boxes provide less intense NB-UVB light and thus require longer treatment times, which is a disadvantage in a busy phototherapy practice. For small phototherapy practices, cheaper options include units without fans, standing platforms, built-in dosimetry and protocols, or panel units. Panel units are typically used for home NB-UVB therapy, but are sometimes sold for clinics as well. NB-UVB phototherapy is also available in hand and foot units, or hand-held units for localized areas, hard-to-reach places, and for the scalp, to be used with a removable comb attachment.

Available since 1989, NB-UVB bulbs are TL-01 fluorescent lamps manufactured by Phillips Company in Holland. They are sold in four sizes: 6 foot bulbs, 2 foot bulbs, 22 inch twin tubes, and 7 inch twin tubes. The requirement for more NB-UVB bulbs compared to BB-UVB translates to higher relamping costs. Bulb prices are shown in Tables 6 and 7. National Biologic sells 6 foot NB-UVB bulbs for $125, or $25 more than BB-UVB. Daavlin offers the two products each for $100. Psoralite Corporation offers

Table 6 NB-UVB Options and Prices Offered By
Psoralite Corporation

Unit	Number of lamps	Price ($)
Model 57000-44 NB	44	15,595
Model 57000-36 NB	36	13,995
Model 57000-24 NB	24	11,995

the 6 foot bulbs for $105. The running lifespan of the TL-01 has not yet been well quantified, and sales corporations offer varying estimates from 300 to 500 h. In practice, the life expectancy seems to be shorter than UVB or UVA bulbs, thus requiring more frequent replacements, which also increases the cost of NB-UVB over to BB-UVB.

Measuring light output is an important part of safe and effective phototherapy. Some machines are sold with built-in dosimetry meters so that output is machine-monitored and calibration needs to be done only once yearly. Daavlin offers a meter for UVA, BB-UVB, and NB-UVB, $2399 or a 3 year plan in which maintenance personnel perform the measurement for a package price of $1500. National Biologic offers UVB meters for $690. Since a measuring device for NB-UVB output is not yet available, the current standard of care is to use a BB-UVB device and multiply by a factor of

Table 7 NB-UVB Options and Prices Offered By
Daavlin Corporation

Unit	Number of lamps	Price ($)
Spectra 311 48	48	17,500
Spectra 311 36	36	16,000
Spectra 311 24	24	14,500
Spectra 311-350	24 NB/24 BB	16,500
Spectra 311-305	36 NB/12 BB	18,500
Theraflex 311-48	48	16,000
Theraflex 311-36	36	14,500
Theraflex 311-24	24	13,000
Theraflex 311-350	24 NB/24 BB	15,000
Theraflex 311-305	36 NB/12 BB	17,500
NB-UVB TL-01 6 foot lamp	Single bulb	100
BB-UVB TL-01 6 foot lamp	Single bulb	100
NB-UVB TL-01 2 foot lamp	Single bulb	80
NB-UVB TL-01 2 foot lamp	Single bulb	68

0.75. Manufacturers recommend replacing the bulbs when energy output drops to 0.75 mW/cm^2.

I. Summary

NB-UVB is an important advancement in the field of dermatology, not only for psoriasis but also for other skin diseases. Although more data are needed in this field, physicians and their patients have welcomed an additional, effective treatment option as a first-line agent, a new choice for resistant psoriasis, or for use in combination with other treatments.

IX. LOCALIZED PHOTOTHERAPY FOR PSORIASIS

As discussed above, UVB is an effective treatment for patients with even severe psoriasis. Since even long-term follow-up studies detect no increased risk of skin cancer following UVB phototherapy (75), it probably offers among the best risk/benefit ratios of any of the treatments for severe psoriasis. While there are few head-to-head trials comparing different treatments, the clearance rate reported for UVB treatment is among the highest of all these treatments (76). Clearance rates for UVB can be as high as > 80% (in combination with topicals), while reported clearance rates for PUVA and methotrexate are 70–80% and 60–70% for cyclosporine A (clearance rates across different studies must be interpreted with caution. Some experienced clinicians believe that cyclosporine clearance rates are better than that observed with UVB phototherapy.) Another advantage of UVB phototherapy is the potential for inducing remissions in psoriasis. Narrow-band UVB provides an even higher efficacy level. For patients with extensive psoriasis, the first line of treatment is UVB phototherapy, unless contraindicated.

Most patients with psoriasis, however, have relatively localized disease. They are treated primarily with topical agents. Topical agents are safer than phototherapy and systemic therapy, but they are also considerably less effective. Moreover, while patients with generalized disease are often quite satisfied with a reduction in the disease and associated symptoms, patients who present for treatment of very localized disease are often unsatisfied unless full clearance of the lesions is achieved.

The use of UVB phototherapy on a localized basis offers the potential of greater efficacy than topical therapy. While localized phototherapy can be achieved with the use of standard phototherapy equipment and careful blocking of surrounding skin, the use of a UVB laser makes this procedure much more amenable to clinical practice. Other forms of localized UV and other lasers offer patients with localized psoriasis additional options. These are also potentially of value for treatment of specific, perhaps more resistant, lesions in patients with more extensive disease.

A. Unmet Need for Localized Psoriasis Treatment

Patients with psoriasis desire a treatment that provides high efficacy, including both clearance of the lesions and a long-term, treatment-free remission of the disease (77). Patients also seek therapies that are safe. Other very important considerations are that therapies not be messy (patients certainly do not want treatments that are worse than the disease), but that they be convenient and low cost. Compared to topical therapies, localized UV therapy meets many of these goals.

B. UV Laser

The most information on localized UVB treatment comes from studies with the excimer laser. This laser is based on a xenon–chloride lasing medium that produces UV light at a wavelength of 308 nm. At high fluences, 308 nm light can be used to ablate tissue, such as cornea or atherosclerotic plaque, or other materials (78, 79). At the relatively low fluences used to treat psoriasis, the laser acts not to destroy tissue but rather as a form of localized UVB phototherapy. The 308 nm peak provides a very narrow band (far narrower than narrow-band UVB) near the peak of the psoriasis improvement spectrum. This, and perhaps the coherence of laser light, may provide some benefit over other forms of UV phototherapy (80).

The excimer laser device is a major technical achievement. It requires an optically pure quartz fiberoptic cable to deliver the monochromatic 308 nm UV light from the machine to the patient. The spot size of this laser is far larger than that typically encountered in dermatology, measuring approximately 3.2 cm^2 (slightly larger than a nickel), allowing practical treatment of several large plaques at a single session. The excimer laser may be used in either paint or a tile mode. In paint mode, UV is delivered continuously as the handpiece is moved over the plaques. In tile mode, the handpiece is held in place, a predetermined amount of UV is given, and the handpiece is then moved to an adjacent area of the plaque. While paint mode is more rapid, tile mode provides greater reproducibility in dosing.

Localized treatment with UVB offers the potential to meet a number of patients' needs. UVB is highly effective and induces remissions. It has a risk of acute sunburn-like reactions, but these are generally better tolerated than standard phototherapy burns because they are local: only the plaques are exposed. There is also a low potential for increased risk of skin cancer with UVB phototherapy, but it is expected that this risk will be lower with localized therapy because the normal skin unaffected by psoriasis is not exposed to UV radiation. Laser phototherapy is not messy, although plaques should be treated with mineral oil or other moisturizer to clarify the scale and facilitate UV penetration into the plaque. Finally, localized laser phototherapy is quicker and more convenient than broadband UV; fewer treatments are required because much higher initial dosages of UV can be given to the plaques. Normal skin, which is not exposed to the laser light, would not tolerate the high dosages that can be used to clear the plaques.

C. UV Laser Efficacy

The efficacy of the 308 nm excimer UVB laser was tested in several studies (81–85). Initial promising case reports were followed by a multicenter study performed in 5 dermatology offices (86). Patients with stable plaque psoriasis (n = 124) covering less than 10% body surface area (BSA) were enrolled and 80 completed the study. In clinical practice, there are no hard guidelines on how much area is appropriate to treat, although if patients have more than 10% BSA it is probably more practical to treat them with standard whole-body phototherapy. The treatment protocol used in the study is described in Table 8. Seventy-two percent of patients achieved at least 75% clearing in an average of 6.2 treatments. Thirty-five percent achieved 90% clearing in an average of 7.5 treatments. In a follow-up study of subjects in this multicenter trial, 25% of subjects reported that the laser treatments were better than any other treatment they had tried; 55% reported overall satisfaction with the treatments. The most common side effects were erythema, blisters, hyper-pigmenetation, and erosion, and these were well tolerated.

While no head-to-head data are available to compare with other treatments, a greater percentage of patients achieved 75% improvement with the excimer laser than has been reported for other forms of phototherapy or systemic therapy. However, the patient populations treated with these forms of therapy are very different: photo- and systemic therapy are for patients with extensive disease, whereas the primary use of the excimer laser is in patients with localized psoriasis. When compared with topical therapies, excimer laser treatment is reported to have an efficacy equal to topical calcipotriene and greater than tazarotene or fluocinonide, and the efficacy is achieved in less time. In clinical practice, it seems sensible to use the excimer laser in combination with one or more of these topical therapies to achieve faster and more extensive clearing, although clinical trial results are not yet available.

D. Other Local UV Treatment

Local delivery of UV light can be achieved by more conventional means. In addition to hand and foot units and UV combs, localized phototherapy can be delivered by hot quartz lamp, shielding the normal skin that surrounds the

Table 8 Excimer Laser Protocol

The following protocol was used in the clinical trial assessing the efficacy of 308nm excimer laser treatment of localized psoriasis. The laser was used in tile mode. This mode is preferred for the research setting since it permits greater standardization between operators and centers. For clinical practice, paint mode is faster and more convenient.

1. MED determined on unexposed, uninvolved skin.
2. Immediately prior to laser irradiation, a small amount of mineral oil was applied to the area to be treated to clarify the scale (12% ammonium lactate [Lac-Hydrin] lotion or equivalent was applied as a descaling agent twice daily for several days prior to laser treatment if needed to reduce scale).
3. Initial UV dose administered based on the MED and the physical characteristics (location, size, thickness) of the plaque.
   a. 3 MED was generally used
   b. Plaques on the ankles or intertriginous areas were treated with 2 MED
   c. Tanned plaques were treated with 1 additional MED
4. Initial dose was maintained until plaques thinned or flattened considerably or pigment appeared
5. Over the course of treatment, dose was continually reduced by 1 MED as plaque became thin and/or hyperpigmented
6. The dose was continually increased by 1 MED at each session of no visual response in the lesion was observed.
7. If blistering occurred, Vaseline or Aquaphor healing ointment was applied, the dose of the subsequent treatment was reduced by 1 multiple of the MED, and the blistered plaque was not treated on the next scheduled treatment.

plaque. While this is another effective means to deliver UV therapy, it is less convenient, and there are no head-to-head studies exploring relative efficacy. A new device that delivers local narrow band UV light using a light guide and handpiece may offer yet another way to treat localized lesions of psoriasis with UV phototherapy. The value of a combination of these forms of UV delivery with topical therapy, topical or systemic PUVA, or oral retinoids has not yet been explored.

E. Other Lasers

The use of the pulsed-dye laser in the treatment of psoriasis was published in 1996 (87). Long-term remission of disease was reported. Nevertheless, widespread use of the pulsed dye-laser did not quickly follow. Limitations included pain with treatment, a small treatment spot size, and high cost that made the therapy impractical. Recent improvements in pulsed-dye lasers including larger spot size and tissue cooling to reduce pain may make this a more practical treatment option for patients with localized psoriasis plaques. Still, multiple treatments may be required, and complete clearing is not always achieved (88).

F. Coding for and Regulation of Laser Treatment of Psoriasis

The standard code used for UVB phototherapy is 96900. Although narrow-band UVB is more expensive to the physician administering it than is broadband UVB, the phototherapy codes used are the same. This phototherapy code covers only administration of the treatment. For Medicare reimbursement, a physician must be "present" at the time of phototherapy. This requirement has resulted in the closure of some phototherapy centers that did not have an on-site physician. Use of an evaluation and management office visit code (99201-5 for new patients or 99211-5 for return patients) in addition to the phototherapy code is appropriate if distinct evaluation and management services are provided at the visit. Evaluation of the patient's progress and signs and symptoms of phototoxicity by a nurse or phototherapist may justify the use of the 99211 code. Using these office visit codes often results in a copayment charge to the patient.

New CPT codes have been developed for laser treatment of psoriasis, which apply to all forms of laser treatment used to treat psoriasis. Because they are new, they may not be recognized by all insurers. The use of medical lasers is regulated on a state-by-state basis. Some states require laser treatments to be delivered by a physician. Physicians should consult with their state medical board to determine their local regulations.

X. LIMITATIONS

Despite many years of advancement in psoriasis treatment, UVB phototherapy remains among the safest, most effective, and most versatile treatments for psoriasis. Nevertheless, the limitations of phototherapy need to be recognized. First and foremost, office UV phototherapy can be a major inconvenience. There is time spent in the office preparing for and undergoing the phototherapy treatment, and traffic and parking time needs to be included in the expected time lost from work. While day treatment programs may be extremely safe and effective, they are perhaps the least convenient way to manage psoriasis. The cost of phototherapy is also not inconsequential. Under some forms of insurance, patients are required to pay a copayment at each visit. The disincentive this places on patients may account in part for the less frequent use of phototherapy in the United States (89). For some patients, the inconvenience of phototherapy (and the cost as well) may be ameliorated through the use of home UVB phototherapy. If office UVB phototherapy is not available, tanning bed treatments may be beneficial for some patients (90). As with all other forms of psoriasis therapy, it is essential to consider the impact of the treatment on the patient's life when determining the treatment plan.

XI. PRACTICAL RESOURCES

A number of practical resources are available to support physicians interested in providing phototherapy to their patients. The National Psoriasis Foundation (NPF, *www.psoriasis.org*) provides very helpful patient-oriented materials, including a specific brochure on phototherapy. Providing a patient with this brochure not only educates the patient on the benefits and risks of (and alternatives to) phototherapy, it also provides the physician a ready way to document that this information has been provided in writing. Through the NPF's *Psoriasis Forum* newsletter, physicians can gain access to sample letters that may be used to help patients gain insurance coverage for phototherapy. The NPF has also produced and distributes an educational resource for insurers to increase their understanding of psoriasis as a disease and the treatments that that fall within the standard of care. The NPF will even assist individual patients with difficulties they may encounter in finding a phototherapy center or obtaining coverage from their insurer. Another valuable NPF service is its course, "Phototherapy from the ground up: How to give light treatment correctly." This is a 2 1/2 day course that offers training and tips to help nurses and phototherapy technicians. It is held three times a year, and participants receive educational credits (through the American Nurses Association) for their attendance. A practical textbook of phototherapy is also available that provides detailed protocols, flow sheets, and consent forms (74).

REFERENCES

1. Koo J, Lebwohl M. Duration of remission of psoriasis therapies. J Am Acad Dermatol 1999; 41(1):51–59.
2. Birt AR, Davis RA. Hereditary polymorphic light eruption of American Indians. Int J Dermatol. 1975; 14:105–111.

3. Gshnait G, Honigsmann H, Brenner W, et al. Induction of UV light tolerance by PUVA in patients with polymorphous light eruption. Br J Dermatol. 1978;99:293–295.
4. Elmets CA. Drug induced photoallergy. In: DeLeo VA, ed. Photosensitivity Diseases Dermatol Clin. 1986; 4(2):231–241.
5. Valerie K, Delers A, Bruck C, et al. Activation of human immunodeficiency virus type 1 by DNA damage in human cells. Nature. 1988;333:78–81.
6. Stein B, Kramer M, Rahmsdorf HJ, Ponta H, Herrlich P. UV-induced transcription from the human immunodeficiency virus type 1 (HIV-1) transcription in nonirradiated cells. J Virol. 1989;63:4540–4544.
7. Legrand-Poels S, Vaira D, Pincemil J, Van de Vorst A, Piette J. Activation of human immunodeficiency virus type1 by oxidative stress. AIDS Res Hum Retroviruses. 1990;6:1389–1397.
8. Osborn L, Kunkel S, Nabel GJ. Tumor necrosis and interleukin 1 stimulate the human immunodeficiency virus enhancer by activation of the nuclear factor kB. Proc Natl Acad Sci USA. 1989; 86:2336–2340.
9. Meola T, Soter NA, Ostreicher R, et al. The safety of UVB phototherapy in patients with HIV infection. J Am Acad Dermatol. 1993;29:216–220.
10. Adrian RM, LeVine MJ, Parrish JA. Treatment frequency for outpatient phototherapy of psoriasis. A comparative study. Arch Dermatol. 1981;117: 623–626.
11. LeVine MJ, Parrish JA. Outpatient phototherapy of psoriasis. Arch Dermatol. 1980;116:552–554.
12. Menkes A, Stern RS, Arndt KA. Psoriasis treatment with suberythemogenic ultraviolet B radiation and a coal tar extract. J Am Acad Dermatol. 1984;12:21–25.
13. Morison WL. Phototherapy and Photochemotherapy of Skin Disease, 2nd ed. New York: Raven Press, 1991:80.
14. Petrozzi JW. Updating the Goeckerman regimen for psoriasis. Br J Dermatol. 1987;98:437–444.
15. Stern RS. Effect of continued ultraviolet B phototherapy on the duration of remission of psoriasis: a randomized study. J Am Acad Dermatol. 1986; 15:546–552.
16. Lowe NJ, Wortzman MS, Breeding J, et al. Coal tar phototherapy for psoriasis reevaluated: erythematous versus suberythemogenic ultraviolet with a tar extract in oil and crude coal tar. J Am Acad Dermatol. 1983;8:781–789.
17. Belsito DV, Kechijian P. The role of tar in Goeckerman therapy. Arch Dermatol. 1982;118:319–321.
18. Petrozzi JW, De los Reyes O. Ultraviolet phototherapy in psoriasis with hydrophilic ointment alone or with crude coal tar. Arch Dermatol Res. 1982;272:257–262.
19. LeVine M, White HAD, Parrish JA. Components of the Goeckerman therapy. J Invest Dermatol. 1979;73:170–173.
20. Frost P. Tar gel-phototherapy for psoriasis. Arch Dermatol. 1979;115:840–846.

21. Pittelkow MR, Perry HO, Muller SA, et al. Skin cancer in patients with psoriasis treated with coal tar. Arch Dermatol. 1981;117:465–468.
22. Alderson MR, Clarke JA. Cancer incidence in patients with psoriasis. Br J Cancer. 1983;47:857–859.
23. Larko O, Swanbeck kG. Is UVB treatment in psoriasis safe? A study of exclusively UVB-treated psoriasis patients compared with a matched control group. Acta Derm Venereol (Stockh). 1982;62:507–512.
24. Olson RL, Sayre RM, Everett MA. Effect of anatomic location and time on ultraviolet erythema. Arch Dermatol. 1996;93:211–215.
25. Chue B, Borok M, Lowe NJ. Phototherapy units; comparison of fluorescent ultraviolet B and ultraviolet A units with a high-pressure mercury system. J Am Acad Dermatol. 1988;18:641–645.
26. Kokelj S, Lavaroni G, Guadagnini A. UVB versus UVB plus calcipotriol therapy for psoraisis vulgaris. Acta Derm Venereol (Stockh). 1995;75:386–387.
27. Ramsay CA, Schwartz BE, Lowson D, et al. Calcipotriol cream combined with twice weekly broad-band UVB phototherapy: a safe, effective and UVB-sparing antipsoriatic combination treatment. The Canadian Calcipotriol and UVB Study Group. Dermatology. 2000;200(1):17–24.
28. Koo J, Lowe N, Lew-Kaya D, Vasilopoulos A, Lue J, Sefton J, Gibson J. Tazarotene Plus UVB phototherapy in the treatment of psoriasis. J Am Acad Dermatol. 2000 Nov; 43(5 Pt 1):821–828.
29. Paul BS, Momtaz K, Stern RS, et al. Combined methotrexate–ultraviolet B therapy in treatment of psoriasis. J Am Acad Dermatol. 1982;7:758–762.
30. Oxholm A, Thomsen K, Menne T. Squamous cell carcinomas in relation to cyclosporin therapy of non-malignant skin disorders. Acta Derm Venereol (Stockh). 1989;69:89–90.
31. Krupp P, Monka C. Side-effect profile of cyclosporin A in patients treated for psoriasis. Br J Dermatol. 1990;122(suppl 36):47–56.
32. Penn I. Cancers following cyclosporin therapy. Transplantation. 1987;43:32–35.
33. Parrish JA, Jaenicke KF. Action spectrum for phototherapy of psoriasis. J Invest Dermatol 1981; 76:359–362.
34. Diffey BL, Farr PM. An appraisal of ultraviolet lamps used for the phototherapy of psoriasis. Br J Dermatol 1987; 117:49–56.
35. Van Weelden H, Young E, van der Leun JC. Therapy of psoriasis: comparison of photochemotherapy and several variants of phototherapy. Br J Dermatol 1980; 103:I.
36. Van Weelden H, van der Leun JC. Improving the effectiveness of phototherapy for psoriasis. Br J Dermatol 1984; 111:484.
37. Van Weelden H, Baart de la Faille H, Young E, van der Leun JC. A new development in UVB phototherapy of psoriasis. Br J Dermatol. 1988; 119:11–19.
38. Coven TR, Burack LH, Gilleaudeau P, Keogh M, Ozawa M, Krueger JG. Narrow band UV-B produces superior clinical and histolpathological resolution of moderate-to-severe psoriasis in patients compared with broad-band UV-B. Arch Dermatol 1997; 133:1514–1522.

39. Karvonen J, Kokkonen EL, Ruotsalainen E. 311 nm UVB lamps in the treatment of psoriasis with the Ingram regimen. Acta Derm Venereol (Stockh) 1989; 69:82–85.

40. Picot E, Meunier L, Picot-Debeze MC. Treatment of psoriasis with a 311-nm UVB lamp. Br J Dermatol 1992; 127:509–512.

41. Green C, Ferguson J, Lakshmipathi T, Johnson BE. 311 nm UVB phototherapy—an effective treatment for psoriasis. Br J Dermatol 1988; 119:691–696.

42. Larko O. Treatment of psoriasis with a new UVB-lamp. Acta Derm Veneorol (Stockh) 1989; 69:357–359.

43. Fischer T, Alsins J, Berne B. Ultraviolet action spectrum and evaluation of ultraviolet lamps for psoriasis healing. Int J Dermatol 1984; 23:633–637.

44. Hofer A, Fink-Puches R, Kerl H, Wolf P. Comparison of phototherapy with near vs. far erythremogenic doses of narrow-band ultraviolet B in patients with psoriasis. Br J Dermatol 1998; 138:96–100.

45. Walters IB, Burack LH, Coven TR, Gilleaudeau P, Krueger JG. Suberythemogenic narrow-band UVB is markedly more effective than conventional UVB in treatment of psoriasis vulgaris. J Am Acad Dermatol 1999; 40:893–900.

46. Behrens S, Grundmann-Kollmann M, Schiener R, Peter RU, Kerscher M. Combination phototherapy of psoriasis with narrow-band UVB irradiation and topical tazarotene gel. J Am Acad Dermatol. 2000;42:493–495.

47. Carrozza P, Hausermann P, Nestle FO, Burg G, Boni R. Clinical efficacy of narrow-band UVB (311nm) combined with dithranol in psoriasis. Dermatology 2000; 200:35–39.

48. Kerscher M, Volkenandt M, Plewig G, Lehmann P. Combination phototherapy of psoriasis with calcipotriol and narrow-band UVB [letter]. Lancet 1993; 342:923.

49. Green C, Ferguson J, Lakshmipathi T, Johnson BE. 311 nm UVB phototherapy—an effective treatment for psoriasis. Br J Dermatol 1988; 119:691–696.

50. Van Weelden H, Baart De La Faille H, Young E, Van Der Leun JC. Comparison of narrow-band UV-B phototherapy and PUVA photochemotherapy in the treatment of psoriasis. Acta Derm Venereol (Stockh) 1990; 70:212–215.

51. Tanew A, Radakovic-Fijan S, Schemper M, Honigsmann H. Narrow-band UV-B phototherapy vs photochemotherapy in the treatment of chronic plaque-type psoriasis: A paired comparison study. Arch Dermatol. 1999; 135:519–524.

52. Hofer A, Fink-Puches R, Kerl H, Wolf P. Comparison of phototherapy with near vs. far erythremogenic doses of narrow-band ultraviolet B in patients with psoriasis. Br J Dermatol 1998; 138:96–100.

53. Gordon PM, Diffey BL, Matthews JNS, Farr PM. A randomized comparison of narrow-band TL-01 phototherapy and PUVA photochemotherapy for psoriasis. J Am Acad Dermatol 1999; 41(5Pt1):728–732.

54. George SA, Bilsland DJ, Johnson BE, Ferguson J. Narrow-band (TL-01) UVB air-conditioned phototherapy for chronic sever adult atopic dermatitis. Br J Dermatol 1993; 128:49–56.

55. Grundmann-Kollmann M, Behrens S, Podda M, Peter RU, Kaufmann R, Kerscher M. Phototherapy for atopic eczema with narrow-band UVB. J Am Acad Dermatol 1999; 40:995–997.

56. Hudson-Peacock MJ, Diffey BL, Farr PM. Narrow-band UVB phototherapy for severe atopic dermatitis. Br J Dermatol 1996; 135:332.

57. Reynolds NJ, Franklin V, Gray JC, Diffey BL, Farr PM. Narrow-band ultraviolet B and broad-band ultraviolet A phototherapy in adult atopic eczema: a randomized controlled trial. Lancet 2001; 357:2012–2016.

58. Pikhammer D, Seeber A, Honigsmann H, Tanew A. Narrow-band ultraviolet B (TL-01) phototherapy is an effective and safe treatment option for patients with severe seborrhoeic dermatitis. Br J Dermatol 2000; 143:964–968.

59. Bilsland D, George SA, Gibbs NK, Aitchison T, Johnson BE, Ferguson J. A comparison of narrow band phototherapy (TL 01) and photochemotherapy (PUVA) in the management of polymorphic light eruption. Br J Dermatol 1993; 129:708–712.

60. Collins P, Ferguson J. Narrow-band UVB (TL-01) phototherapy: an effective preventative treatment for the photodermatoses. Br J Dermatol 1995; 132:956–963.

61. Gupta G, Man I, Kemmett D. Hydroa vacciniforme: a clinical and follow-up study of 17 cases. J Am Acad Dermatol 2000; 42:208–213.

62. Westerhof W, Nieuweboer-Krobotova L. Treatment of vitiligo with UV-B radiation vs topical psoralen plus UV-A. Arch Dermatol 1997; 133:1525–1528.

63. Scherschun L, Kim JJ, Lim HW. Narrow-band ultraviolet B is a useful and well-tolerated treatment for vitiligo. J Am Acad Dermatol 2001; 44(6):999–1003.

64. Njoo MD, Bos JD, Westerhof W. Treatment of generalized vitiligo in children with narrow-band (TL-01) UVB radiation therapy. J Am Acad Dermatol 2000; 42:245–253.

65. Alora MBT, Taylor CR. Narrow-band (311) UVB phototherapy: an audit of the first year's experience at the Massachusetts General Hospital. Photodermatol Photoimmunol Photomed 1997; 13:82–84.

66. Wulf HC, Hansen AB, Bech-Thomsen N. Differences in narrow-band ultraviolet B and broad-spectrum ultraviolet photocarcinogenesis in lightly pigmented hairless mice. Photodermatol Photoimmunol Photomed 1994; 10:192–197.

67. George SA, Ferguson J. Lesional blistering following narrow-band (TL-01) UVB phototherapy for psoriasis: a report of four cases. Br J Dermatol 1992; 127:445–446.

68. Calzavara-Pinton PG, Zane C, Candiago E, Facchetti F. Blisters on psoriatic lesions treated with TL-01 lamps. Dermatol 2000; 200:115–119.

69. Stern RS, Laird N. The carcinogenic risk of treatments for severe psoriasis. Cancer 1994; 73(11):2759–2764.

70. Koo JYM, Fitzpatrick TB, Krueger G, Lebwohl M, Menter A, Taylor JR.

PUVA phototherapy: assessing and optimizing the risk/benefit ratio. Skin Allergy News Suppl 2001; 32(2):1–15.

71. Freeman RG. Data on the action spectrum for ultraviolet carcinogenesis. J Natl Caner Inst 1975; 55:1119–1122.

72. Flindt-Hansen H, McFadden N, Eeg-Larsen T, Thune P. Effect of a new narrow-band UV-B lamp on photocarcinogenesis in mice. Acta Derm Venereol (Stockh) 1991; 71:245–248.

73. Shelk J, Morgan P. Narrow-Band UVB: A practical approach. Dermatol Nurs 2000;12(6):407–411.

74. Zanolli MD, Clark AR, Feldman SR, Fleischer AB, Jr. Phototherapy treatment protocols: for psoriasis and other phototherapy responsive dermatoses. New York: CRC Press-Parthenon Publishing, 2000.

75. Pasker-de Jong PC, Wielink G, van der Valk G, van der Wilt GJ. Treatment with UV-B for psoriasis and nonmelanoma skin cancer: a systematic review of the literature. Arch Dermatol 1999;135:834–840.

76. Al Suwaidan SN, Feldman SR. Clearance is not a realistic expectation of psoriasis treatment. J Am Acad Dermatol 2000; 42:796–802.

77. Rapp SR, Exum ML, Reboussin DM, Feldman SR, Fleischer AB, Clark AR. The physical, psychological and social impact of psoriasis. J Health Psychol 1997;2:525–537.

78. Avrillier S, Ollivier JP, Gandjbakhch I, Delettre E, Bussiere JL. XeCl excimer laser coronary angioplasty: a convergence of favourable factors. J Photochem Photobiol 1990: B 6:249–257.

79. Muller-Stolzenburg N, Muller GJ. Transmission of 308 nm excimer laser radiation for ophthalmic microsurgery—medical, technical and safety aspects. Biomed.Tech.(Berl) 1989:34:131–138.

80. Novak Z, Bonis B, Baltas E, Ocsovszki I, Ignacz F, Dobozy A, Kemeny L. Xenon chloride ultraviolet B laser is more effective in treating psoriasis and in inducing T cell apoptosis than narrow-band ultraviolet B. J Photochem Photobiol B. 2002;67:32–8.

81. Bonis B, Kemeny L, Dobozy A, Bor Z, Szabo G, Ignacz F. 308 nm UVB excimer laser for psoriasis [letter]. Lancet 1997; 350 (9090):1522.

82. Asawanonda P, Anderson RR, Chang Y, Taylor CR. 308-nm excimer laser for the treatment of psoriasis: a dose-response study. Arch Dermatol 2000; 136:619–624.

83. Kemeny L, Bonis B, Dobozy A, Bor Z, Szabo G, Ignacz F. 308-nm Excimer laser therapy for psoriasis. Arch Dermatol 2001; 137:95–96.

84. Housman TS, Pearce DJ, Feldman SR. Case Report: Efficacy of 308 nm excimer laser therapy for psoriasis. Cosmet Dermatol 2001:14:17–20.

85. Trehan M, Taylor CR. High-dose 308-nm excimer laser for the treatment of psoriasis. J Am Acad Dermatol. 2002;46:732–7.

86. Feldman SR, Mellen BG, Housman TS, Fitzpatrick RE, Geronemus RG, Friedman PM, Vasily DB, Morison WL. Efficacy of the 308-nm excimer laser for treatment of psoriasis: Results of a multicenter study. J Am Acad Dermatol. 2002 Jun;46:900–906.

87. Zelickson BD, Mehregan DA, Wendelschfer-Crabb G, Ruppman D, Cook A, O'Connell P, Kennedy WR. Clinical and histologic evaluation of psoriatic plaques treated with a flashlamp pulsed dye laser. J Am Acad Dermatol 1996: 35:64–68, 1996.

88. Hern S, Allen MH, Sousa AR, Harland CC, Barker JN, Levick JR, Mortimer PS. Immunohistochemical evaluation of psoriatic plaques following selective photothermolysis of the superficial capillaries. Br J Dermatol. 2001 Jul;145(1): 45–53.

89. Housman TS, Rohrback JM, Fleischer AB Jr, Feldman SR. Phototherapy utilization for psoriasis is declining in the United States. J Am Acad Dermatol 2002;46:557–9.

90. Fleischer AB Jr, Clark AR, Rapp SR, Reboussin DM, Feldman SR. Commercial tanning bed treatment is an effective psoriasis treatment: results from an uncontrolled clinical trial. J Invest Dermatol 1997;109:170–174.

4
Systemic and Topical PUVA Therapy

Warwick L. Morison
Johns Hopkins Medical School, Baltimore, Maryland, U.S.A.

I. SYSTEMIC PUVA THERAPY

In this section the term PUVA therapy will refer to oral methoxsalen photochemotherapy in which a patient ingests methoxsalen and is subsequently exposed to an indoor artificial source of ultraviolet A (UVA) (320–400 nm) radiation (1–3). This therapy has been used for treating moderate to severe psoriasis for nearly three decades. During this time it has undergone intense scrutiny, and its benefits and risks have been clearly defined. Successful use of PUVA therapy requires a well-informed physician, a trained staff, and an educated, motivated patient. While this can be said of all psoriasis treatment, it is particularly true for PUVA therapy because of the complexity of the regimen.

A. Patient Selection

A careful evaluation of the patient is necessary because PUVA therapy is often a long-term treatment. Good documentation is likewise essential, and an evaluation form ensures that no essential points are missed (Table 1). The absolute and relative contraindications to PUVA therapy need to be kept in mind throughout the evaluation (Table 2) (4). Laboratory investigations are not required except as suggested on the basis of the history and examination. Photosensitizing medications are not a contraindication to treatment, but their use should be noted.

Table 1   Evaluation of the Patient

Patient
  Past and family history
  Pregnancy, lactation, birth control
  Other disease
  Medications
  Photosensitivity
  Social and geographic
  Motivation and intelligence
Psoriasis
  Nature, extent, severity
  Previous treatment and response
  Arthritis
  Effect of exposure to sunlight
Full skin examination
Laboratory investigations
Ophthalmological examination: Repeat yearly

Table 2   Contraindications to PUVA Therapy

Absolute
  Xeroderma pigmentosum
  Lupus erythematosus
  Lactation
Relative
  History or family history of melanoma
  History of nonmelanoma skin cancer
  Extensive solar damage
  Previous treatment with ionizing radiation or arsenic
  Pemphigus and pemphigoid
  Uremia and hepatic failure
  Severe myocardial disease or other infirmity likely to make standing for a
    prolonged period difficult or hazardous
  Immunosuppression
  Pregnancy
  Young age
  Inability to comprehend details of the treatment

The most common indication for PUVA therapy is disabling psoriasis unresponsive to topical therapy. Since the definition of disability can vary among individuals, it is best determined on a case-by-case basis as a consensus between physician and patient. It is unwise to treat minimal disease with PUVA therapy for two reasons. First, such treatment has a poor risk/benefit ratio. Second, PUVA therapy rarely achieves complete clearance: a person with 1% body involvement cleared of 95% of the disease may still be an unhappy patient. In contrast, a person with 50% body involvement who achieves 95% clearance will be delighted. PUVA therapy is indicated in a few patients as the initial treatment because of explosive onset of wide-spread psoriasis. Finally, PUVA therapy is indicated in some patients as they cycle off methotrexate or some other systemic therapy.

When considering the use of PUVA therapy, the alternative treatment considered for most patients is ultraviolet B (UVB) phototherapy. In this decision three important differences must be kept in mind:

PUVA therapy is more effective than UVB phototherapy in clearing psoriasis in most patients.

PUVA therapy is a much more convenient and effective maintenance treatment.

UVA radiation is more penetrating than UVB radiation; that is, UVA penetrates through a greater depth of tissue.

Factors that suggest use of UVB phototherapy include the following:

1. *The disease*
   Psoriasis of recent initial onset. It is possible that long-term maintenance treatment will be unnecessary. The extreme example of this is acute guttate psoriasis, which should always initially be treated with UVB phototherapy.
   Thin, macular psoriasis.
   A history of rapid and easy clearance on exposure to sunlight.
   Psoriasis with a demonstrated photosensitivity to UVA but not UVB radiation.
2. *The patient*
   Pregnancy, lactation, or intention to become pregnant.
   Young age: A child with psoriasis may have a lifetime of disease ahead, and it is best to use the safest treatments first and leave more potent treatments for later.
3. *Skin type I that always burns, never tans; or a past history of x-ray or arsenic treatment.* These patients are prone to PUVA-induced skin cancer.

4. *Illiteracy or low intelligence*
5. *Patient preference for avoiding oral medications*

Factors that suggest use of PUVA therapy include the following:

1. *The disease*

   A long history of psoriasis. This suggests that maintenance therapy will be an almost certain requirement.

   Thick plaques.

   Involvement of the palms and soles. UVB therapy is without significant effect at those sites.

   Nail disease.

   Psoriasis with a demonstrated photosensitivity to UVB but not UVA radiation.

   Failure to respond to UVB phototherapy.

   Active, aggressive disease with a marked inflammatory component. Erythrodermic and pustular psoriasis are the extreme examples of this situation.

2. *The patient*

   Skin types III and higher. Pigmentation appears to be less of an obstacle to successful clearance with PUVA therapy than with UVB phototherapy.

   Geographic, social, or occupational factors that necessitate keeping treatments to a minimum.

In addition to these considerations there are two factors that are not easily quantified: physician and patient preference. Some physicians simply feel more comfortable with one or another treatment. A common reason for a patient's treatment choice is that a relative or friend's disease responded to that particular therapy.

B. Education of Patients

Before the start of PUVA therapy it is essential to inform patients fully about the procedure. This will help to ensure that the treatment is performed correctly and that the patient takes the necessary precautions to avoid adverse effects. It will also prepare the patient for the possibility of adverse side effects. The initial discussion about PUVA therapy usually takes 20–30 min and can be reinforced by providing a handout explaining the treatment and its potential problems. A follow-up discussion between the patient and the nurse or technician prior to the first treatment completes the initial introduction. During the course of therapy the nurse should also regularly question patients about the number and timing of the psoralen capsules they have taken, their use of eye protection, and their avoidance of exposure to sunlight on the days of treatment.

C. Pharmacology and Photobiology

PUVA therapy involves a phototoxic interaction between a psoralen (the photosensitizer) and a waveband of UVA radiation. The exact cellular mechanism of the phototoxic reaction is unknown but is thought to involve formation of monoadducts and crosslinks in DNA as well as damage to cell membranes. Present evidence indicates that psoriasis is an autoimmune disease involving activated T lymphocytes in the skin and these are presumably a target for PUVA therapy either directly or through an effect on keratinocytes.

1. Pharmacology

Psoralens occur naturally in a large number of plants and are responsible for inducing phytophotodermatitis, which is simply a phototoxic reaction in the skin. Several psoralens are used in PUVA therapy, but only methoxsalen (8-methoxypsoralen) is approved for use in treating psoriasis in the United States. Bergapten (5-methoxy-psoralen) is available for treatment in Europe and is now undergoing trials in the United States to confirm its efficacy.

Several features of the pharmacology of psoralens are important in therapy. Psoralens are poorly soluble in water; this limits their absorption from the gastrointestinal tract. Liquid formulations partially overcome this problem and are more completely absorbed than crystalline forms. There is a significant first-pass removal by the liver, however, since this is saturable, as the dose is raised the proportion of active compound reaching the skin rises. Finally, there are large interindividual and smaller intraindividual variations in absorption, and this is reflected in both the height and timing of the peak level in skin and blood.

2. Photobiology

Psoralens must absorb photons in order to photosensitize; they therefore must be exposed to a source of radiation that emits a waveband of radiation that includes their absorption spectrum. Early studies suggested that the peak of the action spectrum for psoralen photosensitization was between 340 and 380 nm, which led to the use of fluorescent bulbs with a peak emission of approximately 355–365 nm. More recent work indicates that the peak of the spectrum is between 320 and 340 nm (5). Since the same fluorescent bulbs have good emission at these shorter wavelengths, they continue to be the most commonly used PUVA lamps. These fluorescent bulbs are usually placed in a cylindrical chamber for whole-body exposure or in a specialized apparatus for hand and foot treatment. Banks of metal halide lamps are also used for whole-body treatment, and single lamps can be used for treating localized disease. Other sources of UVA radiation should not be used for PUVA therapy at this time, since the cutaneous responses to them in combination with psoralens have not been determined. The sun is not a safe source of UVA radiation in combination with methoxsalen, since severe phototoxic reactions are common, even when sophisticated radiometry is used (6).

3. Units of Measurement

The units used in therapy are as follows:

> *Radiant energy* is the amount of radiation and is expressed in joules (J): $1 \text{ J} = 10^3 \text{ mJ}$.
>
> *Radiant power* is the rate of delivery of energy and is expressed in watts (W): $W = J/sec$, $1 \text{ W} = 10^3 \text{ mW}$.
>
> *Irradiance* is the radiant power per unit area (one square centimeter) at a given surface and is expressed in W/cm^2; it is measured by a radiometer.
>
> *Exposure dose* is the radiant energy delivered per unit area of a given surface in a given exposure time and is expressed in J/cm^2; exposure dose = irradiance × exposure time.

4. Cutaneous Responses

PUVA therapy produces erythema and pigmentation of both normal and psoriatic skin. These responses are markedly influenced by several factors: dose; individual susceptibility (e.g., the patient's skin type); prior exposure to UV radiation; and body site (e.g., the limbs can tolerate approximately twice the dose tolerated by the trunk and face).

Erythema from PUVA therapy appears later and lasts longer than sunlight-induced erythema. It usually appears 24–48 h after treatment but may be delayed as long as 72–96 h (Fig. 1). The more intense the erythema, the later it appears and the later it reaches a maximum. PUVA-induced erythema also has a steeper dose–response curve than UVB or sunlight-induced erythema (Fig. 2). Thus, the dose required to produced 4+ erythema with blistering is only a few multiples of the dose that produces 1+ erythema. These features are important in therapy because small alterations in the frequency and timing of treatment or the dose of UVA radiation can result in painful erythema. Erythema is usually associated with a deep, burning pruritus, which may last for weeks.

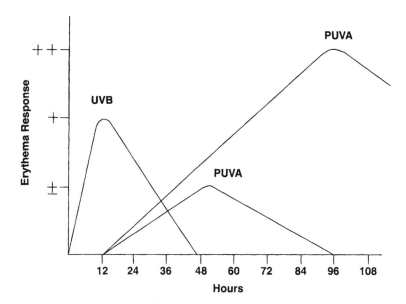

Figure 1 Time course for PUVA and UVB-induced erythema. Note that more intense erythema peaks later.

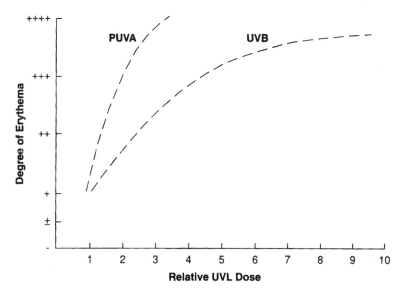

Figure 2 Dose–response curve for erythema following exposure to PUVA and UVB radiation.

Table 3 Dose Schedule for Methoxsalen
(Oxsoralen Ultra)

Patient weight		
(lb)	(kg)	Drug dose (mg)
< 66	< 30	10
66–143	30–65	20
144–200	66–91	30
> 200	> 91	40

Erythema is followed by pigmentation in all patients who possess functioning melanocytes. This pigmentation is darker and lasts longer than the pigmentation following a comparable sunlight-induced erythema.

D. Dosage and Administration

A liquid formulation of methoxsalen is available in 10 mg gelatin capsules (Oxsoralen Ultra, ICN Pharmaceuticals). This formulation is taken at a dosage of 0.4 m/kg body weight (Table 3) 1 h prior to exposure to UVA radiation. It is best to avoid food for an hour before and after ingestion since food slows and diminishes absorption of the drug. Higher dosages of the medication are frequently associated with nausea.

The starting dosages of UVA radiation, the increments of each treatment, and the suggested maximum final clearing doses are usually determined by the skin type of the individual (Table 4). Some centers use a determination of the minimum phototoxic dose (MPD) to decide upon a starting dose of

Table 4 Dosages of UVA Radiation for Bi- and
Triweekly Schedules

Skin type	UVA Radiation Dosage (J/cm^2)		
	Initial	Increments	Final
I	1.5	0.5	5
II	2.5	0.5	8
III	3.5	0.5–1.0	12
IV	4.5	1.0	14
V	5.5	1.0	16
VI	6.5	1.0–1.5	20

UVA radiation (7). Treatments in the clearance phase of therapy are usually given two or three times each week, with 48 h or more between treatments to allow assessment of any erythemal reaction from the last exposure (8). If no erythema occurs following treatment, the UVA dosage should be increased at the next therapy session. If erythema occurs but clears between sessions, the previous exposure dosage should be maintained at the next treatment. If the erythema has not cleared, the treatment should be cancelled unless the erythema is very localized and the area can be shielded with clothing or zinc oxide ointment.

An alternative schedule (more frequently used in Europe) consists of four treatments each week on Monday, Tuesday, Thursday, and Friday with a rest day on Wednesday to assess any cumulative erythema. The starting dosages of UVA radiation for this schedule are lower (Table 5), and the dosage is increased every third treatment. This schedule is more effective in clearing psoriasis but is associated with more phototoxicity. It is most useful in patients with thick plaques who have skin type III or higher or in any patients who have skin type V or VI.

An additional exposure to the limbs is given if there is significant involvement of this area because disease on the limbs (particularly the lower legs) is slower to clear than on the trunk. Disease on the palms and soles is also an indication for additional treatment. The starting dosage for these additional treatments is half the whole-body exposure, but the increments are the same.

When the disease is adequately controlled, the frequency of treatment is reduced to once a week for 4 weeks, then to every other week for 2 months, and finally to monthly treatment to provide maintenance therapy and prevent recurrence of psoriasis. During this progressive reduction in frequency of

Table 5 Dosages of UVA Radiation for Monday, Tuesday, Thursday, and Friday Schedule

| Skin type | UVA radiation dosage (J/cm2) | |
	Initial	Increments
I	0.5	0.5
II	1.5	0.5
III	2.5	0.5
IV	3.5	1.0
V	4.5	1.0
VI	5.5	1.5

treatment, any significant flare of disease is best managed by a return to the previous level of therapy or even to the initial (clearance treatment) level. It is important for the patient to understand that weekly and less frequent treatment seldom produces any clearance of disease and is strictly maintenance therapy.

When the frequency of treatment has been reduced to one exposure each month the decision as to whether to continue maintenance therapy depends on many factors, including the duration and severity of disease, the skin type of the individual, and the personal wishes of the patient. Most patients choose to cease treatment after a few months. Typically, a course of PUVA therapy lasts less than 6 months. However, in the few patients with chronic, active disease, PUVA therapy may be continued for years. There is no upper limit to the amount of treatment that can be given. An individual decision must be made for each patient based upon disability from the disease, adverse effects, and therapeutic alternatives.

E. Precautions

There are three points during treatment at which protection must be considered:

1. During radiation, the eyes require protection by UV-opaque goggles, the male genitalia should be covered by underpants or an athletic supporter unless there is significant disease there, and the face usually should be shielded since it is seldom affected by psoriasis and it receives high ambient exposure to UV radiation.
2. Following ingestion of psoralen, the eyes should be shielded by UV-opaque sunglasses when exposed to sunlight for at least the remainder of that day. Particular attention to eye protection is essential in patients with aphakia. The skin should also be protected by clothing or a broad-spectrum sunscreen. Exposure to sunlight should be minimized.
3. On nontreatment days, patients should be encouraged to minimize exposure to sunlight, since sunlight-induced tanning complicates treatment and increases photoaging. Outdoor use of UV-opaque sunglasses throughout PUVA therapy should be encouraged.

F. Combination Therapy

PUVA therapy is often combined with another treatment to achieve more rapid clearance at a lower dose of UVA radiation. When the disease is clear, the second therapy is usually stopped and control of psoriasis is maintained by PUVA therapy alone. The main indications for combination therapy are listed in Table 6.

1. PUVA and UVB Phototherapy

The patient is exposed to UVA and UVB radiation simultaneously. Fortunately, erythemal reactions from the two treatments are not cumulative. (In fact, the cause of an erythema can be determined from the time course, since a UVB-induced erythema appears on the day of treatment while a PUVA-induced erythema is delayed for at least 24 h.) This combination is useful in two situations. First, as initial therapy on a three times a week schedule using a high-dosage UVB protocol (starting dosage of 70% of minimal erythema dose with increments of 17% each subsequent treatment) and a regular three times a week PUVA schedule (9). Second, UVB therapy may be added to the schedule of a PUVA patient who is showing a slow response to treatment and/ or is near the desired upper limit of the dose of UVA radiation. In this situation, the dosage of UVA radiation is usually held constant, while the starting dosage of UVB is 30–150 mJ/cm^2 for skin types I–VI with increments of 20% each subsequent treatment.

2. PUVA Plus Acitretin

This combination is used widely in Europe although there has been some disagreement as to its efficacy (10, 11). An analysis of the various studies indicates it is useful provided two criteria are met: acitretin is given in a dosage of at least 1 mg/kg body weight, and it is commenced at least 10–14 days before PUVA therapy. The usual limitations on use of acitretin apply (e.g., women of childbearing potential should be strictly excluded), and close monitoring is required. Isotretinoin plus PUVA therapy has been reported to be an alternative combination treatment (12), but the data to support this are not strong.

Table 6 Indications for Combination Therapy

Previous failed or partial response to PUVA therapy
Erythrodermic or generalized pustular psoriasis
Asbestos and coral-plaque psoriasis
Photosensitive psoriasis
Skin types V and VI
Social or geographic limitations on therapy

3. PUVA Plus Methotrexate

Methotrexate is begun 3 weeks before PUVA therapy in a dosage of 2.5–5.0 mg at 12 h intervals for three doses each week. This is continued through the clearance phase of PUVA therapy (13). The usual precaution of methotrexate therapy apply (see Chapter on Methotrexate), and blood tests to monitor the treatment are required before and during therapy. Unexpected and unexplained phototoxic episodes marked the original evaluation of this protocol, but greater experience with the treatment has found that these events are very infrequent.

G. Efficacy

Improvement in disease (flattening of plaques and decreased scaling) usually occurs after 6–10 treatments, followed by clearance of most lesions after 20–30 treatments. If the disease does not respond in this way, the cause of failure must be sought. The most common cause is missed treatments: the patient has been receiving one exposure or less each week, maximizing pigmentation and minimizing clearance. The next most common cause of treatment failure is a low methoxsalen concentration in the skin, which is suggested by a lack of pigmentation of normal skin. Possible reasons for this include a failure to take the medication, low absorption of methoxsalen, and concomitant use of medications such as carbamazepine or phenytoin sodium, which activate microsomal enzymes in the liver. In addition, certain medications such as lithium, antimalarials, and systemic corticosteroids make psoriasis unstable and often result in a failure to respond. Finally, there remains a group of patients whose disease fails to respond to therapy for unknown reasons. For these patients, some other approach to treatment must be found.

Disease of the nails responds in about 70% of affected patients, but usually requires 3–4 months of treatment. Involvement of the scalp and intertriginous areas requires supplemental topical therapy.

H. Side Effects

It is crucially important for patients to know that almost everyone undergoing PUVA therapy experiences some adverse effects from the treatment. It is equally important for them to know what the effects might be. Since most of the problems are short-term, minor, and easily corrected, a full discussion will prepare the patient and help avoid misunderstanding or worse.

1. Short-Term

The short-term side effects of PUVA therapy are listed in Table 7. Nausea from methoxsalen results when a central mechanism is triggered by high serum levels of the drug. The sequential measures to overcome this problem are to ingest the drug with food, to schedule treatments late in the day, and to reduce the dosage by 10 mg. Rarely, use of an antiemetic may be required. Symptoms related to the central nervous system occur in most patients, but few voluntarily complain of them. Headache, dizziness, insomnia, depression, and hyperkinesis are common side effects that seldom interfere with treatment.

The major short-term problem is phototoxicity. At least 10% of patients will have a phototoxic event of sufficient magnitude to warrant interruption of treatment. Patients should be warned of this in advance so they will check for erythema or other changes in their skin. The main causes

Table 7   Short-Term Side Effects

Due to Methoxsalen
  Gastrointestinal disturbance
  CNS symptoms
  Bronchoconstriction
  Toxic hepatitis
  Drug fever
  Exanthema
Phototoxicity
  Erythema
  Pruritus
  Subacute phototoxicity
  Photo-onycholysis
  Friction blisters
  Phytophotodermatitis
  Koebner phenomenon
New rash
  Polymorphous light eruption
  Lupus erythematosus
  Guttate psoriasis
  Seborrheic dermatitis of the face
  Herpes simplex
Nonphototoxic reactions
  Cardiovascular stress
  Hypertrichosis

of phototoxic events are variable absorption of methoxsalen, treatment on a day when erythema has not sufficiently cleared or on consecutive days, and passing the patient's cumulative threshold for erythema. There is no specific treatment for PUVA-induced phototoxicity, and supportive measures such as cool baths, moisturizers, and antipruritics provide only partial relief.

2. Long-Term

The most common long-term problem related to PUVA therapy is photoaging of the skin. Its occurrence depends on the amount of therapy and the skin type of the patient. Dryness and wrinkling of the skin are early changes and largely reversible. Freckling, telangiectasia, and keratoses occur later and are probably irreversible.

Nonmelanoma skin cancer in the form of squamous cell carcinoma or lesions resembling keratoacanthomas occurs in PUVA patients at 10 times the expected frequency in the population (14–16). Patients with skin types I and II account for much of this increase; prior exposure to x-ray, arsenic, or high dosages of sunlight and UVB radiation appears to increase the risk. Prior to development of skin cancer, affected patients almost always have extensive photoaging changes, and such patients should be closely monitored. The lesions are mainly on the trunk and lower limbs; the male genitalia also have a significant incidence (17). Treatment with cyclosporine subsequent to exposure to PUVA therapy appears to increase the risk of skin cancer greatly (18). This agent, and perhaps other immunosuppressants, is relatively contraindicated in patients who have been treated with PUVA therapy.

An increased incidence of melanoma starting about 15 years after treatment with PUVA therapy has been reported in one study (19). The risk is greater in patients exposed to high dosages of PUVA therapy and appears to be increasing with time. An increased frequency of melanoma has not been reported in other cohorts.

The occurrence of cataracts has been a concern since the introduction of PUVA therapy for psoriasis because these were observed in mice and other rodents. However, possibly because eye protection has been used by most patients, cataracts have not occurred with increased frequency (20). Other potential long-term adverse affects that have been looked for but not observed include immune suppression, autoimmune phenomena, systemic neoplasia, and hepatic damage.

II. TOPICAL PUVA THERAPY

Direct application of psoralen to the skin combined with subsequent exposure to UVA radiation has been used for the treatment of psoriasis for almost as long as oral PUVA therapy. The first approach used a dilute solution of trimethylpsoralen (TMP) in a bath (21, 22) and subsequent studies have used methoxsalen and 5-methoxypsoralen in bath solutions as well as creams and lotions. Topical PUVA therapy is used most widely in Europe and it appears to be much less popular elsewhere. In addition, since methoxsalen is the only psoralen available for use in the United States, this section will only discuss treatment with this agent. The suggested advantages of topical PUVA therapy are:

> Marked reduction of systemic exposure to methoxsalen so that gastrointestinal side effects and risk of cataracts are virtually eliminated
> Possible improved efficacy
> Possible reduced risk of skin cancer

The efficacy of any topical PUVA protocol will be determined by how aggressive the dosimetry is in respect of drug and radiation; an aggressive topical PUVA protocol will be more effective than a conservative oral PUVA protocol and vice versa. There is no information on the potential carcinogenicity of topical PUVA therapy using methoxsalen in humans. The lower dosage of UVA radiation required for topical PUVA therapy is often mentioned as an advantage for this treatment, but this is likely to be irrelevant since it is probably the number of adducts formed in DNA that determines therapeutic effect and long-term side effects.

A. Patient Selection

The indications and contraindications are the same as for oral PUVA therapy. Erythrodermic psoriasis is best treated with combination treatment due to the difficulty in differentiating between exacerbations of psoriasis and PUVA-induced erythema. Generalized pustular psoriasis is likewise an indication for combination treatment due to risk of exacerbation by erythema.

B. Pharmacology and Photobiology

Presumably the mechanism of action of topical PUVA therapy is the same as oral PUVA therapy but there is no direct evidence for this. Intraepidermal T lymphocytes appear to be a major target (23).

1. Pharmacology

The kinetics of psoralen absorption and photosensitivity after topical application depend on several variables. When normal skin is immersed in a dilute solution of methoxsalen as in bath or soak PUVA therapy, photosensitivity is maximal in the first 10 min after the immersion and is greatly decreased 40–60 min later; after 4 h no photosensitivity is evident (24, 25). In contrast, maximum photosensitivity is reached 40–60 min after application of methoxsalen in an alcohol/glycerol lotion (26) and can persist for a week or more (27). Psoriatic skin allows faster absorption, while palmoplantar skin has peak photosensitivity 40 min after bathing in a dilute solution and this persists for an hour or more (28). Repeated exposures to bath PUVA produces increased photosensitivity with the MPD reduced by as much as 60% after five exposures (29). Finally, bathing time is important since increasing this time from 5 to 10 min also reduces the MPD by 60% (30). It is assumed that antipsoriatic activity correlates with photosensitivity but this is not definitely established. Plasma levels of methoxsalen are very low or undetectable in most patients treated with topical PUVA therapy. In one study (31) severity of disease correlated with plasma levels after bath PUVA with detectable levels in the half of the patients with the most severe disease. Limited application of a 0.1% solution yielded undetectable levels in all patients (32).

2. Photobiology

The action spectrum for topical methoxsalen photosensitivity is maximal at 330 nm but there is photoreactivity from 313 nm to 350 nm (33). This broad action spectrum probably explains why narrow-band (311 nm) radiation and broadband UVA lamps have similar efficacy in psoriasis in combination with methoxsalen bath treatment (34). The time course of erythema is probably similar for topical and oral PUVA therapy.

C. Dosage and Administration

There are no established protocols for topical PUVA therapy and instead there are various published procedures, some of which have been studied in detail. There are two sources of methoxsalen: Oxsoralen lotion 1% (70% alcohol, propylene glycol, acetone and water) and Oxsoralen Ultra 10 mg capsules (alcohol solution in a soft gelatin capsule).

1. Bath PUVA

Various concentrations of methoxsalen have been used. A 0.5% final concentration in bath water is a conservative dose but appears to be effective (35). This can be achieved by heating five capsules in 3 cups of water or using 10 ml of the 1% Oxsoralen lotion and adding to 100 L of bath water at body temperature. The patient bathes for 15 min, wetting all areas up to the neck, pats dry, and then is immediately exposed to UVA radiation. Higher concentrations of methoxsalen have been used: in one study 30 ml Oxsoralen lotion was added to 80 L bath water to give a final concentration of 3.75 mg/L (36). There is a good correlation between the MPD in a group of individuals and the methoxsalen concentration in bath water (37).

The starting dosage of UVA radiation should be determined by measuring the MPD before initiating whole body treatment. At a bath water methoxsalen concentration of 0.5 mg/L, a suitable range of dosages for testing is 1.0, 2.0, 4.0, 6.0, 8.0, 10.0, 12.0, and 14.0 J/cm^2 with erythema responses read at 72 h; the median MPD will be around 6 J/cm^2 (37). The initial dosage of UVA radiation is one square below the MPD. Treatments are given two or three times weekly and the dosage should not be increased until five treatments are given after which a 1J/cm^2 increase per treatment is usually tolerated. Selecting an initial dosage based on the skin type of the individual can be hazardous since there is a poor correlation between skin type and MPD, particularly for skin types II and III (38).

2. Soak PUVA

This is a topical therapy for treatment of diseases on the palms and soles and the protocols used have been similar to those for bath PUVA. A volume of about 5 L tap water in a basin and concentrations of 0.5 mg/L methoxsalen (39) to as high as 20 mg/L (40) have been used.

3. Cream PUVA

Methoxsalen has been used topically in a cream base for treatment of widespread and local disease (41). The kinetics of photosensitivity are similar to bath PUVA, irradiation is performed immediately after removal of the cream, and photosensitivity is lost within 2 h.

4. Lotion PUVA

Direct application of Oxsoralen lotion to plaques of psoriasis is not an acceptable treatment. This form of PUVA produced prolonged photosensitivity and a high frequency of bullous erythema and intense pigmentation that can persist for a year or more.

D. Precautions

The precautions required with topical PUVA therapy are essentially the same as those for oral PUVA, with minor variations. Following bath PUVA therapy, 4 h avoidance of sun exposure appears to be adequate.

Eye protection should be used since detectable serum levels are found in some patients.

E. Side Effects

1. Short-Term

Phototoxicity is the main adverse effect and its frequency depends on the aggressiveness of the treatment protocol. Erythema, pruritus, and pain are similar in appearance and duration to that seen with oral PUVA. Gastrointestinal disturbances and central nervous system symptoms are not seen with topical PUVA therapy.

2. Long-Term

There is no information in humans on the long-term safety of topical methoxsalen PUVA therapy. A lower risk of skin cancer has been reported with TMP bath therapy than with oral PUVA therapy using methoxsalen (42–44); this may be based on a lower carcinogenic potential of TMP (45). However, based on this mouse study there is no reason to expect bath and oral methoxsalen PUVA to have different risks for skin cancer. Because of the very low serum levels seen with topical PUVA therapy, the potential risk of cataracts should be nonexistent.

III. MONITORING

A. Patient

The nurse or technician must determine the response to the last treatment prior to each exposure. The patient is asked about the occurrence of any erythema and, if the response in doubt, should be examined. Inquiry should also be made about the occurrence of or alteration in any pruritus. An evaluation by the physician is required after every 6–10 treatments (more frequently if problems develop or decision points are reached).

A chart is kept for each patient to record the number of treatments, the dosages given, and what areas were treated (Fig. 3). Remarks about progress and/or problems should be noted for each treatment. Cancelled treatments and no-shows should be prominently recorded. An accurate chart often provides the key to the origin of treatment problems.

Finally, patients need to be sensitized to the need to examine their skin for the development of any new lesions. This educational task is a joint responsibility of the nurse and the physician. During the initial evaluation, at follow-up evaluations, and through newsletters, patients should be encouraged to call the caregiver's attention to freckles, moles,

PUVA TREATMENT SHEET

NAME: Doe, John

DIAGNOSIS: Psoriasis PROTOCOL: B1w

SKIN TYPE: I/2 METHOXSALEN DOSE: 30 mg

Date	Day	Rx#	TRUNK J/cm² Total J/cm²	Time Min.	ARMS/LEGS J/cm² Total J/cm²	Time Min.	HANDS Palms + Dorsa	Feet Soles + Dorsa	Notes
11/27/89	1	1	2		1		1	1	Procedures explained, First Glasses emphasized mwc.
11/30/89	4	2	2						No change, No erythema mwc.
12/5/89	9	3	2.5		1.5		1.5	1.5	No change, No erythema mwc.
12/7/89	11	4	2.5		1.5		1.5	1.5	Less scaling, Some Flattening, No erythema bmc.
12/11/89	15	5	3.0		2.0		2.0	2.0	Still Spotting, improvement mc. No erythema, Saw Dr. Monson
12/13/89	17	6	3.0		2.0		2.0	2.0	Improving mwc.
12/17/89	22	7	3.5		2.5		2.5	2.5	Continued improvement, Still erythema on breasts mwc.
12/21/89	25	8	3.5		2.5		2.5	2.5	No erythema. St. pruritis probably due to dry skin, advised bmc.
1/2/90	31	9	4.0		3.0		3.0	3.0	C
1/4/90	34	9	4.0		3.0		3.0	3.0	C/o legs stinging p last tx. No Erythema today, decrease dose
1/9/90	44	10	4.0		3.0		3.0	3.0	Lesions fading, Flattening, less scaling, Hands not improved mwc
1/11/90	46	11	4.5		3.5		3.5	3.5	No erythema. Elbows stubborn, Still scaling slightly mwc.
1/16/90	51	12	4.5		3.5		3.5	3.5	Continues to improve, No erythema mwc.
1/18/90	55	13	5.0		4.0		No tx given	given 4.0	Telephone Call, from pt c/o erythema, Told to cool bath, antihistamine mwc
1/23/90	58	13	2.5		1.5		1.5	1.5	↓ tx. No erythema today, much improved mwc.
1/25/90	60	14	2.5		1.5		1.5	1.5	Continues to do well, almost clear. nmc.
1/30/90	65	15	3.0		2.0	R/W Hold	2.0	2.0	No erythema, Hand, Feet, Elbows improved, Saw Dr Monson
2/6/90	72	16	3.0		2.0		2.0	2.0	No new lesions, No erythema
2/8/90	80	16	3.0		2.0		2.0	2.0	Holding well mwc.
2/8/90	87	17	3.0		2.0		2.0	2.0	Doing well, staying Clear, No problems nmc.

Figure 3 Sample patient chart for PUVA therapy.

or any other lesions that are new or changed to ensure early detection of long-term problems.

B. Equipment

Safe and effective treatment requires accurate delivery of a measured dose of radiation. The output of bulbs and lamps declines with age and therefore must be monitored. Some radiators are equipped with an internal radiometer that constantly measures the output of the lamps: The dose of radiation is punched into the keyboard and the machine stops when the correct dose is delivered. An alarm that shuts off the machine if it malfunctions is a very useful safety feature with such a system. Other radiators require external monitoring with a hand-held radiometer: The dose is then read off a chart of doses and irradiances. Both systems require periodic checks with another instrument to ensure their accuracy. A log that records dates of relamping and all readings of the output of the system should be kept.

IV. COMPARISONS WITH OTHER THERAPIES

Clinical experience is the only guide for comparing the treatments of moderate to severe psoriasis since controlled studies are not available. Comparisons of the treatments based on personal experience are given in Table 8.

A. Efficacy

Methotrexate is more effective (faster and higher response rate) than PUVA therapy, although combination PUVA therapy makes the treatments almost equal.

Table 8   Comparisons of Treatment Using a 0–10 Scale for Least to Most Desirable Score for Each Parameter (Author's Personal Experience)

	Efficacy	Safety	Cost Time	Cost Money	Cost Monitoring
Ultraviolet radiation					
UVB phototherapy	5	10	4	4	10
Goeckerman therapy	5	10	1	1	10
Oral PUVA therapy	8	7	4	4	8
Bath PUVA therapy	8	7	3	4	8
Systemic					
Methotrexate	10	4	10	7	2
Acitretin	3	4	10	7	4
Cyclosporine	8	2	8	4	2

B. Safety

PUVA therapy causes photoaging of the skin and skin cancer, but these effects are clearly much less toxic than the adverse effects of any of the systemic agents.

C. Cost

A significant disadvantage of PUVA therapy (like other forms of UV therapy) is its cost in terms of time and money. On the other hand, the cost of monitoring for adverse effects is less for UV therapy than for systemic therapy.

D. Other Factors

UV therapy and acitretin are not associated with a rebound of disease when the treatment is stopped. Psoriasis may stay in remission or it may gradually return. Methotrexate frequently alters the nature of psoriasis when it is used for more than a few months so that it becomes more active and inflammatory. When the drug is then stopped, a major flare of disease frequently occurs 4–6 weeks later.

REFERENCES

1. Parrish JA, Fitzpatrick TB, Tanenbaum L, Pathak MA. Photochemotherapy of psoriasis with oral methoxsalen and longwave ultraviolet. N Engl J Med 1974;291:1207-1211.
2. Morison WL. Phototherapy and Photochemotherapy of Skin Disease. 2nd ed. New York, NY: Raven Press, 1991.
3. Abel EA. Photochemotherapy in Dermatology. New York: Igaku-Shoin, 1992.
4. Guidelines of care for phototherapy and photochemotherapy. J Am Acad Dermatol. 1994;31:643-648.
5. Farr PM, Diffey BL, Higgins EM, Matthews JNS. The action spectrum between 320 and 400nm for clearance of psoriasis by psoralen photo-chemotherapy. Br J Dermatol. 1991;124:443-448.
6. Parrish JA, White AD, Kingsbury T, Zahar M, Fitzpatrick TB. Photo-chemotherapy of psoriasis using methoxsalen and sunlight. Arch Dermatol. 1977;133:1529-1532.
7. Wolff K, Gschnait F, Honigsmann H, Konrad K, Parrish JA, Fitzpatrick TB. Phototesting and dosimetry for photochemotherapy. Br J Dermatol. 1977;96: 1-10.
8. Melski JW, Tanenbaum L, Parrish JA, Fitzpatrick TB, Bleich HL, and 28 participating investigators. Oral methoxsalen photochemotherapy for the

treatment of psoriasis: a cooperative clinical trial. J Invest Dermatol. 1977;68:328-335.

9. Momtaz-TK, Parrish JA. Combination of psoralens and ultraviolet A and ultraviolet B in the treatment of psoriasis vulgaris: a bilateral comparison study. J Am Acad Dermatol. 1984;10:481-486.

10. Fritch PO, Honigsmann H, Jaschke E, Wolff K. Augmentation of oral methoxsalen–photochemotherapy with an oral retinoic acid derivative. J Invest Dermatol. 1978;70:178-182.

11. Parker S, Coburn P, Lawrence C, Marks J, Shuster S. A randomized double-blind comparison of PUVA-etretinate and PUVA-placebo in the treatment of chronic plaque psoriasis. Br J Dermatol. 1984;110:215-220.

12. Honigsmann H, Wolff K. Isotretinoin-PUVA for psoriasis. Lancet. 1983;1:236.

13. Morison WL, Momtaz K, Parrish JA, Fitzpatrick TB. Combined methotrexate PUVA therapy in the treatment of psoriasis. J Am Acad Dermatol. 1982; 6:46-51.

14. Stern RS, Thibodeau LA, Kleinerman RA, Parrish JA, Fitzpatrick TB, and 22 participating investigators. Risk of cutaneous carcinoma in patients treated with oral methoxsalen photochemotherapy for psoriasis. N Eng J Med. 1979;300:809-813.

15. Stern RS, Lange R, and members of the photochemotherapy follow-up study. Non-melanoma skin cancer occurring in patients treated with PUVA five to ten years after first treatment. J Invest Dermatol 1988;91:120-124.

16. Henseler T, Christophers E, Honigsmann H, Wolff K, and 19 other investigators. Skin tumors in the European PUVA study. J Am Acad Dermatol. 1987;16:108-116.

17. Stern RS, and members of the photochemotherapy follow-up study. Genital tumors among men with psoriasis exposed to psoralens and ultraviolet A radiation (PUVA) and ultraviolet B radiation. N Engl J Med. 1990;322:1093-1097.

18. Marcil I, Stern RS. Squamous-cell cancer of the skin in patients given PUVA and cyclosporin: nested cohort crossover study. Lancet. 2001;358:1042-1045.

19. Stern RS. The risk of melanoma in association with long-term exposure to PUVA. J Am Acad Dermatol. 2001;44:755-761.

20. Stern RS, Parrish JA, Fitzpatrick TB. Ocular findings in patients treated with PUVA. J Invest Dermatol. 1985;85:269-273.

21. Fischer T, Alsins J. Treatment of psoriasis with trioxsalen baths and dysprosium lamps. Acta Dermatovener (Stockh) 1976;56:383-390.

22. Hannuksela M, Karvonen J. Trioxsalen bath plus UVA effective and safe in the treatment of psoriasis. Br J Dermatol. 1978;99:703-707.

23. Coven T, Murphy F, Gilleaudeau P, Cardinale I, Krueger J. Trimethylpsoralen bath PUVA is a remittive treatment for psoriasis vulgaris. Arch Dermatol. 1998;134:1263-1268.

24. Neumann N J, Kerscher M, Ruzicka T, Lehmann P. Evaluation of PUVA bath phototoxicity. Acta Derm Venereol (Stockholm). 1997;77:385-387.

25. Gruss C, Behrens S, Reuther T, Husebo L, Neumann N, Altmeyer P, Lehmann

P, Kerscher M. Kinetics of photosensitivity in bath-PUVA photochemotherapy. J Am Acad Dermatol. 1998;39:443-446.

26. Meffert H, Andersen K, Sonnichsen N. Phototoxicity and antipsoriatic effect of a topical methoxypsoralen solution in relation to the application time. Photodermatology 1984;1:191-194.
27. Gange RW, Levins P, Murray J, Anderson RR, Parrish J A. Prolonged skin photosensitization induced by methoxsalen and subphototoxic UVA irradiation. J Invest Dermatol. 1984;82:219-222.
28. Diffey B. Time course of activity of topical 8-methoxypsoralen. Br J Dermatol. 1992;127:654-659.
29. Koulu L, Jansen C. Skin phototoxicity variations during repeated bath PUVA exposures to 8-methoxpsoralen and trimethylpsoralen. Clin Exp Dermatol. 1984;9:64-69.
30. Dolezal E, Seeber A, Honigsmann H,Tanew A. Correlation between bathing time and photosensitivity in 8-methoxypsoralen (8-MOP) bath PUVA. Photodermatol Photoimmunol Photomed. 2000;16:183-185.
31. Gomez M, Azana J, Arranz I, Harto A, Ledo A. Plasma levels of 8-methoxypsoralen after bath-PUVA for psoriasis: relationship to disease severity. Br J Dermatol. 1995;133:37-40.
32. Hallman C, Koo J, Omohundro C, Lee J. Plasma levels of 8-methoxypsoralen after topical paint PUVA on nonpalmoplantar psoriatic skin. J Am Acad Dermatol. 1994;31:273-275.
33. Cripps D, Lowe N, Lerner A. Action spectra of topical psoralens: a reevaluation. Br J Dermatol. 1982;107:77-82.
34. Ortel B, Perl S, Kinaciyan T, Calzavara-Pinton P, Honigsmann H. Comparison of narrow-band (311 nm) UVB and broad-band UVA after oral or bath-water 8-methoxypsoralen in the treatment of psoriasis. J Am Acad Dermatol. 1993;29:736-740.
35. Vallat V, Battat L, Heftler N, Hodak E, Krueger J. PUVA bath therapy with 8-methoxypsoralen. In: Weinstein GD, Gottlieb AB, eds. Therapy of Moderate-to-Severe Psoriasis. Portland, OR: National Psoriasis Foundation, 1994:39-55.
36. Lowe N, Weingarten D, Bourget T, Moy L. PUVA therapy for psoriasis: Comparison of oral and bath-water delivery of 8-methoxypsoralen. J Am Acad Dermatol. 1986;14:754-760.
37. Tanew A, Kipfelsperger T, Seeber A, Radakovic-Fijan S, Honigsmann H. Correlation between 8-methoxypsoralen bath-water concentration and photosensitivity in bath-PUVA treatment. J Am Acad Dermatol 2001;44:638-642.
38. Schiener R, Behrens-Williams S, Pillekamp H, Peter R, Kerscher M. Does the minimal phototoxic dose after 8-methoxypsoralen baths correlate with the individual's skin phototype? Photodermatol Photoimmunol Photomed. 2001;17:156-158.
39. Grundmann-Kellmann M, Behrens S, Peter R, Kerscher M. Treatment of severe recalcitrant dermatoses of the palms and soles with PUVA-bath versus PUVA-cream therapy. Photodermatol Photoimmunol Photomed. 1999; 15:87-89.

40. Taylor C, Baron E. Hand and foot PUVA soaks: an audit of the Massachusetts General Hospital's experience from 1994 to 1998. Photodermatol Photoimmunol Photomed. 1999;15:188-192.

41. Grundmann-Kollmann M, Tegeder I, Ochsendorf F, Zollner T, Ludwig R, Kaufmann R, Podda M. Kinetics and dose-response of photosensitivity in cream psoralen plus ultraviolet A photochemotherapy: comparative in vivo studies after topical application of three standard preparations. Br J Dermatol. 2001;144:991-995.

42. Berne B, Fischer T, Michaelsson G, Noren P. Long-term safety of trioxsalen bath PUVA treatment: an 8-year follow-up of 149 psoriasis patients. Photodermatology. 1984;1:18-22.

43. Lindelof B, Sigurgeirsson B, Tegner E, Larko O, Berne B. Comparison of the carcinogenic potential of trioxsalen bath PUVA and oral methoxsalen PUVA. Arch Dermatol. 1992;128:1341-1344.

44. Hannuksela A, Pukkala E, Hannuksela M, Karvonen J. Cancer incidence among Finnish patients with psoriasis treated with trioxsalen bath PUVA. J Am Acad Dermatol 1996;35:685-689.

45. Hannuksela M, Stenback F, Lahti A. The carcinogenic properties of topical PUVA. Arch Dermatol Res. 1986;278:347-351.

5

Therapy of Moderate-to-Severe Psoriasis with Methotrexate

Gerald D. Weinstein
University of California, Irvine, College of Medicine, Irvine, California, U.S.A.

I. INTRODUCTION

A half century has passed since the serendipitous observation by Gubner that the folic acid aminopterin improved the lesions of psoriasis during a trial to assess its anti-inflammatory effects in patients with psoriatic arthritis (2). These observations were transferred into clinical trials utilizing a daily dosage schedule of aminopterin (3). In the late 1950s methotrexate (MTX) replaced aminopterin. During the next two decades alternative dosage schedules were developed based on cell cycle information and cancer chemotherapy concepts. Until the development of psoralen/ultraviolet A treatment (PUVA) in 1975, UVB phototherapy and methotrexate were the only effective treatments for moderate-to-severe psoriasis. Methotrexate was approved for psoriasis by the Food and Drug Administration (FDA) without the usual, at least by current standards, large double-blind clinical trials. Methotrexate usage for psoriasis appeared to be grandfathered in, in part related to guidelines for MTX therapy for psoriasis referred to below. Thus there are no large clinical trials to quantitate the efficacy and safety of the drug for the treatment of psoriasis. Its usefulness is based on many years of clinical experience and numerous clinical retrospective studies with more emphasis on side effects than efficacy (4–7). In recent years it has been estimated that 25,000–30,000 patients were receiving methotrexate therapy in the United States, although current data are not available.

In 1988, MTX was approved for the treatment of rheumatoid arthritis (RA) and has become one of the main choices of therapy for RA in the past decade. With a much larger population of patients with this chronic benign disease being treated with MTX in dosages similar to those used for psoriasis, much more data have become available on the relative safety of this drug. Guidelines developed by rheumatology organizations are similar to dermatology guidelines but have differed by not requiring liver biopsies prior to MTX therapy. This reflects a lack of significant liver toxicity found in RA in comparison to that discussed in detail in the dermatology literature (8).

II. PATIENT SELECTION

Patients with psoriasis involving greater than 15–20% body surface area were usually considered to have moderate-to-severe disease. Further thinking and experience have suggested that many patients may have lesions of a lesser amount but in critical areas of the body (i.e., face, hands, areas of occupational or social importance) that raise the importance of this type of disease to a moderate–severe degree rather than a limited or smaller percentage amount. Examples of patients who may warrant MTX treatment with lesser amounts of skin disease might include salespeople, actors, or young socially involved men and women. It is estimated that this population of patients makes up approximately 20% of psoriatic patients in the United States (9). Thus in recent years the criteria for using therapies like methotrexate have changed from a more rigid percentage body involvement to that of the location of the disease and its impact on quality of life (10). This extent/location of disease warrants more aggressive forms of therapy when topical therapy is not effective. Thus we consider treating these patients with a choice of several modalities including phototherapy, PUVA, retinoids, methotrexate, or possibly cyclosporine, based in part on quality of life concerns. The information in this paper is based in part on the concepts that have evolved in a series of guidelines on the use of methotrexate for psoriasis from 1972 to 1998 (11–14).

III. INDICATIONS

Methotrexate is indicated for the treatment of patients with moderate to severe psoriasis unresponsive to topical therapy. Administration of MTX for psoriasis must be an individualized decision, as we have learned from many years of experience. It is used in patients with moderate to extensive

Table 1 Indications for the Use of Methotrexate in Psoriasis

Erythrodermic psoriasis
Pustular psoriasis (acute and localized)
Psoriatic arthritis
Extensive psoriasis unresponsive to less toxic therapies
Psoriasis that significantly affects a patient's economic or psychological well-being
Lack of response to phototherapy, PUVA, or retinoids

plaque lesions as well as other variants of psoriasis including erythrodermic psoriasis, acute pustular psoriasis (von Zumbusch), psoriatic arthritis, and localized pustular psoriasis (Table 1). Its use is justified in certain other patients when the location or severity of the psoriasis jeopardizes the patient's economic, psychosocial, or physical well-being. While MTX is an extremely effective drug for psoriasis, it is the author's belief that phototherapy modalities (UVB or PUVA) should generally be the initial form of therapy for most patients prior to using MTX. Available information suggests that most patients are treated with UVB or PUVA because these are effective treatment modalities with less serious potential long-term toxicities. If light therapy is ineffective and/or has been used so extensively that the risks of side effects are increasing, then rotating therapy to MTX would be appropriate (3). In many patients, however, MTX may be the initial choice of therapy if the patient is light-sensitive, is unable to take light treatment for physical reasons, or is unable to travel or lives too far away from a physician's office to undergo light therapy. For patients being cared for by a physician other than a dermatologist, dermatological consultation is recommended for considering the use of MTX.

IV. CONTRAINDICATIONS

Relative contraindications to therapy with MTX are, in general, disease processes that may enhance the toxicity of MTX, particularly liver and kidney diseases (Table 2). Absolute contraindications include women who are pregnant or nursing and patients of either gender, who are attempting to conceive. An appropriate history and physical examination should allow the physician to detect any contraindications to therapy with MTX. In selected patients, circumstances may arise in which relative contraindications may be waived when it is considered that benefits of therapy may outweigh potential risks.

Table 2 Relative Contraindications to Methotrexate Therapy

Liver disease
    Significantly abnormal liver function tests
    Cirrhosis or severe degrees of histologically proven fibrosis
    Recent or active hepatitis
    Excessive alcohol consumption
Kidney disease
    Significantly decreased renal function (elevated creatinine and BUN; decreased
        creatinine clearance). Decreased renal function is frequently seen in elderly
        individuals and compensation can be made using lower than standard dosages
        of MTX.
Hematopoietic abnormalities
    Severe leukopenia, anemia, or thrombocytopenia
Active severe infectious diseases
    HIV, tuberculosis, etc.
Concurrent use of trimethoprim–sulfamethoxazole antibiotics (absolute)
Active peptic ulcer
Fertility considerations
    Pregnancy (absolute)
    Male or female patients attempting to conceive (absolute)
Unreliable patient

V. MECHANISM OF ACTION

Methotrexate blocks the synthesis of DNA by inhibiting dihydrofolic acid reductase, preventing the donation of methyl groups during synthesis of purine and pyrimidine nucleotides and, particularly, thymidylate (15). Thymidylate, one of the four DNA precursors, is necessary for DNA synthesis and the cell division that follows within hours.

    Methotrexate may exert a therapeutic effect in psoriasis by directly interfering with epidermal cell proliferation. Psoriatic skin contains twice as many proliferating cells and eight times as many cells in the S (synthesis) phase of cell division as normal skin. In addition, the proliferating cells have a cell cycle of 36 h, which is eight times faster than normal (16). Previous studies of MTX's mechanism of action indicate that after systemic or intralesional administration MTX inhibits DNA synthesis in psoriatic epidermal cells, followed within several hours by the cessation of mitoses (17). These data for many years suggested a direct effect of MTX on decreasing the rapidly proliferating psoriatic keratinocyte population.

    With the discovery that cyclosporine, an immunologically active drug, was effective for the treatment of psoriasis (another serendipitous observation in psoriasis therapy), much evidence has accumulated for an immunological basis for psoriasis. Based on that information, research in our laboratory has suggested an effect of MTX on both lymphocytes and keratinocytes. In vitro studies have revealed that keratinocytes are relatively resistant to MTX in culture at clinical concentrations reached in low-dosage MTX therapy (18). In comparison, activated lymphocytes are sensitive to MTX at concentration about 100-fold lower than those needed to affect keratinocytes. One may infer from these and other data that MTX may have a major immunosuppressing effect on psoriatic disease at levels that do not appear to produce a clinically immunosuppressive side effect profile in patients, based on the long experience with this drug.

VI. THERAPEUTIC EVALUATION/CONTRAINDICATIONS

The pretherapy evaluation starts with an appropriate history and physical examination that concentrates mainly on the patient's renal and liver function (Table 3). Methotrexate is excreted mainly by the kidneys; therefore, any underlying renal disease must be detected. This is especially important in older individuals who are more likely to have decreased renal excretory function, which could cause both higher and extended MTX blood levels resulting in increased toxicity at otherwise usual doses. A routine urinalysis, serum creatinine, and blood urea nitrogen (BUN) analysis are the standard tests for renal function. A more sensitive test of kidney excretion is the creatinine clearance over 24 h and may be especially important for older individuals whose renal function may be diminished significantly. Creatinine clearance less than 50 ml/min is indicative of at least moderate renal failure and may be a relative contraindication to therapy. In patients with decreased 24 h urine creatinine clearance rates, lower dosages of MTX should be used at

Table 3 Pretherapy Evaluation

History (including risk factors for liver and kidney disease) and physical examination
Liver function tests (SGOT, SGPT,[a] alkaline phosphatase)
Renal function tests (serum creatinine, BUN, 24 h urine or creatinine clearance)
CBC with platelet count
Chest x-ray (optional based on history)
Liver biopsy (before or shortly after initiation of therapy in patients with risk factors for liver disease)
HIV antibody determinations for patients at risk for acquired immunodeficieny syndrome

---

[a] Now AST and ALT, respectively.

the beginning of therapy and may be adequate. In these patients more vigilant monitoring for methotrexate toxicity will be necessary.

VII. PRETREATMENT OR EARLY LIVER BIOPSY

In all the years of MTX use for psoriasis, the issue of liver toxicity risk has received the most discussion and concern. In the 1998 guidelines for MTX (14), this issue was discussed in detail and is summarized below. While a history and physical examination and liver function tests may identify some patients with pre-existing risk factors for liver disease, the liver biopsy still remains the most reliable test for liver damage. In most studies in which patients *had no significant risk factors*, liver biopsies have found very few patients with fibrosis or cirrhosis.

Controversy exists as to the need for an early liver biopsy, but the current consensus (14) appears that it is not generally needed in patients *without* risk factors of liver disease.

The risk factors of concern are the following:

History of current excessive alcohol consumption (MTX toxicity is associated with a history of total lifetime alcohol intake before MTX therapy. The exact amount of alcohol that confers risk is unknown and differs among persons.)

Persistent abnormal liver chemistry studies

History of liver disease including chronic hepatitis B or C

Family history of inheritable liver disease

Diabetes mellitus, obesity (probably of secondary importance)

History of significant exposure to hepatotoxic drugs or chemicals

A. No Risk Factors

If there is no evidence of significant risk factors, it is rare for life-threatening liver disease to occur within the first 1–1.5 g of cumulative MTX. On this basis the guidelines have been **revised** to recommend *not obtaining* a liver biopsy until a patient has received this amount of MTX or is developing risk factors such as persistent elevated results of liver function tests (14).

B. Patients with Risk Factors

If risk factors are found prior to initiating MTX, it is advisable that a liver biopsy be done, when feasible, at or near the beginning of MTX treatment. Since it is possible that some patients will not continue taking MTX after the first few months because of adverse effects, lack of effectiveness, or other reasons, it is reasonable to postpone the biopsy until after this initial period. If the drug is effective and its use will continue for long-term therapy, it provides more incentive for a patient to accept the decision for a liver biopsy. There is no information available that short-term use of MTX will cause clinically significant liver disease. Clinical experience has also suggested that a liver biopsy may not be warranted in the following situations:

Elderly patients
During acute illness and/or severe exacerbation of psoriasis
In the presence of medical contraindications for a biopsy (e.g., cardiac instability, bleeding problems, etc.)
In patients with limited life expectancy

VIII. DOSAGE/ADMINISTRATION

Dosage regimens for MTX in the treatment of psoriasis have gone through several stages of evolution. Initially, an empirically derived schedule was based on daily small dosages of aminopterin and, later, MTX (19). This daily schedule was subsequently found to produce greater liver toxicity. Using experience from oncological therapy schedules with MTX, weekly schedules of intramuscular MTX were found to be effective in the treatment of psoriasis (20). This regimen was then adapted for use as a single weekly oral dose (12).

The triple-dose schedule (MTX at 12 h intervals for three doses each week) was proposed in 1971 to provide a therapeutic level of MTX for approximately 36 h which is the duration of the psoriatic cell cycle (21).

Today, MTX is administered for psoriasis principally by two schedules: the triple-dose regimen or a single weekly dose, either orally or intramuscularly. A majority of surveyed dermatologists use the triple-dose schedule (Table 4) (9). The triple-dose regimen is initiated with a test dose of 5 mg (2.5

Table 4   Dermatologists' Preferences for Methotrexate Dosing Schedules: Results of a 1984 Survey

Dosing schedule	Percentage
Weekly divided oral doses	74
Weekly single oral dose	16
Weekly intramuscular dose	3
Other dosing schedule	7

Source: Data from Ref. 9.

mg every 24 h for two doses) (Table 5). The concept of a small test dose was initiated when weekly doses were first used to avoid possible serious side effects if a patient had a hidden or undiscovered medical or allergic sensitivity to MTX. Early use of MTX was given with much larger doses than are currently used and severe side effects were being found. A complete blood count (CBC) is repeated after 7 days. If these results are normal and there is no unusual sensitivity to the test dose, the first triple dose is started at a dosage of one 2.5 mg tablet every 12 h for three doses (1/1/1), totaling 7.5 mg for the week. One week later, if there are no adverse effects, the dosage is increased to 4 tablets (2/1/1), for a total of 10 mg. Over the following weeks the dosage is increased by one 2.5 mg tablet per week every 2–3 weeks, depending on the effectiveness of the drug and the patient's ability to tolerate a given dosage regimen. In the typical 70 kg patient, the dosage is usually plateaued at 2/2/2 (15 mg/wk), although larger patients or those with more resistant psoriasis may require a higher dosage. This schedule is continued until the patient's psoriasis is under adequate control. Most patients begin to see improvement in 6–8 weeks.

To minimize the risk of side effects (in particular, severe liver toxicity), MTX dosages should be kept as low as possible to achieve and maintain what is termed adequate control of the disease. Total clearing of lesions is *not* the intended goal of therapy since that may require continuing increases in weekly dosages approaching toxicity. At the point of optimal response, the dosage is titrated down every month by 1 tablet per week until the lowest effective maintenance dosage, perhaps 1–3 tablets per week, is achieved. When possible, attempts should be made to discontinue therapy for several months at a time, the summer often being a good time. This limits the cumulative dosage, extends the time interval between potential liver biopsies, and permits longer-term use of MTX. New MTX patients are seen weekly for 2–3 weeks, then biweekly, and finally monthly as they develop a response pattern (Table 5). Clinical responses are titrated by 1 tablet up or down at monthly visits, reflecting very sensitive responses to changes of only one tablet.

Table 5   Drug Dosage Schedules

Divided oral dose schedule
2.5 to 5.0 mg at 12-hr intervals for 3 doses each week
Gradually increase by 2.5mg/wk every 2–4 weeks with appropriate monitoring of laboratory tests
Total dosage generally not to exceed 6–9 tablets per week (15–22.5 mg)
Weekly single oral dosage ranges from 7.5 to 30 mg/wk
If single weekly doses are used by intramuscular or IV administration, the dosages can go as high as 50 mg/wk . Intravenous drips of MTX should not be used. As the dosages are increased, the CBC should be monitored more frequently.

The dosage schedule using single weekly oral doses is initiated with a 5.0–7.5 mg test dosage and is subsequently increased by 2.5 mg per week. The total weekly maintenance dosage is usually between 7.5 and 25.0 mg. However, dosages as high as 37.5 mg per week may be required. Occasionally MTX is administered in weekly intramuscular (IM) doses, usually for unreliable patients. The IM route may also be used when the effectiveness of oral MTX has diminished, or when gastrointestinal (GI) side effects are limiting treatment. Doses are somewhat higher than weekly oral doses because the half-life of MTX in plasma is shorter when given via the IM route.

Alternative methods of administration have been explored by rheumatologists, which include the use of subcutaneous injections of MTX, which can be self-administered by patients, and oral usage of injectable MTX preparations (22). If oral administration of a MTX solution is used, the parenteral solution is usually in 50 mg/2 ml aqueous vial. A syringe would be used to withdraw 0.1 ml or more of this solution, which is equal to a 2.5 mg tablet, and put into a small amount of water or other drink. According to available information, administration by tablet or the equivalent carefully measured solution has equal effectiveness. Regardless of the dosage schedule or route of administration, the same principles previously described for adjusting dosages for individual patients to minimize the cumulative MTX dosage should be followed (Table 6).

Table 6   Instructions to Patients Taking Methotrexate for Psoriasis

---

Great care is needed when taking methotrexate

Methotrexate is usually taken only three times per week (*not* daily). Each pill is taken 12 hours apart. Sometimes methotrexate is given as single weekly doses orally or by injection.

Take only the prescribed, correct dose of methotrexate at the *same time and day* each week.

Do *not begin or change* the dosage of *any medication* (including nonprescription medications) unless your physician has approved it.

Avoid alcoholic beverages.

If you have side effects or any symptoms of dehydration, notify your physician before the next dose.

If you develop cough, fever, and shortness of breath or have any problems with sore throat; infections, including skin infections; or skin or mouth ulcers, STOP METHOTREXATE AND CALL YOUR PHYSICIAN.

See your physician regularly, usually every 4 weeks (more frequently at the beginning of therapy).

Do not miss doctor's appointments or blood tests.

Notify your physician at once if an accidental overdose has occurred.

Table 7 Duration of Methotrexate
Treatments to Achieve a Cumulative
Dose of 1.5 g

Weekly dosage (mg)	Months to 1.5 g
7.5	50
15.0	25
22.5	17

How long can or should a patient be maintained on MTX? As clearing is obtained, weaning of dosages is started, with the goal of achieving the *lowest* possible long-range dosing schedule. If a patient can be maintained with as little as 2–3 tablets per week, the calculated cumulative dosage would be 260–400 mg/year. Using a 1.0–1.5 g cumulative dose as the range within which liver changes may develop (Table 7), a patient could receive low-dosage MTX *continuously* for over 3 years. If rest periods off MTX consisting of several months each year were successful, even longer durations of MTX could be utilized before reaching this cumulative dose range. However, if a patient were to require higher maintenance dosages, such as 15 mg/week (2/2/2), then a cumulative dosage warranting concern about liver toxicity could be reached in 1.5–2.0 years. At that time we would recommend stopping MTX and rotating the patient to another form of therapy. At some future time the patient could restart therapy with MTX, it is hoped, with some reversal of any cumulative liver toxicity (23–25). If MTX needs to be continued, a liver biopsy would have to be considered.

IX. MONITORING THERAPY

Patients receiving MTX are monitored for the drug's effect on hematopoietic and liver function as they are reflected in laboratory tests (Table 8). During the first several weeks of initial therapy a CBC is obtained every week initially, then biweekly, and thereafter at the time of each visit, usually monthly. The CBC should be obtained at least 7 days after the last dose since MTX causes a maximal depression in the leukocyte and platelet counts 7–10 days after drug administration. Dosage reduction or a brief interruption of therapy is warranted when the counts drop below the minimum normal levels. The appearance of oral mucosal ulcerations, previously used to clinically monitor MTX toxicity, is now infrequently observed due to the use of lower-dosage regimens and careful monitoring of hematopoietic function.

Table 8 Monitoring Therapy

CBC and platelet count (every 1–4 weeks, drawn at least 1 week after the last dose).
Serum chemistries, including routine liver and renal function tests (every 3–4 months, at least 1 week after the last dose).
Chest x-ray (annual) if there are pulmonary symptoms.
Liver biopsy:
  In patients without risk factors:
    First biopsy at 1.0–1.5 g cumulative MTX
  In patients with risk factors
    First biopsy after 2–4 months of therapy
    Subsequent biopsies after each 1.0 g cumulative dose

It is now recommended to obtain liver function tests (LFTs) every 2–3 months during therapy (see below). Since MTX can cause a transient and clinically unimportant elevation in liver enzymes 1–3 days after drug administration, these tests should also be obtained at least 7 days after the last dose. If liver enzymes are significantly elevated at that time, MTX therapy should be interrupted for 1–2 weeks and the tests repeated before restarting therapy. In most cases, the LFTs will return to normal. However, if significant elevations persist, a liver biopsy should be considered before continuing MTX therapy.

In the absence of abnormal liver enzymes, the 1998 Guidelines recommend liver biopsy after each cumulative MTX dose of 1.5 g (14). In patients who have one or more risk factors for cirrhosis, signs of liver disease, or significant liver enzyme abnormalities a liver biopsy should be considered after each 1.0 g MTX or more frequently. It is suggested that this procedure be performed at least 2 weeks after the last dose of MTX to minimize any acute histological liver changes. Liver biopsy may not be in the best interest of older patients or patients with acute diseases or other contraindications to liver biopsy. The risk of liver biopsy versus the risk of continued MTX therapy must be carefully assessed in these patients. There are also occasional reluctant patients who refuse to allow a liver biopsy. In the absence of evidence of liver changes, it then becomes the option of the physician to continue using MTX or consider the availability of other therapies, using benefit/risk considerations. It is recommended that the patient's chart reflect the discussions on this point and the patient's decision not to undergo liver biopsy. We would suggest that the patient sign such a notation in the chart.

Additional monitoring of patients on long-term MTX therapy includes hemoglobin/hematocrit and renal function tests every 3–4 months. A chest x-ray should be performed in the event of acute or chronic pulmonary changes that might suggest a so-called MTX pneumonitis, seen rarely in psoriatics but more frequently in rheumatoid arthritis patients taking MTX.

X. SIDE EFFECTS

Short-term side effects of MTX such as nausea, anorexia, and fatigue are dose-related and rapidly reversible with a decrease in dosage or brief interruption in therapy. As an alternative, rotating between triple-dose and weekly oral or IM dosage may alleviate severe symptoms that may otherwise cause a patient to discontinue therapy with MTX. However, utilizing the IM route does not necessarily reduce GI side effects. In patients receiving higher dosages of MTX, nausea may be psychologically triggered in anticipation of the next dose. Food and occasional antiemetic drugs may be necessary to permit drug administration. Re-evaluation of renal function is prudent, especially in the older patient, or in a patient who suddenly develops symptoms after adequately tolerating a specific dosage regimen. A decline in renal function can result in persistent blood levels of MTX, leading to greater toxicity at a given dosage. A review of the patient's concurrent medications might likewise reveal a potential drug interaction causing increased MTX toxicity (see discussion of Drug Interactions below).

A. Folic and Folinic Acid Supplements

Several reports have suggested that concomitant administration of folic acid (1–5 mg/day) can reduce side effects such as nausea and megaloblastic anemia without affecting the effects of MTX. Folinic acid, the direct anti-dote for MTX, if given on days when MTX is not administered (the other 5 days of the week), will also reduce side effects such as nausea (26, 27).

B. Liver Toxicity

The major limitation in the use of MTX is the potential for severe drug-induced liver fibrosis and cirrhosis. Even with lower dosage regimens, long-term use of MTX can cause life-threatening cirrhosis (28). Data from several studies suggest that MTX's effects on the liver are mainly related to the cumulative dose. The incidence of cirrhosis is 3% in the range of 1.5–2.0 g cumulative dose, and as high as 20–26% with a cumulative dose of 4.0 g (12). The incidence of MTX-induced cirrhosis in the United States appears to be lower than in Scandinavian populations, although the reasons for this are unclear (29, 30). As mentioned previously, potential candidates for MTX therapy must be questioned about underlying risk factors for liver disease that may be present prior to therapy. The prevalence of fibrosis and cirrhosis in patients with psoriasis could be the same as that for the population at large, as estimated from autopsies in the general public. A history of heavy alcohol consumption or intravenous drug use, or the presence of diabetes mellitus, obesity, suboptimal renal function, or pre-existing liver pathology, is a risk factor for the development of severe liver toxicity (31). It is recommended that any patient with moderate-to-severe psoriasis avoid or at least minimize alcohol consumption prophylactically to maintain the option for MTX treatment use in the future.

Fibrosis or cirrhosis due to methotrexate can be detected and may improve once therapy with MTX is discontinued, as demonstrated by repeat liver biopsies (24). Some researchers believe that MTX-related cirrhosis is not aggressive, as evidenced by little or no progression of liver histopathological findings in patients with documented cirrhosis who continued taking MTX (23). A few of these patients with cirrhosis even showed improvement. However, most would agree that if the liver biopsy shows grade III B or grade IV (moderate-to-severe fibrosis or cirrhosis), MTX should be discontinued (Table 9). Severe liver disease, as well as a few deaths, have occurred in patients receiving long-term methotrexate. To the author's knowledge, most have occurred in situations of significant deviations from appropriate patient/doctor safeguards (28).

Liver toxicity can often be detected by monitoring liver enzymes as recommended. Unfortunately, these tests are not always reliable; in fact, severe liver disease, including cirrhosis, can be present in the absence of elevated liver enzymes (32). As a result, other tests of liver function have been investigated as an indicator of liver disease that might obviate the need for liver biopsies. Levels of serum amino terminal propeptide of type III procollagen (PIIINP) have been correlated with liver histological findings

Table 9 Classification of Liver Biopsy Findings

Grade I	Normal; mild fatty infiltration/portal inflammation
Grade II	Moderate-to-severe fatty infiltration/portal tract inflammation
Grade III	A: Mild fibrosis
	B: Moderate-to-severe fibrosis
Grade IV	Cirrhosis
Clinical Interpretation of Liver Biopsy Results	
Grade I or II	Continue MTX therapy
Grade III A	May continue MTX therapy. Repeat biopsy after 6 months of continuous MTX therapy.
Grade III B	Discontinue MTX therapy.
Grade IV	Discontinue MTX therapy.

(33). In psoriatic patients without arthritis, high levels of PIIINP appear to be an indicator of liver fibrosis. Patients with coexistent arthritis often have high levels of PIIINP in the absence of liver fibrosis. In addition, the test has a high rate of false negatives: 25–33% of patients in the study had fibrosis, albeit mild, in the presence of normal PIIINP levels. On a more practical note, this test is not widely available in the United States.

Attempts have been made to correlate imaging modalities with liver pathology. Magnetic resonance imaging and static radionuclide scanning have been unreliable (34, 35). Comparison studies of liver ultrasound and liver biopsy have demonstrated varied results, with a sensitivity in detecting liver fibrosis or cirrhosis as low as 11% and as high as 100% (36, 37). In a recent analysis, one investigator concluded that given the risks of liver biopsy, ultrasound, if performed by an experienced specialist, is a justified screening method and urged re-evaluation of the guidelines for routine liver biopsy (38). Imaging procedures have still not replaced the liver biopsy as a reliable indicator of fibrosis or cirrhosis.

To date, liver biopsy remains the gold standard for evaluating MTX-induced liver toxicity. Unfortunately, this procedure is not without risk and carries a general complication rate of 2.2% and a mortality rate of 9/100,000 (39). The risks of liver biopsies have tended to be lower in patients with psoriasis than with other diseases. Most adverse events occur in patients with internal hepatic problems related to other diseases. Notwithstanding, most would agree that, although uncommon, the risk of severe and life-threatening liver damage due to MTX outweighs the risk of liver biopsy. A qualified gastroenterologist who performs frequent liver biopsies should be consulted for appropriate patients. In addition, the pathologist should be familiar with the liver pathology classifications in MTX-treated patients as described in the 1998 Guidelines to provide the best clinicopathological correlations (14).

C. Hematological Complications

Methotrexate can suppress bone marrow function when high or incorrect dosages are used. Dosage errors by medical staff or patients have been reported. Specific directions, orders, and prescriptions should be legibly written and discussed with the patient. Periodic monitoring of the CBC should alert the physician to any significant changes. In rare cases, MTX can cause reversible agranulocytosis or pancytopenia at low dosages (40).

D. Methotrexate Overdosage

Causes of MTX overdosage include patient/physician/nurse/pharmacist errors, impaired renal function, or concomitant administration of drugs such as trimethoprin or trimethoprim–sulfamethoxazole (Bactrim, Septra, and generics). If MTX overdosage is suspected, leukovorin calcium (citrovorum factor or folinic acid) should be administered immediately to prevent hematological toxic effects (Table 10). In overdoses of MTX used for cancer chemotherapy, the success of antidote administration greatly decreases if the last dose of MTX was received more than 24–48 h prior to rescue (41).

When MTX toxicity develops secondary to decreased renal function, leukovorin administration may be prolonged. If serum creatinine concentration has increased to > 50% of baseline, leukovorin should be given intravenously at 100 mg/m^2 every 3 h until MTX concentration is less than 0.01 μmol/L. Alkalinization of the urine by means of sodium bicarbonate and fluid administration may be necessary to prevent precipitation of MTX in the renal tubules. All cases of suspected overdosage require vigilant monitoring for development of hematological or other toxic effects. Laboratory tests for MX blood levels should be obtained for guidance but these tests may not be readily available.

E. Drug Interactions

Reports of interactions between MTX and other drugs have been observed but, fortunately, are not common. Mechanisms of some drug interactions include interference with protein binding, renal tubular secretion, or intracellular transport of methotrexate (42). Other drugs may affect the efficacy or increase the toxicity of methotrexate. Barbiturates, phenylbutazone, phenytoin, probenecid, salicylates, and sulfonamides can displace MTX from serum albumin, causing elevated levels of free MTX and enhancing potential toxicity. Nonsteroidal anti-inflammatory agents, phenylbutazone, probenecid, salicylates, and sulfonamides can compete with MTX for active renal tubular secretion, thus increasing the half-life of MTX. Dipyridamole can interfere with intracellular transport of MTX and also prolong the effects of

Table 10 Leukovorin Rescue After Methotrexate Overdose

Serum MTX Level (μmol/L)	Leukovorin Dose (mg)
5×10^{-7}	20[a]
1×10^{-6}	100
2×10^{-6}	200
$> 2 \times 10^{-6}$	Proportionately increased

[a] The initial 20 mg dose of leukovorin is given parenterally, with subsequent doses given every 6 h either orally or parenterally.

MTX. The combination of MTX and trimethoprim can cause severe suppression of bone marrow function and is best avoided (43). Methotrexate can be ineffective if given concomitantly with folic acid or vitamin preparations that contain folic acid. Folic acid, or more specifically folinic acid, may bypass MTX inhibition of the dihydrofolic acid pathway. In a patient not responding to MTX, concurrent medications should be reviewed for any vitamin preparations that may contain folic acid.

Methotrexate in combination with other systemic therapies for psoriasis should be used with caution. Historically, many of the early cases of severe side effects and deaths occurred with the concomitant use of systemic corticosteroids and MTX. Many of these patients had severe disease or pustular psoriasis. Methotrexate-induced leukopenia together with steroid suppression of immune function led to overwhelming infections. It is thus well appreciated that the combination of MTX and systemic corticosteroids should be avoided as much as possible.

In one report, 2 of 10 patients receiving combined therapy with MTX and etretinate developed life-threatening drug-induced hepatitis (23). Cyclosporine and MTX, through their respective renal and liver toxicities and metabolic pathways (liver and renal, respectively), can cause elevated levels of both drugs, thereby increasing the risk of severe side effects from both drugs (44). However, rheumatologists have used this combination successfully to treat rheumatoid arthritis (45).

F. Fertility

Methotrexate is a known abortifacient and possible teratogen even at the low dosages commonly used in psoriasis. A report of 10 pregnancies occurring in 8 women receiving MTX for rheumatic disease included 5 normal infants delivered at full-term, 3 spontaneous abortions, and 2 elective abortions (46). The authors conclude that MTX may have strong abortifacient properties even at low weekly dosages. However, their results do not demonstrate an association between low-dosage weekly MTX and teratogenicity. Another report of normal offspring born to women who had previously received higher dosages of MTX for choriocarcinoma does not show any increase in congenital malformations (47). One patient received high-dosage MTX for choriocarcinoma during pregnancy starting at 27 weeks and went on to deliver a normal infant (48). Nonetheless, female patients should take all precautions to avoid pregnancy while taking MTX and for at least 1 month (or, more conservatively, 3–4 months) after discontinuing MTX.

Oligospermia (49) and sperm abnormalities have been reported in men receiving MTX, yet we are aware of five male patients receiving MTX who fathered normal offspring. Nonetheless, it is recommended that male patients taking MTX avoid fathering offspring during therapy and for 3–4 months after discontinuing therapy.

G. Pulmonary Complications

Pneumonitis due to methotrexate has been reported in at least 20 patients with rheumatoid arthritis (50). One patient, a 39-year-old woman, also had psoriasis and had been treated with MTX 15 mg/wk on a triple-dosage regimen for 5 months prior to developing symptoms of nonproductive cough and progressive dyspnea (51). The occurrence of MTX pneumonitis in psoriatics appears rarely in contrast to rheumatoid arthritis patients receiving MTX. Nonetheless, unexplained pulmonary symptoms in MTX-treated patient should be evaluated for MTX pneumonitis and the drug discontinued, at least temporarily.

H. Infectious Complications

A review of case reports of infectious complications of low-dosage MTX therapy includes varicella zoster, *Pneumocystis carinii* pneumonia, nocardiosis, and cryptococcosis (52). The patients described were all receiving low-dosage MTX for arthritic conditions. Three cases of disseminated histoplasmosis in patients receiving low-dosage MTX for psoriasis were also reported. Two had received a total of 7 and 8 g of MTX, respectively, and the third had received only 160 mg. Opportunistic infections should be considered in patients receiving MTX therapy who have unexplained prolonged fever. In the early years of MTX use some patients were treated with combinations of MTX and corticosteroids orally, which led to frequent infections and several deaths.

XI. COST

In the decision process of therapy today, one must consider the cost/benefit ratio as well as the benefit/risk ratios of different therapies. The limitations of health care resources have restricted access to some forms of therapy for many patients. For patients with moderate to severe psoriasis, the treatments available include phototherapy, PUVA, MTX, retinoids, and cyclosporine. In the near future it is likely that several biologicals will be available that will be significantly more expensive than the treatments listed above. Recently we quantitated the costs of several treatments (53). UVB phototherapy and MTX were significantly lower in cost than the other treatments. In 1997 the average annual cost for UVB was approximately $1850 and MTX costs ranged from $1500 to $2150. For comparison, PUVA and etretinate were approximately $3000 and cyclosporine was $4000. These estimates did not include physicians fees.

Combination therapies tend to shorten the duration of therapies, (e.g., PUVA plus retinoid or MTX and cyclosporine). Ellis et al. created a simulation of treatment over 10 years of MTX alone compared with a rotational scheduled use of MTX and cyclosporine (54). For MTX alone, the cost was $33,000 ($3,300/year), which is higher than estimated above (53). When using MTX rotated with cyclosporine over 10 years, the cost was approximately $38,000. For the additional amount the rotated MTX/cyclosporine produced 4 years of clearing while MTX alone produced only 2 years of clearing. Assuming the efficacy and comparative safety of these two schedules over 10 years, one would have to decide whether the additional 2 years of clearing are worth an additional $5,000. In effect, this is another benefit, albeit economic, of the rotational approach to psoriasis therapy of which the major benefit is safety for long-term chronic therapy of psoriasis (25).

XII. CONCLUSION

We have been fortunate to have had access to MTX for the past approximate half a century. It is amazing that no other folic acid antagonists (after aminopterin) have become available to improve on the effectiveness and safety of MTX for the treatment of psoriasis as well as for cancer chemotherapy. We have learned that the drug is quite effective: producing at least 70% good improvement in at least 70% of patients being treated. Psoriasis has not developed resistance in most patients to intermittent or continued therapy, in contrast to what happens in some forms of leukemia.

Adverse events resulting from the short-term or continuing use of MTX have been relatively limited, with the exception of the concern for hepatic toxicity. In the early years of MTX use more problems were found when there was inadequate information on how to use the drug safely. In recent years, the prior problems of liver damage have been minimized because we have selected patients more carefully for this drug; tested patients more frequently for liver disease; and perhaps most importantly, treated psoriasis by rotating the additional new therapies so that MTX is not used as frequently or for so long at any time (55). In our experience the number of episodes of severe liver disease in recent years has been rare. This does not mean that MTX cannot cause problems. However from knowledge acquired from other physicians and malpractice litigation, these difficulties appear to arise in situations where there is misuse or abuse by patients (28), or inappropriate use. Given this long and fortuitous experience, it remains an important drug for the therapy of moderate to severe psoriasis.

REFERENCES

1. Bukaty LM, Weinstein GD. The therapy of moderate-to-severe psoriasis with methotrexate. In: Weinstein GD, Gottlieb AB, eds. Therapy of Moderate-to-Severe Psoriasis. Portland, OR: National Psoriasis Foundation, 1995; 1–148.
2. Gubner R. Effect of aminopterin on epithelial tissues. Arch Dermatol 1951;64: 699–699.
3. Rees RB, Bennett JH, Bostwick WL. Aminopterin for psoriasis. Arch Dermatol. 1955;72:133–143.
4. Kuijpers AL, van de Kerkhof PC. Risk-benefit assessment of methotrexate in the treatment of severe psoriasis. Am Jrnl Clin Dermatol. 2000;27–39.
5. Wollina U, Stander K, Barta U. Toxicity of methotrexate treatment in psoriasis arthritis—short and long-term toxicity in 104 patients, 2001;20(6): 406–410.
6. Kumar B, Saraswat A, Kaur I. Short-term methotrexate therapy in psoriasis: a study of 197 patients. Int J Dermatology; 2002;41(7):444–448.
7. Van Dooren-Greebe RJ, Kiujpers AL, Mulder J, De Boo T, Van de Kerkhof PC. Methotrexate revisited: effects of long-term treatment in psoriasis. Br J Dermatol. 1994;130(2):204–210.
8. Roenigk HH Jr, Mibach HI, Weinstein GD. Guidelines on methotrexate therapy for psoriasis. Arch Dermatol 1972;105:363–365.
9. Peckham PE, Weinstein GD, McCullough JL. The treatment of severe psoriasis. A national survey. Arch Dermatol 1972;123;1303–1307.
10. Krueger GG, Feldman SR, Camisa C, Duvec M, Elder JT, Gottlieb AB, Koo J, Krueger JG, Lebwohl M, Lowe N, Menter A, Morison WL, Prystowsky JH, SHupack JL, Taylor JR, Weinstein GD, Barton TL, Rolstad T, Day RM. Two considerations for patients with psoriasis and their clinicians: what defines mild, moderate and severe psoriasis? What constitutes a clinically significant improvement when treating psoriasis? J Am Acad Dermatol, 2000 Aug; 43(2 pt 1):281–285.
11. Roenigk HH Jr, Maibach HI, Weinstein GD. Guidelines on methotrexate therapy for psoriasis. Arch Dermatol. 1972;105:363–365.
12. Roenigk HH, Auerbach R, Maibach HI, Weinstein GD. Methotrexate guidelines revised. J Am Acad Dermatol. 1982;6:145–155.
13. Roenigk HH, Auerbach R, Maibach HI, Weinstein GD. Methotrexate in psoriasis: revised guidelines. J Am Acad Dermatol. 1988;19:145–156.
14. Roenigk HH, Auerbach R, Maibach H, Weinstein GD, Lebwohl M. Methotrexate in psoriasis: consensus conference, Am Acad Dermatol. 1998; 38:478–485.

15. Olsen EA. The pharmacology of methotrexate. J Am Acad Dermatol. 1991;25:306–316.
16. Weinstein GD, McCullough JL, Ross PA. Cell kinetic basis for pathophysiology of psoriasis. J Invest Dermatol. 1985;85:579–583.
17. Weinstein GD, Goldfaden G, Frost P. MTX: mechanism of action on DNA synthesis in psoriasis. Arch Dermatol. 1971;104:236–243.
18. Zanolli MD, Sheretz EF, Hedberg AE. Methotrexate: anti-inflammatory or antiproliferative? J Am Acad Dermatol. 1990;22:523–524.
19. Rees RB, Bennett JH, Maibach HI, Arnold HL. Methotrexate for psoriasis. Arch Dermatol. 1967;95:2–11.
20. Van Scott EJ, Auerbach R, Weinstein GD. Parenteral methotrexate in psoriasis. Arch Dermatol. 1964;95:2–11.
21. Weinstein GD, Frost P. MTX for psoriasis: a new therapeutic schedule. Arch Dermatol. 1971;103:33–38.
22. Zackheim HS. Subcutaneous administration of methotrexate. J Am Acad Dermatol. 1992;26:1008.
23. Zachariae HS. Methotrexate side effects. Br J Dermatol. 1990;12(suppl 36)L127–L133.
24. Newman M, Auerbach R, Feiner H, Holzman R, Shupack J, Migdall P, et al. The role of liver biopsies in psoriatic patients receiving long-term methotrexate treatment, improvement of liver abnormalities after cessation of treatment. Arch Dermatol. 1989;125:1218–1224.
25. Weinstein GD, White GM. An approach to the treatment of moderate to severe psoriasis with rational therapy. J Am Acad Dermatol. 1993;28:454–459.
26. Ortiz, Shea B, Suarez-Almazor ME, et al, The efficacy of folic acid and folinic acid in reducing methotrexate gastrointestinal toxicity in rheumatoid arthritis. A metanalysis of randomized controlled trials. J Rheumatol 1998;25:36–43.
27. Duhra P. Treatment of gastrointestinal symptoms associated with methotrexate therapy for psoriasis. J Am Acad Dermatol. 1993;28:466–469.
28. Gilberg SC, Klintmalm G, Menter A, Silverman A. Methotrexate-induced cirrhosis requiring liver transplantation in three patients with psoriasis. A word of caution in light of the expanding use of the steroid sparing agent. Arch Intern Med. 1990;150:889–891.
29. Zachariae H, Kragballe K, Sogaard H. MTX induced liver cirrhosis. Br J Dermatol. 1980;102:407–412.
30. Nyfors A. Liver biopsies from psoriatics related to MTX therapy. Acta Pathol Microbiol Scand. 1976;84:262–270.
31. Roenigk HH, Auerbach R, Maibach HI, Weinstein GD. Methotrexate in psoriasis: revised guidelines. J Am Acad Dermatol. 1988;19:145–156.
32. Weinstein GD, Roenigk H, Maibach HI, Cosmides J, Halprin K, Millard M. Psoriasis–liver–MTX interactions. Arch Dermatol. 1973;108:36–42.
33. Zachariae H, Aslam HM, Bjerring P, Sogaard H, Zachariae E, Heickendorff L. Serum Aminoterminal propeptiede of type III procollagen in psoriasis and psoriatic arthritis: relation to liver fibrosis and arthritis. J Am Acad Dermatol. 1991;25: (1pt1):50–53.

34. Rademaker M, Webb JAW, Lowe DG, Meyrick-Thomas RH, Kerby JD, Munro DD. Magnetic resonance imaging as a screening procedure for methotrexate-induced liver damage. Br J Dermatol 1987;117:311–316.

35. Geronemus RG, Auerbach R, Tobias H. Liver biopsies versus liver scans in methotrexate-treated patients with psoriasis. Arch Dermatol 1982;118: 649–651.

36. Mitchell D, Johnson RJ, Testa HJ, Haboubi NY, Chalmers RJ. Ultrasound and radionuclide scans-Poor indicators of liver damage in patients treated with methotrexate. Clin Exp Dermatol. 1987;116:491–495.

37. Coulson IH, McKenzie J, Neild VS, Joseph AE, Marsden RA. A comparison of liver ultrasound with liver biopsy histology in psoriatics receiving long-term methotrexate therapy. Br J Dermatol. 1987;116:491–495.

38. Verschuur AC, van Everdingen JJ, Cohen EB, Chamuleau RA. Liver biopsy versus ultrasound in methotrexate-treated psoriasis: a decision analysis. Int J Dermatol. 1992;31(6):101–109.

39. Piccinino F, Sagnelli E, Pasquale G, Giusti G. Complications following percutaneous liver biopsy: a multicentre retrospective study on 68,276 biopsies. J Hepatol. 1986;2:165–173.

40. Shupack JL, Webster GF. Pancytopenia following low-dose oral methotrexate therapy for psoriasis. JAMA 1988;259:3594–3596.

41. Bertino JR. Rescue techniques in cancer chemotherapy: use of leucovorin and other rescue agents after methotrexate treatment. Semin Oncol. 1977;4: 203–216.

42. Evans WE, Christensen ML. Drug interactions with methotrexate. J Rheumatol Suppl 1985;12:15–20.

43. Groenendad H, Rampen FHJ. Methotrexate and trimethoprim/sulfamethoxazole—A potentially hazardous combination. J Am Acad Dermatol. 1990; 23(2pt1):320–321.

44. Korstanje MJ, van Breda Vrissman CJ, van de Staak WJ. Cyclosprine and methotrexate—a potentially hazardous combination. Clin Exp Dermatol. 1990; 15:358–360.

45. Tugwell P, Pincus T, Yocum D, et al, Combination therapy with cyclosporine and methotrexate in severe rheumatoid arthritis. The Methotrexate Cyclosporine Combination Study Group. N Engl J Med 1995;333:137–141.

46. Kozlowski RD, Steinbrunner, JV, MacKenzie AH, Clough JD, Wilke WS, Segal AM. Outcome of first-trimester exposure to low dose methotrexate in eight patients with rheumatic disease. J Am Acad Dermatol 1990;88:580–592.

47. Ayhan A, Ergeneli M, Yuce K, Yapar E, Kisnisci A. Pregnancy after chemotherapy for trophoblastic disease. J Reprod Med 1990;35:522–524.

48. Nabers J, Spliner TAW, Wallenburg HCS, Tenkate FJW, Oosterom R, Hilvering C. Choriocarcinoma with lung metastases during pregnancy with successful delivery and outcome after chemotherapy. Thorax. 1990;15(5): 116–118.

49. Sussman A, Leonard JM. Psoriasis, methotrexate and oligospermia. Arch Dermaol. 1980;115:215–217.

50. Ridly MG, Wolfe CS, Mathews JA. Life threatening acute pneumonitis during low dose methotrexate treatment for rheumatoid arthritis: a case report of the literature. Ann Rheum Dis. 1988;47:784–788.

51. Schwartz GF. Anderson St. Methotrexate induced pneumonitis in a young woman with psoriasis and rheumatoid arthritis (letter). J Rheumatol. 1990; 7:980.

52. Witty LA, Steiner F, Curfman M, Webb D, Wheat LJ. Disseminated histoplasmosis in patients receiving low-dose methotrexate therapy for psoriasis. Arch Dermatol. 1992;128:91–93.

53. Lee GC, Weinstein GD. Comparative cost-effectiveness of different treatments for psoriasis. In: Rajagopalan R, Scherertz EF, Anderson RT, eds. Care and Management of Skin Diseases. New York: Marcel Dekker, 1998:269–298.

54. Ellis CN, Reiter KL, Bandekar RR, Fendrick AM. Cost-effectiveness comparison of therapy for psoriasis with a methotrexate-based regimen versus a rotation regimen of modified cyclosporine and methotrexate. 2002 (2) J Am Acad Dermatol;242–250.

55. Weinstein GD, White GM. An approach to the treatment of moderate to severe psoriasis with rotational therapy. J Am Acad Dermatol 1993;28:454–459.

6
Systemic Retinoids

Paul S. Yamauchi, Dalia Rizk, Tanya Kormeili, Rickie Patnaik, and Nicholas J. Lowe
Clinical Research Specialists, Santa Monica, and UCLA School of Medicine, Los Angeles, California, U.S.A.

I. INTRODUCTION

The systemic retinoids possess a remarkable range of activities and clinical applications. They are an important form of therapy for patients with more severe and resistant types of psoriasis. In general, systemic retinoids are used most effectively in the treatment of plaque psoriasis in combination with other forms of therapy, such as phototherapy or other systemic agents. With generalized pustular psoriasis, they are effective as monotherapy and are frequently helpful for the control of exfoliative psoriasis.

The U.S. Food and Drug Administration (FDA) has approved four derivatives of systemic retinoids. Isotretinoin, whose main indication is for cystic acne, has been found to be ineffective for plaque-type psoriasis as monotherapy (1). However, clinical responses were observed with isotretinoin for pustular psoriasis (1) and in conjunction with phototherapy for psoriasis (2, 3). Bexarotene is approved for the treatment of cutaneous T-cell lymphoma. One report showed that bexarotene at 0.5–2 mg/kg/day reduced lesions in patients with moderate to severe psoriasis (4).

This chapter will focus on the treatment of psoriasis with acitretin, the only systemic retinoid approved for psoriasis and will also briefly discuss its predecessor, etretinate which was replaced by acitretin in 1997 and is no longer available. Combination acitretin therapy with phototherapy and other therapeutic agents will also be described. In addition, new retinoid analogs undergoing clinical investigation at the time of preparation of this article will be mentioned. Finally, potential toxicities and adverse effects associated with systemic retinoids will be discussed

II. CHEMISTRY AND PHARMACOLOGY

Figure 1 shows the chemical structures of acitretin and etretinate. Acitretin is the principal active metabolite of the prodrug etretinate. They are very similar, except that etretinate is the ethylester form of acitretin. However, because of this modification, under physiological conditions, etretinate is in an uncharged state and is 50 times more lipophilic than acitretin, which carries a negative charge (5). Consequently, etretinate is accumulated in adipose tissue because of its high lipophilicity as opposed to acitretin, which is not stored in fat. This is the main pharmacokinetic reason why acitretin has a much shorter half-life (approximately 50 h) than etretinate (approximately 120 days). In light of the highly teratogenic effects associated with systemic retinoids (to be discussed later) and because of its long half-life and detection in the serum up to 2 years after discontinuing treatment, etretinate was withdrawn from the market in 1997 following the introduction of acitretin.

Studies have demonstrated that the concurrent ingestion of ethanol with acitretin results in the transesterification conversion of acitretin to etretinate (6, 7). Furthermore, higher alcohol consumption was linked to higher etretinate concentrations. This is clinically significant because the ingestion of alcohol will extend the half-life of acitretin to the same as that of etretinate because of the enzymatic conversion. There are no data documenting the spontaneous conversion of acitretin to etretinate in the absence of alcohol consumption.

It is also important to instruct to patients that systemic retinoids, including acitretin, have higher absorption and improved bioavailability when ingested with food (8).

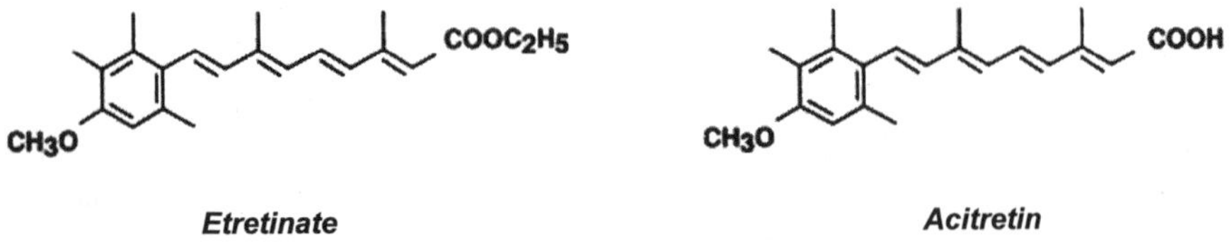

Etretinate   **Acitretin**

Figure 1 Chemical structures of etretinate and acitretin.

III. MECHANISM OF ACTION

The exact molecular mechanism by which retinoids are able to exert their effects on psoriasis is unknown. It has been demonstrated that acitretin modulates the cellular differentiation of the epidermis, which results in deceased scaling, erythema, and thickness of the plaques. There is also histological evidence that acitretin decreases the thickness of the stratum corneum and the inflammation in the epidermis and dermis associated with psoriasis.

Two classes of nuclear retinoid receptors have been identified: the retinoic acid receptor (RAR) and retinoid X receptor (RXR). The RARs and RXRs are each composed of three different subtypes, labeled α, β, and γ (9). Nuclear retinoid receptors exists as dimers, and RARs are known to form heterodimers with RXRs (10). Acitretin has been shown to activate all three subtypes of RAR, despite the absence of measurable binding to any of the subtypes (10). To date, the function of these RAR–RXR heterodimers is unknown in the skin. Such data indicate that further studies are necessary to understand the interaction of acitretin with nuclear receptors.

IV. MONOTHERAPY WITH SYSTEMIC RETINOIDS

Several studies have confirmed the efficacy of acitretin treatment for different types of psoriasis (11–18). Pustular forms of psoriasis are more responsive to systemic retinoid monotherapy than plaque-type psoriasis, which responds more slowly. With plaque-type psoriasis, it is possible to enhance the response to therapy by combining retinoids with other treatments.

A. Pustular Psoriasis

When acitretin is used as monotherapy for generalized pustular psoriasis, the initial dosage is 25–50 mg/day, but higher dosages may be required in some patients. A rapid resolution of generalized pustular psoriasis is achieved usually within 10 days of initiating acitretin, which is probably the drug of first choice for the treatment of this condition.

One advantage of acitretin for the treatment of pustular psoriasis over methotrexate is the absence of acute effects on the peripheral blood count. Methotrexate may occasionally produce acute leukopenia in patients with generalized pustular psoriasis, which can lead to a major toxicity risk in these patients. Pustular psoriasis leads to rapid proliferation of monocytes in the S-phase of the cell cycle. Methotrexate, which blocks DNA synthesis in these cells, may lead to failure of maturation of cells beyond mitosis that leads to myelosuppression (19). This phenomena is not clinically evident with acitretin.

After the clearance of pustulation, the psoriasis can continue to be controlled by reducing the dosage of acitretin (for example, from 25 mg/day to 25 mg every other day or to 10 mg/day). However, some patients' disease will relapse and they will develop plaque-type psoriasis. In such patients, alternative forms of therapy such as phototherapy can gradually be instituted in combination with acitretin. When the psoriasis improves, the retinoid dosage then can be tapered down.

In women of childbearing age, acitretin should probably be avoided whenever possible, even for the treatment of pustular psoriasis. If acitretin is required, strict birth control must be adhered to and alcohol must be avoided. In such situations, oral isotretinoin, with its shorter half-life of 10–20 h may be used as an alternative to control the pustulation. Starting dosages range from 1 to 1.5 mg/kg per day. If necessary, phototherapy may be initiated to control the psoriasis.

Another situation in which acitretin is effective is in the treatment of palmoplantar pustular psoriasis, particularly where there is significant hyperkeratosis or severe pustulation. Isotretinoin may be used as an alternative in women of childbearing age. Retinoid therapy reduces the degree of hyperkeratosis and pustulation. If monotherapy with acitretin is not achieving the desired results, then combination with psoralen/ultraviolet A (PUVA) phototherapy is extremely useful. As an alternative, hydrea at 500 mg twice a day in conjunction with acitretin is another way of controlling palmoplantar pustular psoriasis.

B. Exfoliative Erythrodermic Psoriasis

In the treatment of exfoliative erythrodermic psoriasis, acitretin is useful at starting dosages of 25–50 mg/day. It is advantageous to use emollients liberally along with the application of mild topical corticosteroids, for example, triamcinolone acetonide (0.025% cream or ointment) under occlusion to achieve more rapid resolution of psoriasis.

In rare cases, patients with severe exfoliative erythrodermic psoriasis may need to use a combination of acitretin with methotrexate. This combination should only be rarely used and, when it is, only with careful monitoring of the peripheral blood count and liver function tests.

Another option for the treatment of exfoliative psoriasis is to use methotrexate or cyclosporine therapy to achieve a rapid improvement, after which the methotrexate or cyclosporine dosage is reduced and low dosages of acitretin (10–25 mg/day) are introduced.

V. COMBINATION THERAPY FOR MODERATE-TO-SEVERE PLAQUE PSORIASIS

In patients with severe plaque psoriasis, especially if the condition is extensive with hyperkeratosis, the use of a retinoid plus other forms of treatment, particularly phototherapy, has been shown to be highly effective. The dosage of the retinoid or the amount of alternative therapy required when used separately can be reduced if used in combination with each other.

A. Acitretin and PUVA Phototherapy

For combination therapy, the optimum dosage for acitretin is 0.3 mg/kg/day, either 2 weeks prior to starting phototherapy or at the same time. The increases in ultraviolet radiation should be more gradual and cautious than in patients not taking systemic retinoids because of an increased risk of ultraviolet radiation-induced erythema. This is not a true photosensitivity, but probably represents increased epidermal transmission of the ultraviolet radiation due to altered optical properties of the stratum corneum caused by the retinoid.

The concomitant use of PUVA with acitretin has been studied by several investigators (20–26). The majority of patients receiving the combination improve more quickly than with PUVA or acitretin alone. In addition, the total number of ultraviolet radiation exposures can be reduced. Following clearance of psoriasis, various maintenance regimens may be employed. Acitretin administered in low maintenance dosages can be effective, or acitretin therapy can be stopped and maintenance therapy undertaken solely with PUVA.

In a double-blind comparative study, patients with severe, widespread psoriasis were randomized to receive either PUVA alone or PUVA in combination with acitretin (20). Eighty percent of patients with PUVA alone demonstrated marked or complete clearing of psoriasis while 96% of patients who received adjunctive therapy with PUVA plus acitretin exhibited the same degree of improvement. The mean cumulative UVA dose given to patients who received combination therapy was 42% less than that required for patients who received PUVA alone.

When patients with psoriasis were initially treated with acitretin at 50 mg/day for 2 weeks followed by a decrease in the amount to 25 mg/day in conjunction with PUVA for up to 10 weeks, there was a 40.5% reduction in the total cumulative UVA dose, a decrease of the overall duration of treatment by almost 18 days, and a reduction in the number of PUVA treatments by nearly six sessions compared to treatment with PUVA alone (21).

Bath PUVA together with acitretin is another option for treatment of patents with pustular, plaque-type, or erythrodermic psoriasis (23). After 4 weeks of treatment, patients had greater than a 90% response rate with no relapse after 3 months.

The safety of PUVA is now of concern because of the risk of melanoma and nonmelanoma skin cancer. Whether acitretin alters this risk is unknown at this stage.

B. Acitretin and UVB Phototherapy

Acitretin plus UVB therapy is another combination form of therapy to treat psoriasis that has been investigated (27–29). This option can be used for those patients who are intolerant of side effects associated with oral psoralens such as gastrointestinal toxicity.

Treatment with UVB combined with acitretin at 50 mg/day or placebo resulted in greater clearance with fewer treatments and smaller amounts of UVB radiation when acitretin was used compared to placebo (28). A 74% improvement in the psoriasis score was noted in patients treated with acitretin plus UVB compared to 35% with UVB only. In addition, in the same study, when only acitretin was used there was a 42% reduction in psoriasis. There was a decrease in the total number of hours of exposure time to UVB therapy by approximately 6 h when acitretin was used to attain clearance compared to light treatment alone. Another study demonstrated that when patients with psoriasis were initially treated with 35 mg/day of acitretin during the first 4 weeks of therapy followed by concomitant therapy with UVB radiation plus 25 mg/day acitretin and compared with the placebo group, there was a 79% decrease in the psoriasis severity index in the acitretin and UVB group and a 35% reduction in the UVB only group (27). In addition, the median cumulative dose to achieve 75% clinical improvement was 41.5% lower when acitretin was combined. Finally, the number of treatments to attain 80–100% clearance of psoriatic plaques was decreased by 5.6 sessions with UVB plus acitretin vs. UVB only (29). The total UVB dose and minimal erythema dose was reduced by approximately 20%.

In summary, reasons for combining PUVA or UVB with systemic retinoids include:

1. Better clearance
2. Decreased cumulative ultraviolet doses

3. Reduced number of treatments and duration of PUVA therapy
4. Possibility of reduction or cessation of acitretin therapy before the occurrence of side effects such as hyperlipidemia or alopecia

C. Combination Therapy with Other Agents

Combination therapy of acitretin with other modalities other than light therapy can be used to control psoriasis. Concomitant treatment with acitretin and topical calcipotriene may help to reduce psoriatic plaques better than with either alone (30, 31). In addition, acitretin at 25 mg/day together with hydroxyurea 500 mg twice daily has been effective for some patients with chronic plaque psoriasis and pustular psoriasis. When using combination therapy with acitretin and hydroxyurea, the complete blood count should be carefully monitored.

D. Combination Therapy with Immunomodulatory Agents

New-generation drugs are being developed that selectively target key cytokines and receptor molecules on T cells and antigen-presenting cells involved in the pathogenesis of psoriasis. These immunomodulators are in the form of monoclonal antibodies or fusion proteins administered as injections subcutaneously, intramuscularly, or intravenously.

One biological agent currently on the market and FDA approved for the treatment of rheumatoid arthritis and psoriatic arthritis is etanercept. Etanercept is currently undergoing clinical trials as monotherapy for psoriasis. Etanercept is a fusion protein that acts as a soluble tumor necrosis factor (TNF) and competitively binds to TNF, thereby preventing TNF from binding to cell surface receptors on target cells. Because TNF is involved in the pathogenesis of psoriasis, through such inhibition etanercept serves as an anti-inflammatory agent that is beneficial in the treatment of psoriasis. A recent report demonstrated that combination therapy with etanercept and various systemic agents such as cyclosporine, methotrexate, acitretin, or hydroxyurea in patients with severe recalcitrant psoriasis resulted in marked improvement and reduction in the psoriasis area severity index (PASI) score (32). More important was that, no added toxicity was seen in these patients when etanercept was combined with a systemic agent. Figure 2 shows a patient with refractory psoriasis who responded well to combination therapy with 25 mg/day acitretin plus twice-weekly 25 mg subcutaneous injections of etanercept.

Combination treatment with systemic agents and immunomodulators underscores the significance of treating psoriasis in the future. With the advent of new biological agents and the existing systemics, this new

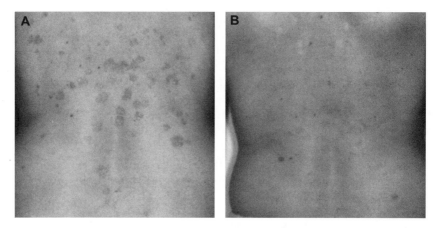

Figure 2   Patient with recalcitrant plaque-type psoriasis (A) before and (B) after treatment with 25 mg acitretin each day plus etanercept 25 mg twice a week subcutaneously for 8 weeks. (Refer to the color insert.)

approach to combination therapy may provide an impetus in controlling psoriasis that previously was difficult to treat.

VI.   OTHER SYSTEMIC RETINOIDS: ORAL TAZAROTENE

An oral form of tazarotene (a topical retinoid approved for treatment of plaque psoriasis and acne) has recently been developed that is currently not available on the market. Tazarotene is converted to its active metabolite, tazarotenic acid, which has a short elimination half-life of 7–12 hr (data on file, Allergan, Inc).

In a dosage escalation study, 181 patients with moderate to severe plaque psoriasis received daily doses of oral tazarotene (0.4–6.3 mg) or placebo (unpublished results). Optimal efficacy was seen with the 4.2 mg dose. At this dose, the body surface area involvement was reduced by 17% at week 12 and 82% of patients were satisfied or very satisfied with oral tazarotene. Figure 3 shows a patient who had good clearance of psoriatic plaques by week 12 with oral tazarotene at 4.2 mg/day.

The only significant adverse effect noted was cheilitis at doses of 2.8 mg or higher. There were no other dose-related adverse events such as increased liver function enzymes, hyperlipidemia, or changes in the hematological profile. The shorter half-life of oral tazarotene may potentially be a useful alternative for systemic retinoid treatment in women of childbearing age with psoriasis.

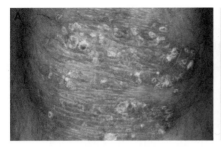 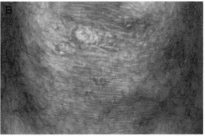

Figure 3 Patient with plaque-type psoriasis (A) before and (B) after treatment with oral tazarotene 4.2 mg each day for 12 weeks. (Refer to the color insert.)

VII. TOXICITIES AND ADVERSE REACTIONS

A. Teratogenicity

All systemic retinoids are highly teratogenic, with a pregnancy category of X rated by the Food and Drug Administration (FDA). Major human fetal abnormalities associated with retinoids include meningomyelocele, meningoencephalocele, multiple bony malformations, facial dysmorphia, low-set ears, high palate, decreased cranial volume alterations, and cardiovascular malformations.

In light of its teratogenicity, acitretin must not be used by women who are pregnant or who intend to become pregnant during therapy or at any time for at least 3 years following discontinuation of therapy. In addition, acitretin must not be used by women who may not be using reliable contraception while taking acitretin or for at least 3 years following cessation of treatment. In addition, the current guideline states that ethanol must not be ingested by women patients either during treatment with acitretin or for 2 months after discontinuing acitretin to avoid conversion into etretinate, which carries a much longer elimination half-life. This is due to the transesterification of acitretin to etretinate by ethanol, as previously discussed.

B. Mucocutaneous Toxicity

Mucocutaneous toxicity occurs with all of the systemic retinoids (33). The common mucocutaneous side effects, in order of frequency, are cheilitis, skin peeling, alopecia, xerosis, rhinitis, nail dystrophy, epistaxis, sticky skin, retinoid dermatitis, and xerophthalmia. Hair loss may occur a few weeks after initiation of treatment and ceases 6–8 weeks after discontinuation of therapy. In rare cases, chronic hair loss has occurred. Patients frequently find these symptoms extremely difficult to accept. Rapid reduction in retinoid therapy is desirable to reduce the impact on patients of these toxicity problems. Some studies have suggested that 800 IU vitamin E daily may reduce some of the mucocutaneous effects of systemic retinoids (34).

C. Arthralgias and Myalgias

Some patients experience muscle pain and myalgias with or without an elevation in creatine phosphokinase levels. In general, it is wise for patients to avoid excessive muscle exercising, particularly excessive weight lifting and contact sports as these forms of activity may increase such risks. Arthralgias occur in a small percentage of patients and disappear upon discontinuation of therapy.

D. Pseudotumor Cerebri

Acitretin and other systemic retinoids have been associated with cases of pseudotumor cerebri (benign intracranial hypertension). Such symptoms and signs include papilledema, severe headaches, nausea and vomiting, and visual disturbances. If pseudotumor cerebri is suspected, ophthalmological evaluation for papilledema should be conducted, and if present, the retinoid should be discontinued immediately. Oral retinoids should not be taken with tetracycline or tetracycline derivatives due to increased risk of pseudotumor cerebri.

E. Ophthalmological Effects

Ocular toxicity does not appear to be a major problem with acitretin, although rare cases of disturbances of color vision have been recorded. Most of the ocular symptoms have been mucocutaneous: dry eyes, irritation of eyes, and loss of brow and lashes. Other side effects such as blurred vision, cataracts, decreased night vision, and diplopia are much less common.

F. Skeletal Toxicity

There is some concern that long-term high-dosage acitretin therapy is associated changes that resemble diffuse idiopathic skeletal hyperostosis (DISH), including anterior spinal ligamentous calcification and the formation of osteophytes and bony bridges. Disk space narrowing is not evident in DISH. There appears to be a cumulative threshold dose of 25–30 g etretinate below which skeletal toxicity is not seen radiographically.

G. Psychiatric Effects

There are no recorded incidents of suicide or depression linked to patients receiving systemic retinoid therapy for the treatment of psoriasis. There is clearly a background of depression with some psoriasis patients but this has not been noted to be aggravated by acitretin (Lowe NJ, unpublished observations).

H. Hyperlipidemia

Hyperlipidemia occurs in 25–50% of patients. Occasionally, severe levels reaching five to eight times the normal value occur, but usually levels are increased two to three times over normal. The incidence of pancreatitis or eruptive xanthomas with increased triglyceride levels is uncommon. In addition, levels of high-density lipoproteins (HDL) decrease with oral retinoid treatment. These abnormal levels are reversible upon cessation of therapy. Patients with an increased tendency to hypertriglycedemia include those with diabetes mellitus, obesity, increased alcohol intake, or a familial history of these conditions. There are number of ways to manage hyperlipidemia including low-fat diets, reduced alcohol intake, physical activity, the use of polyunsaturated fish-oil supplements, and lipid-lowering drugs.

I. Hepatotoxicity

All the systemic retinoids have the potential for liver toxicity. Elevations of the transaminases AST (serum glutamic exaloacetic transaminase [SGOT]), ALT (serum glutamic pyruvic transaminase [SGPT]), GGT (GGTP), along with lactic dehydrogenase (LDH) and alkaline phosphatase have occurred in 33% of patients treated with acitretin. During the clinical trials in the United States for acitretin, 3.8% of patients had sufficient elevation of liver function tests that they were discontinued from further treatment. If hepatotoxicity is suspected with acitretin, the drug should be discontinued and a liver work-up should be conducted.

VIII. FOLLOW-UP

Blood investigations should include a full blood count, a complete metabolic panel including measurement of liver enzymes, renal function tests, creatine phosphokinase, and a lipid panel including triglycerides, cholesterol, and HDL. Of course in all women of childbearing age, a monthly pregnancy test must be conducted. These investigations should be carried out initially every 2 weeks while patients are receiving clearance doses, reducing to monthly or 2-monthly assessments depending on the maintenance dose required. There is presently no requirement for liver biopsy.

IX. GUIDELINES FOR USE

1. Acitretin can be prescribed for male patients or postmenopausal female patients. It is up to the clinician's discretion to prescribe acitretin in women of childbearing age, keeping in mind the strict guidelines associated with acitretin's teratogenicity. If there is any suggestion that a woman desires to become pregnant, or suspicion that adequate birth control methods will not be practiced, or abstinence from alcohol cannot be avoided, acitretin should not be prescribed for that woman.

2. Careful pretreatment screening should be carried out to exclude the possibility of hyperlipidemia and hepatotoxicity. Risk factors for hyperlipidemia (diabetes mellitus, obesity) should be looked for and a history of alcohol use and hepatitis sought in every patient.

3. Retinoids should be considered as monotherapy in generalized pustular psoriasis.

4. Combination therapy of acitretin with PUVA or UVB is advised in patients with severe plaque psoriasis and localized palmoplantar psoriasis, including local pustular psoriasis of the palms and soles.

5. Combination therapy of acitretin with hydrea may be beneficial in some patients with plaque or pustular psoriasis. In addition, combination therapy with the retinoids and the new immunomodulatory biological agents may play pivotal roles in the future treatment of psoriasis.

6. New retinoids such as oral tazarotene seems to have a good safety profile. Longer-term studies and combination studies with this drug are eagerly awaited.

REFERENCES

1. Moy RL, Kingston TP, Lowe NJ. Isotretinoin vs etretinate therapy in generalized pustular and chronic psoriasis. Arch Dermatol 1985;121:1297–301.
2. Roenigk RK, Gibstine C, Roenigk HH Jr. Oral isotretinoin followed by psoralens and ultraviolet A or ultraviolet B for psoriasis. J Am Acad Dermatol. 1985;13:153–155.

3. Honigsmann H, Wolff K. lsotretinoin-PUVA for psoriasis. Lancet. 1983;1: 236.
4. Lowe MN, Plosker GL. Bexarotene. Am J Clin Dermatol. 2000;1:245–50.
5. Wiegand UW, Chou RC. Pharmacokinetics of acitretin and etretinate. J Am Acad Dermatol. 1998;39:S25–33.
6. Jensen BK, Chaws CL, Huselton CA. Clinical evidence that acitretin is esterified to etretinate when administered with ethanol [Abstract]. FASEB J 1992;6:A1570
7. Larsen FG, Jakobsen P, Knudsen J, Weismann K, Kragballe K, Nielsen-Kudsk F. Conversion of acitretin to etretinate in psoriatic patients is influenced by ethanol. J Invest Dermatol 1993;100:623–7.
8. McNamara PJ, Jewell RC, Jensen BK, Brindley CJ. Food increases the bioavailability of acitretin. J Clin Pharmacol 1988;28:1051–5.
9. Chambon P. The retinoid signaling pathway: molecular and genetic analysis. Semin Cell Biol 1994;5:115–25.
10. Saurat JH. Retinoids and psoriasis: novel issues in retinoid pharmacology and implications for psoriasis treatment. J Am Acad Dermatol. 1999;41:S2–6.
11. Ling MR. Acitretin: optimal dosing strategies. J Am Acad Dermatol. 1999;41: S13–7.
12. Lowe NJ, Lazarus V, Matt L. Systemic retinoid therapy for psoriasis. J Am Acad Dermatol. 1988;19:186–91.
13. Goldfarb MT, Ellis CN, Gupta AK, Tincoff T, Hamilton TA, Voorhees JJ. Acitretin improves psoriasis in a dose-dependent fashion. J Am Acad Dermatol 1988;18 (suppl 4, pt 1):655–62.
14. Olsen EA, Weed WW, Meyer CJ, Cobo LM. A double-blind, placebo-controlled trial of acitretin for the treatment of psoriasis. J Am Acad Dermatol 1989;21(suppl 4, pt 1):681–6.
15. Torok L, Kadar L, Geiger JM. Acitretin treatment of severe psoriasis. Acta Dermatol Venereol Suppl (Stockh) 1989;146:104–6.
16. Murray HE, Anhalt AW, Lessard R, et al. A 12-month treatment of severe psoriasis with acitretin: results of a Canadian open multicenter trial. J Am Acad Dermatol 1991;24:598–602.
17. Geiger JM Czarnetzki BM. Acitretin (Ro 10-1670, etretin): overall evaluation of clinical studies. Dermatologica 1988;176:182–90.
18. Lassus A, Geiger JM, Nyblom M, Virrankoski T, Kaartamaa M, Ingervo L. Treatment of severe psoriasis with etretin (Ro 10-1670). Br J Dermatol 1987; 117:333–41.
19. Hoffman TE, Watson W. Methotrexate toxicity in the treatment of generalized pustular psoriasis. Cutis. 1978;21:68–71.
20. Tanew A, Guggenbichler A, Hönigsmann H, Geiger JM, Fritsch P. Photo-chemotherapy for severe psoriasis without or in combination with acitretin: a randomized, double-blind comparison study. J Am Acad Dermatol 1991; 25:682–4.
21. Saurat J-H, Geiger J-M, Amblard P, Beani J-C, Boulanger A, Claudy A, et al. Randomized double-blind multicenter study comparing acitretin–PUVA,

etretinate–PUVA, and placebo–PUVA in the treatment of severe psoriasis. Dermatologica 1988;177:218–24.

22. Laurahanta J, Geiger J-M. A double-blind comparison of acitretin and etretinate in combination with bath PUVA in the treatment of extensive psoriasis. Br J Dermatol 1989;121:107–12.

23. Muchenberger S, Schoff E, Simon JC. The combination of oral acitretin and bath PUVA for the treatment of severe psoriasis. Br J Dermatol 1997;137:587–9.

24. Rosén K, Mobacken H, Swanbeck G. PUVA, etretinate, and PUVA-etretinate therapy for pustulosis palmoplantaris: a placebo-controlled comparative trial. Arch Dermatol 1987;123:885–9.

25. Parker S, Coburn P, Lawrence C, Marks J, Shuster S. A randomized double-blind comparison of PUVA-etretinate and PUVA-placebo in the treatment of chronic plaque psoriasis. Br J Dermatol 1984;110:215–20.

26. Lawrence CM, Marks J, Parkers S, Shuster S. A comparison of PUVA–etretinate and PUVA–placebo for palmoplantar pustular psoriasis. Br J Dermatol 1984;110:221–6.

27. Ruzicka T, Sommerburg C, Braun-Falco O, Koster W, Lengen W, Lensing W, et al. Efficiency of acitretin in combination with UV-B in the treatment of severe psoriasis. Arch Dermatol 1990;126:482–6.

28. Lowe N, Prystowsky JH, Bourget T, Edelstein J, Nychay S, Armstrong R. Acitretin plus UVB therapy for psoriasis: comparisons with placebo plus UVB and acitretin alone. J Am Acad Dermatol 1991;24:591–4.

29. Iest J, Boer J. Combined treatment of psoriasis with acitretin and UVB phototherapy compared with acitretin alone and UVB alone. Br J Dermatol 1989;120:665–70.

30. Scott LJ, Dunn CJ, Goa KL. Calcipotriol ointment. A review of its use in the management of psoriasis. Am J Clin Dermatol. 2001;2:95–120.

31. Ashcroft DM, Li Wan Po A, Williams HC, Griffiths CE. Combination regimens of topical calcipotriene in chronic plaque psoriasis: systematic review of efficacy and tolerability. Arch Dermatol. 2000;136:1536–43.

32. Iyer S, Yamauchi P, Lowe NJ. Etanercept for severe psoriasis and psoriatic arthritis: observations on combination therapy. Br J Dermatol. 2002;146:118–21.

33. Lowe NJ, David M. New retinoids for dermatologic diseases. Uses and toxicity. Dermatol Clin. 1988;6:539–52.

34. Lebwohl M, Ali S. Treatment of psoriasis. Part 2. Systemic therapies. J Am Acad Dermatol. 2001;45:649–61.

7

Cyclosporine in the Treatment of Severe Psoriasis

Charles N. Ellis* and Madhu Battu
University of Michigan Medical School, Ann Arbor, Michigan, U.S.A.

I. INTRODUCTION

Since the cause of psoriasis is still unknown, no single therapy directed at a specific causative factor has been developed. Indeed, it is unlikely that there is a single biochemical abnormality in psoriasis that could be corrected. Nevertheless, cyclosporine has had a major impact on psoriasis therapy and research. Besides being extremely effective itself (1–24) in the treatment of psoriasis, cyclosporine has inspired the search for other compounds that act in the same way. In addition, the efficacy of cyclosporine in the treatment of psoriasis (Fig. 1) has caused a substantial proportion of psoriasis research to shift from investigations into keratinocyte abnormalities to studies of the immune system (25).

II. PHARMACOLOGY

A. Mechanism of Action

Cyclosporine prevents the activation of T cells, which is important in the immune system-induced propagation of psoriasis. Cyclosporine, by inhibiting the intracellular enzyme calcineurin, prevents the transcription of the

---

* Dr. Ellis has served as a principal investigator and consultant for Novartis Pharmaceuticals Corporation.

A   B

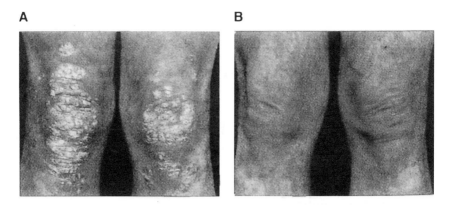

Figure 1   A typical optimal response to cyclosporine therapy for psoriasis. (A) Pre-therapy. (B) After 8 weeks of cyclosporine, 3 mg/kg/day. (Refer to the color insert.)

interleukin-2 (IL-2) gene. Therefore, the IL-2 cytokine is not released into the skin. Because IL-2 is a major factor in the activation and proliferation of other T cells, T-cell-mediated immune activity is inhibited. Thus, cyclosporine reduces a specific part of inflammation in the skin thought to be involved in the maintenance of psoriasis. This is the same mechanism by which cyclosporine prevents the immune system from rejecting transplanted organs.

Inhibiting IL-2 production reduces the release of other T-cell cytokines including interferon-γ (IFN-γ). Thus, cellular immune reactivity is dampened and the driving factors of psoriasis may be reduced. The T cell has secondary effects on a number of other cells in the immune cascade; in addition, cyclosporine may directly affect antigen presentation, mast cells, and possibly even keratinocyte activity.

Various molecules expressed on the surface of cells are important in the regulation of the immune process. Some of these molecules (such as intercellular adhesion molecule-1 [ICAM-1]) affect adhesion of cells to each other. Cyclosporine reduces the production of cytokines (particularly IFN-γ) that cause adhesion molecules to be expressed by various cells. Thus, cyclosporine prevents the egress of various inflammatory cells from the vascular system by reducing adhesion molecules on the vessel surface. Furthermore, reduction of adhesion molecules in the skin means that the inflammatory cells that traverse the area are less likely to stay in the skin and be activated. For a more detailed discussion, see the article by Wong et al. (25).

B. Metabolism

Cyclosporine is primarily eliminated by the liver and the parent compound has a terminal half-life of approximately 20 h (26). Many of the metabolites of cyclosporine circulate in the blood, and some of them have immuno-suppressive activity.

III. CLINICAL USE IN PSORIASIS

A. Patient Selection

1. Typical Patient

Cyclosporine therapy should be limited to the treatment of patients with moderately severe to severe psoriasis. This encompasses patients who have substantial portions of their body surface area affected (at least 20%, but likely in practice greater than 30%) and patients who are disabled by psoriasis. Current data suggest that cyclosporine is effective for all types of psoriasis (10, 27–31). Therefore, it should be considered for appropriate patients with erythrodermic and pustular psoriasis. The drug has also been shown to improve the condition of patients with psoriatic arthritis (32).

The main reason for restricting cyclosporine from systemic use in mild psoriasis is its side effects (discussed below). If, in future, these side effects can be overcome by some method, cyclosporine might be used in the treatment of milder forms of psoriasis as well.

Because cyclosporine is recommended for short-term use (see sections on Dosage and Duration of Use below), it is appropriate for patients who, for whatever reason, are not able to continue their previous therapy, either temporarily or permanently. For example, a patient may have changes in liver histology that mandate stopping methotrexate therapy. Because cyclo-sporine is not known to cause liver fibrosis or to exacerbate methotrexate-induced liver damage, such a patient could be transferred to cyclosporine treatment in the absence of severe hepatic function impairment. Weinstein has suggested rotational therapy as a way of reducing toxicities from sys-temic agents used in the therapy of psoriasis (see Chapter 1). Cyclosporine could be used as one of many short-term treatments in rotation to try to reduce the serious side effects that might accumulate during prolonged use of any one of the treatments (see also section on Comparison with Other Therapies, below).

2. Flaring Psoriasis

Cyclosporine may also be useful for patients who have a sudden, severe flare of psoriasis. With dosages in the top range of 5 mg/kg/day, cyclo-sporine usually has a rapid onset of action that may be desirable for treat-ing patients with acute flaring of psoriasis. Cyclosporine therapy may also help patients whose disease is unresponsive to other treatments. In many cases, cyclosporine may allow a patient to achieve sufficient clearing such that a previously ineffective therapy may become more useful in maintaining the remission.

3. Short-Term Use

Another use for cyclosporine may be in patients who are experiencing major life events. Substantial clearing of psoriasis for a wedding or similar major event may be an important use of cyclosporine when used with discretion by dermatologists. However, careful explanation is required to ensure that the patient does not later demand long-term cyclosporine therapy. Most dermatologists are familiar with this quandary, which also occurs with the use of systemic corticosteroids for the treatment of various dermatoses.

4. Prepare the Patient

Careful explanation to the patient of the short-term nature of cyclosporine therapy is required. Patients and their physicians should expect to use cyclosporine until the psoriasis is nearly cleared or cleared, and shortly thereafter begin to taper the dosage while an alternative therapy is instituted. Normally, this process takes about 6 months and should not exceed approximately 1 year. Patients who are unlikely to accept the eventual discontinuation of the drug may represent poor candidates for therapy.

B. Contraindications

1. General Advice

Because cyclosporine can produce nephrotoxicity, patients who take it should have adequate renal function and should not be taking other drugs concurrently that reduce kidney activity, such as nonsteroidal anti-inflammatory agents. Cyclosporine may increase serum uric acid levels, resulting in difficulty for patients with gout. Cyclosporine is an immunosuppressive. Therefore, patients should not receive cyclosporine if they have substantial, active infections; known cancers, or a history of lymphoma or related nonsolid malignancies; or if they would be harmed by being immunosuppressed for any other reason. Furthermore, patients who routinely use immune-stimulating drugs or products, such as echinacea or goldenseal—and who are unwilling to stop use of such agents—would not be considered good candidates for cyclosporine therapy.

Patients with high blood pressure, migraines, or other vascular-related medical problems (e.g., strokes) have relative contraindications to cyclosporine use. Because cyclosporine causes vasoconstriction, these problems may be exacerbated. Hypertension, whether pre-existing or induced by cyclosporine therapy, should be controlled; patients with hypertension may be at increased risk for nephrotoxicity from cyclosporine.

Elderly patients require special consideration. Renal function declines with age and elderly patients are more likely to have some of the problems listed in the previous paragraphs. Therefore, the risk-to-benefit ratio must be considered in treating elderly patients.

Cyclosporine would be contraindicated in patients previously proved to have a hypersensitivity to any of the components of the medication, although this is extremely rare. If a patient has a pre-existing condition that could be made worse by the known side effects of cyclosporine, such relative contra-indications must be considered. These are discussed in more detail in the sections on Patient Selection and Side Effects.

2. Pregnancy

As with other medications, cyclosporine should not be given to pregnant women unless clearly necessary. However, it is reassuring that in over 100 pregnancies in women receiving cyclosporine (most of whom took the drug throughout the entire pregnancy because they were transplant recipients), the only consistent findings were premature birth at 28–36 weeks and low birth-weight even after taking into consideration the shortened gestation (26). The drug is not known to be mutagenic or teratogenic when it is administered at the appropriate dosage; it was only shown to be teratogenic in rodents at dosages five time the normally administered dosage (26).

Patients taking cyclosporine should not nurse because the drug is excreted in breast milk. Cyclosporine has been used in infants and children for nondermatological indications without any unexpected side effects (26).

Patients who are given cyclosporine should be available for follow-up as discussed below. Table 1 summarizes contraindications to cyclosporine therapy for psoriasis.

C. Drug Interactions

Because many patients use other drugs or substances at any given time, drug interactions need to be considered to evaluate for possible contraindications in the administration of cyclosporine.

Cyclosporine is metabolized in the gut and liver by CYP3A4 (formerly called cytochrome P-450IIIA4) enzymes, which also metabolize numerous other drugs (33). (See Table 2 for specific examples that utilize this system.) Any drug or substance that also utilizes CYP3A4 enzymes may change the bioavailability of cyclosporine. Some agents inhibit the CYP3A4 enzymes, causing higher cyclosporine blood levels, while the reverse is true for other

Table 1 Contraindications to Cyclosporine Therapy for Psoriasis

Strong contraindications
  Uncontrolled hypertension
  Renal disease
  Infections, including zoster
  Sensitivity to components of the medication
  Pregnancy, nursing
  Cancer (or history of cancer especially lymphoma)[a]
  Migraines, strokes, other major vascular-related problems (especially in the central
    nervous system or critical organs, e.g., cardiac angina)
  Patients requiring vaccinations during therapy
  Patient unavailable for regular follow-up
  Active infection

Relative contraindictions
  Patient who is unlikely to agree to the intermittent use of the drug
  Patient with treated hypertension
  Gout
  Patients taking nephrotoxic drugs (see Table 2)
  Elderly patients
  Drug interactions (see Table 2)
  Significant hepatic disease
  Gingivitis or excessive dental plaque
  Immunodeficiency of any cause, including due to other psoriasis therapy

[a] Usually treated basal cell carcinomas do not represent contraindications.

agents (33). Therefore, patients should be instructed to report all medications taken over the course of cyclosporine therapy, so that physicians can address any potential interactions.

Patients using cyclosporine therapy should avoid drugs that cause renal damage. Because immunosuppression beyond that caused by cyclosporine is undesirable, patients should not be receiving other immunosuppressive agents unless the combination is specifically designed to reduce the side effects of both agents without causing excessive immunosuppression. Immune stimulants might contravene the desired effects of cyclosporine.

D. Dosage

1. Dosage Forms

Novartis Pharmaceuticals Corp. produces two forms of cyclosporine—Sandimmune (cyclosporine USP) and Neoral (cyclosporine USP modified)—both of which are available in 25 mg or 100 mg soft gelatin capsules,

Table 2   Selected Interactions of Other Medications with Cyclosporine

Medications or dietary agents that inhibit hepatic CYP3A4 activity and may increase the blood concentration of cyclosporine
Erythromycin, clarithromycin, cephalosporins, doxycycline
Quinupristin/dalfopristin
Ketoconazole, fluconazole, itraconazole
Oral contraceptives
Cimetidine
Diltiazem, nicardipine, verapamil
Danazol
Androgenic steroids
Methylprednisolone
Allopurinol
Bromocriptine
Metoclopromide
Cochicine
Amiodarone
Disulfiram or acute alcohol use
Norfloxacin, ciprofloxacin
Valproic acid
Low-sedating antihistamines (?)
Grapefruit and grapefruit juice
HIV protease inhibitors (e.g., indinavir, nelfinavir, ritonavir, saquinavir)

Medications that cause potential synergistic nephrotoxicity
Nonsteroidal anti-inflammatory drugs: azapropazon, diclofenac, naproxen,
   sulindac
Colchicine
Diuretics
Gentamycin, tobramycin, vancomycin
Cimetidine, ranitidine
Aminoglycosides
Melphalan
Amphotericin B
Ketoconazole
Trimethoprim–sulfamethoxazole
Tacrolimus

Medications or dietary agents that increase the risk of hyperkalemia
Nonsteroidal anti-inflammatory agents, especially indomethacin
Certain antihypertensives
   Potassium-sparing diuretics
   Angiotensin-converting inhibitors
   Beta-adrenergic blockers
Digitalis

(*continued on next page*)

Table 2 (continued)

Heparin
Potassium-containing products
  Salt substitutes
  Potassium in penicillins
  Potassium iodides
  Certain foods and food supplements

Drugs that increase or decrease immunosuppression
Various

Other drug interactions with cyclosporine
Digitalis levels elevated (risk: digitalis toxicity)
Lovastatin levels elevated (risk: rhabdomyolysis)
Vaccines (if substantial immunosuppression exists, could reduce efficacy of
  vaccine or the patient receiving or exposed to persons receiving live vaccines
  could be infected)

*Medications or dietary agents that induce hepatic CYP3A4 activity and may
decrease the blood concentration of cyclosporine*[a]
Griseofulvin
Nafcillin
Carbamazepine
Chronic alcohol use
Octreotide
Orlistat
Phenobarbital
Phenytoin
Pioglitazone, rosiglitazone
Rifampin
St. John's wort
Ticlopidine

[a] These agents are of less medical concern in the treatment of psoriasis than the others in this table because the risk of cyclosporine toxicity is reduced; however, the psoriasis may not respond as well.

or in 50 ml bottles of an oral solution containing 100 mg cyclosporine per ml. The solution requires the patient to follow specific instructions for mixing with a beverage (26).

Generic versions of cyclosporine USP modified are available. Although generics meet Food and Drug Administration (FDA) tests for bioavailability equivalent to the reference drug Neoral, some uncertainty exists as to whether the formulations are interchangeable in practice. While variations in bioavailability are more critical in the treatment of transplant rejection, patients with psoriasis should be instructed to notify their physicians if they receive different capsules than usual from their pharmacists. In such cases, changes in clinical or laboratory results may be related to drug absorption.

Oral cyclosporine should be divided into two doses daily, which is thought to reduce the side effect profile. Whether dividing the dose so that the drug is taken three or four times a day would provide any additional benefit is unknown. Cyclosporine is erratically absorbed even within the same patient over time. However, Neoral has been shown to yield more consistent absorption within a single person and in the population at large than Sandimmune. Furthermore, Neoral has a 10–54% greater bioavailability than Sandimmune (34–38). Thus, physicians may need to adjust the dosage of drug if converting among Neoral, its generic versions, or Sandimmune. Typically, the patient may start on the initial dose and adjustments made if indicated by clinical changes or abnormal laboratory results.

In general, patients' responses to cyclosporine represent a combination of the dosage and time on therapy. For example, in our study of Sandimmune about two-thirds of the patients receiving 5 mg/kg/day were clear or nearly clear of psoriasis after 2 months of therapy (19). However, only about one-third of the patients receiving 3 mg/kg/day had achieved that response in the same period. Longer periods of treatment tend to achieve continued clearing in many patients.

2. Dosage Regimens

The recommended starting dosage for cyclosporine USP modified is 2.5 mg/kg/day. Table 3 provides a conversion chart to determine the dosage based on the patient's weight. Patients' clinical responses at approximately monthly intervals will suggest how to modify the dosage. If their condition has improved, the dosage may be held constant and reassessed in another month. If the response has been clearly insufficient, the dosage may be increased by 0.5–1 mg/kg to the maximum dose. In the United States, the labeled maximum dosage is 4 mg/kg/day for Neoral. However, many authorities recommend a maximum dosage of 5 mg/kg/day for Neoral; with proper monitoring, this may help more patients achieve the desired results without adverse effects. Even higher dosages may result in faster clearing, but the risk of side effects increases. Although Sandimmune is not marketed for psoriasis in the United States, the recommended maximum dosage is 5 mg/kg/day.

If the patient shows no improvement after receiving 4–5 mg/kg/day (or the patient's own highest tolerated dosage if lower) for 3–4 months, cyclosporine should be stopped by tapering off over the next month. Such a period

Table 3 Total Cyclosporine Dosage (mg/day) Based on Patient Weight and Daily Dose[a]

Weight		Dosage								
lbs	kg	1	1.5	2	2.5	3	3.5	4	4.5	5
80	36	36	54	73	91	109	127	145	163	181
90	41	41	61	82	102	123	143	163	184	204
100	45	45	68	91	113	136	159	181	204	227
110	50	50	75	100	125	150	175	200	225	250
120	54	54	82	109	136	163	191	218	245	272
130	59	59	88	118	147	177	206	236	265	295
140	64	64	95	127	159	191	222	254	286	318
150	68	68	102	136	170	204	238	272	306	340
160	73	73	109	145	181	218	254	290	327	363
170	77	77	116	154	193	231	270	309	347	386
180	82	82	123	163	204	245	286	327	368	408
190	86	86	129	172	216	259	302	345	388	431
200	91	91	136	181	227	272	318	363	408	454
210	95	95	143	191	238	286	333	381	429	476
220	100	100	150	200	250	300	350	400	450	500
230	104	104	157	209	261	313	365	417	470	522
240	109	109	163	218	272	327	381	436	490	544
250	113	113	170	227	284	340	397	454	510	567
260	118	118	177	236	295	354	413	472	531	590
270	123	123	184	245	306	368	429	490	551	613
280	127	127	191	254	318	381	445	508	572	635
290	132	132	197	263	329	395	461	526	592	658
300	136	136	204	272	340	408	476	544	613	681

[a] Cyclosporine is available in 25 and 100 mg capsules. For dosages over 75 mg/day, I recommend rounding up or down to the nearest 100 mg.

of maximal dosing should be sufficient to determine that the patient will not be successfully treated with cyclosporine and there is little point in continuing. The recommended maximum dosage should not be exceeded unless there is documented poor absorption of the drug (39).

In our experience, most patients require 3–4 mg/kg/day of Neoral to achieve and maintain a desired clearing. Once near-clearing is achieved, the daily dosage may be reduced by 0.5 mg/kg/day every month until recurrence becomes apparent. For most patients, 2.5–3.0 mg/kg/day is an effective dosage in the maintenance period (40–42). In a fashion similar to methotrexate usage, it is reasonable to adjust the dosage so that the patient maintains a small amount of psoriasis; if the psoriasis were completely cleared, the patient might be receiving more cyclosporine than necessary. However, the concept of maintaining patients with small amounts of psoriasis is not easily accomplished with cyclosporine. First, initial therapy with cyclosporine may clear the patient's disease completely. Second, as the dosage is tapered, patients often reach a point where psoriasis begins to recur and continues to progress; a dosage often cannot be found that maintains minimum psoriasis. Usually the dosage will have to be increased to the last previously effective one.

An alternative administration scheme begins at 1 mg/kg/day. The dosage is increased every month or two by 0.5–1 mg/kg/day until sufficient clearing or the maximum dosage is achieved. Such a regimen may result in lower total exposure to cyclosporine during a treatment period, but the patient is likely to have more psoriasis during the earlier stages of therapy. The dosage schemes have not been compared directly (7, 8, 19). Thus, they cannot be compared easily for relative efficacy, side effects, and total dose administered.

In the case of persistent and intolerable side effects, the dosage should be decreased by 1 mg/kg. If the side effects persist, further dosage reduction is required. Throughout maintenance administration, side effects should be judged reasonable and therapeutic response adequate or cyclosporine should be discontinued.

E. Duration of Usage

Cyclosporine is recommended as an intermittent therapy for psoriasis; the US labeling recommends that treatment courses not exceed 1 year. Most studies suggest that effective results can be achieved with a short-term course of cyclosporine that lasts from 6 months to no more than 1 year (34, 40, 43, 44). If a patient has been on therapy for one year, it is time to taper off cyclosporine and begin a different treatment. Cyclosporine may then be used again later. Continuous use over many years should be avoided due to the long-term side effects. In a few select cases, patients have been able to extend therapy for over 5 years, but this requires vigilant monitoring because of the increasing risk of side effects (45–49). For patients unwilling to comply with such stringent measures, short-term cyclosporine therapy or an alternative long-term therapy should be pursued.

Cyclosporine should be considered a switch for psoriasis. When cyclosporine is administered, the disease is turned off. When cyclosporine is stopped, the disease will recur; the drug does not permanently alter the natural course of the disease (50). Breakthrough of psoriasis while the patient is receiving an adequate dosage of cyclosporine rarely occurs. After a period of approximately 6 months, tapering of cyclosporine may begin and if necessary an alternative treatment begun. Because of the natural course of psoriasis in patients, some will be in remission and may not require additional therapy for varying lengths of time (43). Others will require a direct transition to another treatment. It is hoped that patients whose psoriasis begins to recur after cyclosporine treatment is discontinued will be able to control their limited disease with alternative therapies.

F. Recurrence of Psoriasis After Cyclosporine Treatment

Predictions may be made about the rate of recurrence of psoriasis after cyclosporine administration is stopped. In our experience, recurrence reflects the severity and intensity of the patient's psoriasis when untreated. Thus, patients with stable, chronic plaque psoriasis are likely to have a gradual recurrence, while patients with brittle, highly inflammatory, and active psoriasis should expect a quicker recurrence. Recurrence of psoriasis to an extent beyond that of the patient's pretherapy condition is unusual.

Psoriasis therapies may be categorized into those that are remittive and those that are not; usually this is a function of whether the therapy depletes the pathogenic T cells or merely suppresses them. Cyclosporine is not remittive; rather, it turns the switch off or on. However, the relapse rate after stopping cyclosporine is probably not significantly different from that when other major nonremittive therapies are discontinued in patients with moderate to severe psoriasis (50).

G. Side Effects of Cyclosporine

1. Miscellaneous Side Effects

Side effects of cyclosporine are usually dose-dependent (see Table 4) (19). Cyclosporine is remarkably well tolerated when used in low dosages for the treatment of dermatological disease. If they occur, cyclosporine-induced headaches, tremors, paresthesias, nausea, and malaise tend to resolve without treatment after several weeks of therapy. Hypertrichosis is of minimal concern to most patients; however, women may find it more troublesome than men. Gingival hyperplasia may be minimized by careful dental hygiene. Hyperbilirubinemia is typically asymptomatic and does not require dosage reduction. Hyperuricemia and gout are not usually problems in nontransplant patients.

Hyperlipidemia and hypertension require intervention, which should begin with dietary changes and an increase in physical activity. If these measures are unsuccessful, pharmacological intervention may be necessary

Table 4 Side Effects of Relatively Common
Frequency when Cyclosporine Is Used in
Dermatologic Dosages

Clinical symptoms
Early onset, tends to resolve during therapy
    Malaise, fatigue
    Nausea
    Headaches
    Achiness in muscles and joints
    Hand tremor
    Paresthesias
    Distal sensitivity to hot or cold
Onset at any time, persists during therapy
    Hypertrichosis
    Gingival hyperplasia[a]
Clinical signs
Onset at any time
    Hypertension[b]
Laboratory changes
Increased
    Creatinine[c]
    Urea nitrogen
    Lipids[b]
    Bilirubin[d]
    Uric acid
    Potassium[c]
Decreased
    Magnesium[e]
    Glomerular filtration rate[c]

Side effects in **bold** represent the most important
ones (including nephrotoxicity).
[a] May improve with increased dental hygiene.
[b] May require cyclosporine dosage adjustment or
addition of specific therapy.
[c] May require cyclosporine dosage adjustment.
[d] Usually asymptomatic and does not require
intervention.
[e] May require replacement therapy.

if cyclosporine dosage reduction is not feasible. Isradipine or nifedipine
therapy usually returns blood pressure to normal levels (51) and these
agents are the first choice for antihypertensive treatment in patients taking
cyclosporine. Hyperkalemia may respond to reduced potassium in the diet
or a thiazide diuretic. Low serum magnesium levels may require replacement therapy.

2. Renal Toxicities

Cyclosporine-induced renal toxicity remains a major concern (52–60). Indeed, serum creatinine levels may increase within a few weeks of beginning cyclosporine as a result of its early, reversible, vasoconstrictive effect (19). As a general rule, renal effects can be minimized by low-dosage cyclosporine, and by adjusting the dosage if the serum creatinine rises 25–30% above baseline (61). Fish oil supplements (62) or amlodipine (63, 64) may be able to minimize renal toxicity. Measurements of glomerular filtration rate may be useful in following renal function in patients who have abnormal creatinine levels. Renal biopsies are unlikely to be needed in patients treated with intermittent dosing.

Nevertheless, there remains concern that cyclosporine could induce progressive renal failure in some patients. A number of considerations are implicit in this concern and few have been tested adequately in the population with psoriasis. In our experience and in the literature (65), no patients treated as described for less than 1 year have developed any renal dysfunction that has affected their normal daily lives. Although most of the patients received therapy for 6 months or less, some were treated for as long as 3 years. Nevertheless, histological changes in the kidney of tubular atrophy and interstitial fibrosis do occur after 1 year or more of treatment (61, 66, 67).

If we assume that a patient has normal kidney function prior to beginning cyclosporine therapy, one concern is to what degree his or her normal renal reserve is expended following cyclosporine treatment. If renal reserve is diminished, to what degree is this an issue? A full assessment of the impact of intermittent cyclosporine therapy on patients' kidneys over their lifetimes cannot be judged definitively at this time. It is known that everyone has reduced kidney function with aging; in addition, some people receive drugs or other agents that reduce or that cause kidney damage. How all these factors interact requires further study.

There is a point in renal damage that is irreversible and leads to a very slow but progressive decline of renal function. In the intermittent treatment of psoriasis with cyclosporine, it is expected that this point would not be reached. However, patients' kidney function must be monitored so that therapy may be stopped if laboratory tests exceed those recommended. This should prevent progressive declines in renal function.

3. Cancer and Infection Risk

The risk of lymphoma or other cancer as a direct result of cyclosporine therapy for psoriasis is low (39). Because cyclosporine is used at low, intermittent dosages in patients with psoriasis, and additional immunosuppression such as with systemic corticosteroids is not used simultaneously as it is in transplant patients, the risk of tumors is much lower than in graft recipients (39). However, if patients have received psoralen and ultraviolet A (PUVA) prior to cyclosporine therapy, there is an increased risk of squamous cell carcinoma of the skin equivalent to that associated with 200 PUVA treatments (68).

In one case, cyclosporine therapy was associated with the onset of cutaneous T-cell lymphoma (CTCL) that disappeared when the cyclosporine was stopped (69). Some patients who appear to develop CTCL during cyclosporine therapy are found in retrospect likely to have had the condition prior to beginning cyclosporine (70). Patients with atypical psoriasis or psoriasis that has been thought to be spongiotic dermatitis or eczema clinically or histologically in the past may actually have CTCL. Because cyclosporine may exacerbate CTCL, such patients should probably avoid cyclosporine.

Benign lymphocytic infiltrates have been reported during cyclosporine treatment of psoriasis (71). Increased infections (including warts, impetigo, and tineas) are not encountered, (19) perhaps because T-cell immunity is sufficient for these situations and non-T-cell immune responses are unaffected.

H. Monitoring

The most laboratory test is measurement of the serum creatinine (39). Before initiating therapy, it is imperative to establish a baseline creatinine level for each patient (see Table 5 for a suggested protocol). If creatinine levels ever exceed the baseline reading by 25–30%, the patient's cyclosporine dosage needs to be reduced.

Blood levels of cyclosporine are rarely useful, except to demonstrate poor absorption or noncompliance (72–74). In the rare person who fails to respond adequately to cyclosporine, a blood level may provide information that the patient is a nonresponder as opposed to not absorbing or taking the drug. At the dosage used in the treatment of psoriasis, it is extremely unlikely that a patient would achieve such a high blood level of cyclosporine that the dosage would be reduced on this account alone. Expected blood levels are lower than those desired in transplant patients, and therefore may be lower than the "normal" values given by the laboratory (72). Nevertheless in most patients the dosing is titrated by renal function or clinical response, and blood levels usually provide little helpful information.

I. Combination Therapy

Using topical drugs, such as anthralin, topical corticosteroids, or vitamin D analogs such as calcipotriene, concurrently with cyclosporine improves clearance rates, often at lower cyclosporine dosages (12, 75–77). In one study,

Table 5 Suggested Monitoring of Patients Taking Cyclosporine and Responses to Findings

---

Obtain at least two pretherapy measurements of serum creatinine to determine
  a baseline; the values should be within 20 percent or additional measures should
  be obtained
At baseline, after 2 and 4 weeks, and then monthly, obtain measurements of
  Blood pressure
  Serum
      Creatinine (for baseline, see above)
      Urea nitrogen
      Lipids (once stable, may be assessed less often)
      Bilirubin, liver function tests
      Uric acid
      Magnesium
      Electrolytes
  A review of any new medications
For hypertension; reduce cyclosporine dosage if possible or treat the high
  blood pressure.
Reduce the cyclosporine dosage if serum creatinine exceeds baseline by 25–30%.
Give replacement therapy if serum magnesium below normal range.
Although bilirubin usually increases, therapy is rarely warranted and dosage
  reduction usually not needed.
Other laboratory abnormalities should be addressed if significantly abnormal.
Outpatient creatinine clearance tests tend to be unreliable; creatinine clearance can
  be calculated from formulas based on the serum creatinine but this often adds
  little additional information. Glomerular filtration rates (GFRs) may be
  measured by qualified physicians, usually nephrologists; a rate significantly
  below expected for a patient would serve as a contraindication for cyclosporine
  therapy. However, there is no consensus that routine measurements of GFR are
  necessary when cyclosporine is used at dermatological dosages.

---

improvement rate was four times higher when patients used cyclosporine and calcipotriene ointment than cyclosporine and placebo; furthermore, clearance rates were achieved by using a dosage as low as 2.0 mg/kg/day of cyclosporine USP (78).

Because most systemic therapies for psoriasis would provide additive immunosuppression (e.g., methotrexate, phototherapy, or biological response modifiers such as alefacept), they appear to be inappropriate to use with cyclosporine. In most patients, cyclosporine is so effective that other therapies are not required unless they can be clearly shown to reduce side effects of both agents. However, in a few cases, coadministration of mycophenolate mofetil (MMF) with cyclosporine has helped clear psoriasis in patients unresponsive to cyclosporine alone (79). Combining methotrexate and cyclosporine allowed for lower dosages of each in the treatment of 19 patients with severe psoriasis (80); the combination may have significant risks, however.

Phototherapy has the risk of inducing skin cancers during the modest immunosuppression of cyclosporine. Furthermore, cyclosporine with PUVA was of less benefit than an oral retinoid with PUVA in one study (81).

While not a specific immunosuppressive therapy, oral retinoids often cause lipid elevations. Because cyclosporine does likewise, the two may be difficult to use together (82, 83), and such combination therapy did not provide substantial benefit (84). Nevertheless, acitretin is a useful follow-on therapy after cyclosporine.

J. Transitioning Off Cyclosporine

Moving a patient from cyclosporine therapy to another treatment can be difficult, in part because of patient satisfaction with cyclosporine. Patients taking cyclosporine tend to have more severe psoriasis and therefore are likely to demonstrate recurrences when cyclosporine is discontinued or shortly thereafter. In our experience, a taper of cyclosporine is easier to accomplish than stopping the therapy abruptly. Although some patients' disease can be controlled for a while with topical treatment alone, often a new systemic therapy must be instituted during the cyclosporine taper.

Perhaps the best choice for the new treatment is acitretin. Short-term overlapping therapy with acitretin is usually possible without significant side effects (65). Although there is some concern about transitioning from cyclosporine directly to irradiation with ultraviolet, acitretin can provide a buffer period before beginning ultraviolet and, if ultraviolet is later added to the acitretin, the retinoid theoretically may inhibit skin malignancies that might occur from any residual immunosuppression combined with ultraviolet.

Following cyclosporine with methotrexate or similar agents seems reasonable because of their different organ toxicities, as long as the overlap period is short. Sulfasalazine, were it to be effective in a higher percentage of patients, would also be a good choice. Biological agents that inhibit tumor necrosis factor might be useful, although experience is lacking at present. It is unclear whether therapies directed at activated T cells, such as alefacept, would be appropriate immediately after cyclosporine; there might not be enough activated T cells for such treatments to work. However, it is also possible that the T cells would be highly susceptible to the biological therapy when released from their inhibition by cyclosporine.

There is no definitive opinion as to when a patient who previously took cyclosporine may take it again. It seems reasonable to wait a year if possible between courses, particularly if the cyclosporine treatment course lasted near

Table 6 Authors' Opinion Comparing Various Systemic Therapies for Psoriasis with Regard to Selected Parameters

| | Efficiency | Patients' perspective on ease of use | Patient Appears Normal | Side effects | | | | | Overall quality |
				Liver toxicity	Kidney toxicity	Hyperlipidemia	Bone changes	Risk of serious side effect	
Cyclosporine	++++ Very high percentage of patients respond	++++ Oral medicine; blood tests	++++	+/– May reduce liver enzyme elevations in many patients	–––– Requires monitoring and intermittent dosing	– Often increased lipids, but rarely significant	? May cause reduced density after long use (unproved) (85,86)	–– Kidney (see text)	+++
Methotrexate	++++ High percentage of patients respond	++ Oral medicine; blood tests; liver biopsy	++++	––––	– If present, may lead to overdosing	0	0	–– Liver toxicity over time; acute methotrexate toxicity can be serious but clinically overlooked	+++
Acitretin	++ Often requires UV therapy as well	++++ Oral medicine; blood tests	+ Many muco-cutaneous side effects	–– Rare, idiosyncratic hepatitis	0	–––– May be cause for stopping therapy	–––– Long use frequently associated with hyper-ostosis	– Rare, idio-syncratic hepatitis or ascites	++

Sulfasalazine	+ 25% of patients have good results	++++ Oral medicine; blood tests	++++ Early-onset rash common, but such patients should stop therapy	--	0	0	- Agranulocytosis	+++ In the small percentage of patients who respond well
UVB Phototherapy	+++ Most patients achieve substantial clearing	++ Frequent treatments required	++ Deep tan; may be desirable to some	0	0	0	0	++
PUVA	+++ Most patients achieve substantial clearing	++ Oral medicine; blood tests; frequent treatments required	++ Deep tan; may be desirable to some; protective glasses required	- Psoralen adds slight risk over UV alone	0	0	0	++

Each + sign indicates a degree of advantage; each − sign indicates a degree of disadvantage. Under side effects, 0 indicates rare or not reported which is an advantage; ? indicates further information is needed.

Note: There is insufficient information at the time of this writing to comment on the biological therapies.

the recommended maximum of 1 year. The patient's serum creatinine level should be near its original baseline before resuming cyclosporine.

IV. COMPARING CYCLOSPORINE WITH OTHER THERAPIES

Cyclosporine USP modified costs at retail about $175 per mg/kg/day for 1 month for an average 70 kg patient; thus, drug costs alone for such a patient treated at 4 mg/kg/day would cost $700 per month. Depending on a patient's insurance, this may not be an issue for the patient. Of course, medication costs alone do not represent the full cost of therapy or time away from the patient's other activities. To compare with other treatments, one must consider all the costs (such as doctor visits, laboratory tests, value of time missed from school or work, etc.) as well as the agent's efficacy (Table 6).

From the patient's point of view, cyclosporine is one of the easiest, if not the easiest, systemic antipsoriatic therapy to take. At the dosages used in dermatology, the patient-recognized side effects are few and well tolerated, the treatment is convenient, and the efficacy is usually high and of quick onset. Routine renal biopsies and measurements of glomerular filtration rates are not required.

Oral retinoid treatment may be the most similar to cyclosporine with regard to administration and monitoring; however, retinoids are not as effective as a monotherapy and are often used in conjunction with phototherapy. Sulfasalazine is inexpensive and requires only modest routine monitoring. However, it is effective in only about one-quarter of the patients who begin treatment, and even among those patients sulfasalazine therapy rarely yields a thorough clearing of psoriasis (87). Thus, cyclosporine is much more likely to result in control of psoriasis.

Low-dosage systemic methotrexate is effective treatment for psoriasis. However, its monitoring requires liver biopsies while cyclosporine does not require any organ biopsies, which makes methotrexate therapy less convenient. We projected that using cyclosporine in rotation with methotrexate provides more years clear of psoriasis over 10 years at a modestly higher cost than methotrexate alone (88).

Because cyclosporine is given orally while phototherapy (UVB or PUVA) requires administration of ultraviolet radiation in the confines of a specific set up, the two treatment approaches cannot be compared easily. Although both can be expected to provide a thorough clearing, cyclosporine does so for a greater percentage of patients. However, phototherapy provides a longer remission.

The biological response modifiers, such as alefacept, etanercept, or infliximab, do not appear to provide thorough clearing in as high a percentage of patients as does cyclosporine. Convenience of subcutaneous or intramuscular injection is slightly less than for cyclosporine, and some of the newer treatments are given intravenously in a doctor's office or infusion center. However, in some patients remissions may be longer than with cyclosporine. The long-term side effect profile for the biological therapies remains to be determined. Biologicals may be able to be used more continuously than cyclosporine, which could be an advantage (89–91).

Systemically administered tacrolimus (Prograf) has also been used for psoriasis; it has the same mechanism of action: inhibition of calcineurin. In limited studies, it appears to be of comparable efficacy to and there is likely a similar side effect profile to systemic cyclosporine (92, 93). Sirolimus (formerly rapamycin, Rapamune) binds to the same intracellular binding-protein as tacrolimus, but does not inhibit calcineurin; sirolimus inhibits T-cell activation and proliferation through a different mechanism. Used as a monotherapy, sirolimus did not appear to be as effective as cyclosporine, although limited numbers of patients have been treated. Cases of cytokine release syndrome have been reported among patients with psoriasis taking sirolimus (94). Sirolimus and very-low-dosage cyclosporine have been used together to treat psoriasis (95).

No consistently effective formulation of topical cyclosporine has been developed; the drug does not penetrate well through skin. Although an intravenous formulation of Sandimmune exists and has been diluted and injected intralesionally directly into psoriatic plaques, the discomfort involved and the required three times per week injections for 1 month make this treatment relatively impractical (96–98). Topical tacrolimus (Protopic) and pimecrolimus (Elidel) do not have much benefit when applied to typical plaques of psoriasis, but may be useful for psoriasis on the face, genitals, axillae, or other areas of thin skin.

REFERENCES

1. Mueller W, Herrmann B. Cyclosporin A for psoriasis. N Engl J Med 1979; 301:555 [letter].
2. Ellis CN, Gorsulowsky DC, Hamilton TA, Billings JK, Brown MD, Headington JT, Cooper KD, Baadsgaard O, Duell E, Annesley TM, Turcotte J, Voorhees JJ. Cyclosporine improves psoriasis in a double-blind study. J Am Acad of Dermatol 1986;256:3110–3116.

3. Muller W, Graf U. Die behandlung der Psoriasis-Arthritis mit Cyclosporin A, einem neuen Immunosuppressivum. Schweiz Med Wochenschr 1981;111:408–413.
4. Harper JI, Keat ASC, Staughton RCD. Cyclosporine for psoriasis. Lancet 1984;2:981–982.
5. van Hooff JP, Leunissen KML, Staak WVD. Cyclosporin and psoriasis. Lancet 1985;1:335.
6. Marks J. Psoriasis. Br Med J 1986;293:509.
7. Griffiths CEM, Powles AV, Leonard JN, Fry L, Baker BS, Valdimarsson H. Clearance of psoriasis with low dose cyclosporin. Br Med J 1986;293:731–732.
8. Brookes DB. Clearance of psoriasis with low dose cyclosporin. Br Med J 1986;293:1098–1099.
9. van Joost T, Heule F, Stolz E, Beukers R. Short-term use of cyclosporin A in severe psoriasis. Br J Dermatol 1986;114:615–620.
10. Wentzell JM, Baughman RD, O'Connor GT, Bernier GM Jr. Cyclosporine in the treatment of psoriasis. Arch Dermatol 1987;123:163–165.
11. Picascia DD, Garden JM, Freinkel RK, Roenigk HH Jr. Treatment of resistant severe psoriasis with systemic cyclosporine. J Am Acad Dermatol 1987;17:408–414.
12. Griffiths CEM, Powles AV, Baker BS, Fry L, Valdimarsson H. Combination of cyclosporine A and topical corticosteroid in the treatment of psoriasis. Transplant Proc 1988;20:Suppl 4:50–52.
13. van Joost T, Bos JD, Heule F, Meinardi MMHM. Low-dose cyclosporin A in severe psoriasis: A double-blind study. Br J Dermatol 1988;118:183–190.
14. Meinardi MMHM, Bos JD. Cyclosporine maintenance therapy in psoriasis. Transplant Proc 1988;20:Suppl 4:42–49.
15. Finzi AF, Mozzanica N, Cattaneo A, Chiappino G, Pigatto PD. Effectiveness of cyclosporine treatment in severe psoriasis: a clinical and immunologic study. J Am Acad Dermatol 1989;21:91–97.
16. Heule F, Bousema MT, Laeijendecker R, van Joost T. Three long-term regimens with cyclosporin for psoriasis vulgaris. Acta Derm Venereol Suppl (Stockh) 1989;146:171–175.
17. Meinardi MMHM, de Rie MA, Bos JD. Oral cyclosporin A in the treatment of psoriasis: an overview of studies performed in the Netherlands. Br J Dermatol 1990;122:Suppl 36:27–31.
18. Timonen P, Friend D, Abeywickrama K, Laburte C, von Graffenried B, Feutren G. Efficacy of low-dose cyclosporin A in psoriasis: results of dose-finding studies. Br J Dermatol 1990;122:Suppl 36:33–39.
19. Ellis CN, Fradin MS, Messana JM, Brown MD, Siegel MT, Hartley AH, Rocher LL, Wheeler SM, Hamilton TA, Parish TG, Ellis-Madu M, Duell E, Annesley TM, Cooper KD, Voorhees JJ. Cyclosporine for plaque-type psoriasis. Results of a multidose, double-blind trial. N Engl J Med 1991;324:277–284.
20. Powles AV, Baker BS, Valdimarsson H, Hulme B, Fry L. Four years of

experience with cyclosporin A for psoriasis. Br J Dermatol 1990;122:Suppl 36: 13–19.

21. Tegelberg-Stassen MJAM, Lammers A, Van Floten WA, Meinardi MMHM, De Rie MA, Bos JD, Faber WR, Smeenk G, Hamminga L, Velthuis PJ, Rompelman-Schiere S, Van Der Veen JPW, Van Duren JA, Den Hengst CW. Responsiveness of moderate psoriatic skin lesions to 1, 2, or 3 mg/kg/day cyclosporin A: a multicenter study. Eur J Dermatol 1992;2:147–150.

22. Dubertret L, Grossman R, Perrussel M, Robbiola O, Abiraced J, Bernnazzedine S, Reigneau O. Low-dose cyclosporin A in psoriasis. In: Wolff K, ed. Cyclosporin A and The Skin, International Congress and Symposium Series No. 192. London: Royal Society of Medicine Services Limited, 1992:13 [abstract].

23. Christophers E, Mrowietz U, Henneicke HH, Farber L, Welzel D. Cyclosporin A in psoriasis: Interim results of a multicentre dose-finding study in severe chronic plaque-type psoriasis. In: Wolff K, ed. Cyclosporin A and The Skin, International Congress and Symposium Series No. 192. London: Royal Society of Medicine Services Limited, 1992:21–26.

24. Mahrle G, Schulze HJ, Farber L. Cyclosporin A vs. etretinate in the treatment of psoriasis: Preliminary results. In: Wolff K, ed. Cyclosporin A and The Skin, International Congress and Symposium Series No. 192. London: Royal Society of Medicine Services Limited, 1992:27–28.

25. Wong RL, Winslow CM, and Cooper KD. The mechanisms of action of cyclosporin A in the treatment of psoriasis. Immunol Today 1993;14;69–74.

26. Novartis Pharmaceuticals Corporation. Neoral; Sandimmune. Physician's Desk Reference, 2002.

27. Nogita T, Mitsuishi T, Terajima S, et al. Efficacy of ciclosporin in two cases of erythrodermic psoriasis (letter). J Dermatol 1991;18:302–304.

28. Reitamo S, Mustakallio KK. Cyclosporin in erythrodermic psoriasis. Acta Derm Venereol 1989;Suppl 146:140–141.

29. Korstanje MJ, Bessems PJMJ, van de Staak WJBM. Combination therapy ciclosporin-etretinate effective in erythrodermic psoriasis (letter). Dermatologica 1989;179:94.

30. Sutthipisal N, Sriwatsantsak J, Sirimachan S, et al. The use of low dose cyclosporin A in a case of recalcitrant erythrodermic psoriasis. J Int Med Res 1988;16:485–488.

31. Korstanje MJ, Bessems PJMJ, Hulsmans RFHJ. Pustular psoriasis and acrodermatitis continua (Hallopeau) need high doses of systemic ciclosporin A (letter). Dermatologica 1989;179:90–91.

32. Gupta AK, Matteson EL, Ellis CN, Ho VC, Tellner DC, Voorhees JJ, McCune WJ. Cyclosporine in the treatment of psoriatic arthritis. Arch Dermatol 1989; 125:507–510.

33. Watkins PB. The role of cytochromes P-450 in cyclosporine metabolism. J Am Acad Dermatol 1990;23:1301–1311.

34. Koo J. A randomized, double-blind study comparing the efficacy, safety and

optimal dose of two formulations of cyclosporin, Neoral and Sandimmun, in patients with severe psoriasis. OLP302 Study Group. Br J Dermatol 1998; 139:88–95.

35. Somerville MF, Scott DG. Neoral—new cyclosporin for old? Br J Rheumatol 1997;36:1113–1115.

36. Berth-Jones J, Henderson CA, Munro CS, Rogers S, Chalmers RJ, Boffa, MJ, Norris PG, Friedmann PS, Graham-Brown RA, Dowd PM, Marks R, Sumner MJ. Treatment of psoriasis with intermittent short course cyclosporin (Neoral). Br J Dermatol 1997;136:527–530.

37. Gulliver WP, Murphy GF, Hannaford VA, Primmett DR. Increased bioavailability and improved efficacy, in severe psoriasis, of a new micro-emulsion formulation of cyclosporin. Br J Dermatol 1996; 135 Suppl 48:35–39.

38. Elder CA, Moore M, Chang CT, Jin J, Charnick S, Nedelman J, Cohen A, Guzzo C, Lowe N, Simpson K. Efficacy and pharmacokinetics of two formulations of cyclosporine A in patients with psoriasis. J Clin Pharmacol 1995;35:865–875.

39. Fradin MS, Ellis CN, Voorhees JJ. Management of patients and side effects during cyclosporine therapy for cutaneous disorders. J Am Acad Dermatol 1990;23:1265–1275.

40. Shupack J, Abel E, Bauer E, Brown M, Drake L, Freinkel R, Guzzo C, Koo J, Levine N, Lowe N, McDonald C, Margolis D, Stiller M, Wintroub B, Bainbridge C, Evans S, Hilss S, Mietlowski W, Winslow C, Birnbaum JE. Cyclosporine as maintenance therapy in patients with severe psoriasis. J Am Acad Dermatol 1997;36:423–432.

41. Ellis CN, Fradin MS, Hamilton TA, Voorhees JJ. Duration of remission during maintenance cyclosporine therapy for psoriasis. Relationship to maintenance dose and degree of improvement during initial therapy. Arch Dermatol 1995; 131:791–795.

42. Mahrle G, Schulze HJ, Farber L, Weidinger G, Steigleder GK. Low-dose short-term cyclosporine versus etretinate in psoriasis: improvement of skin, nail, and joint involvement. J Am Acad Dermatol 1995;32:78–88.

43. Ho VC, Griffiths CE, Berth-Jones J, Papp KA, Vanaclocha F, Dauden E, Beard A, Puvanarajan L, Paul C. Intermittent short courses of cyclosporine microemulsion for the long-term management of psoriasis: a 2-year cohort study. J Am Acad Dermatol 2001;44:643–651.

44. Finzi AF. Individualized short-course cyclosporin therapy in psoriasis. Br J Dermatol 1996;135 Suppl 48:31–34.

45. Powles AV, Hardman CM, Porter WM, Cook T, Hulme B, Fry L. Renal function after 10 years' treatment with cyclosporin for psoriasis. Br J Dermatol 1998;138:443–449.

46. Lowe NJ, Wieder JM, Rosenbach A, Johnson K, Kunkel R, Bainbridge C, Bourget T, Dimov L, Simpson K, Glass E, Grabie MT. Long-term low-dose cyclosporine therapy for severe psoriasis: effects on renal function and structure. J Am Acad Dermatol 1996;35(5 Pt 1):710–719.

47. Grossman RM, Chevret S, Abi-Rached J, Blanchet F, Dubertret L. Long-term safety of cyclosporine in the treatment of psoriasis. Arch Dermatol 1996; 132:623–629.
48. Mrowietz U, Farber L, Henneicke-von Zepelin HH, Bachmann H, Welzel D, Christophers E. Long-term maintenance therapy with cyclosporine and post-treatment survey in severe psoriasis: results of a multicenter study. German Multicenter Study. J Am Acad Dermatol 1995;33:470–475.
49. Peluso AM, Bardazzi F, Tosti A, Varotti C. Intermittent cyclosporin A treatment of severe plaque psoriasis. Long-term follow-up of 26 patients. Acta Derm-Venereol Suppl 1994;186:90–91.
50. Higgins E, Munro C, Marks J, Friedmann PS, Shuster S. Relapse rates in moderately severe chronic psoriasis treated with cyclosporin A. Br J Dermatol 1989;121; 1:71–74.
51. Nakayama J, Koga T, Furue M. Long-tern efficacy and adverse event of nifedipine sustained-release tablets for cyclosporin A-induced hypertension in patients with psoriasis. Eur J Dermatol 1998;8:563–568.
52. Feutren G, Mihatsch MJ. Risk factors for cyclosporine-induced nephropathy in patients with autoimmune diseases. N Engl J Med 1992;326:1654–1660.
53. Powles AV, Carmichael D, Hulme B, et al. Renal function after long-term low-dose cyclosporin for psoriasis. Br J Dermatol 1990;122:665–669.
54. Gilbert SC, Emmett M, Menter A, Silverman A, Klintmalm G. Cyclosporine therapy for psoriasis: serum creatinine measurements are an unreliable predictor of decreased renal function. J Am Acad Dermatol 1989;21:470–474.
55. Messana JM, Rocher LL, Ellis CN, Fradin MS, VanGurp JR, Cantu-Gonzalez G, Parish TG, Wheeler SM, Voorhees JJ. Effects of cyclosporine on renal function in psoriasis patients. J Am Acad Dermatol 1990;23:1288–1293.
56. Feutren G, Laburte C, Krupp P. Safety and tolerability of cyclosporin A in psoriasis. In: Wolff K, ed. Cyclosporin A and The Skin, International Congress and Symposium Series No. 192. London: Royal Society of Medicine Services Limited, 1992:3–12.
57. Feutren G, Abeywickrama K, Friend D, Von Graffenried B. Renal function and blood pressure in psoriatic patients treated with cyclosporin A. Br J Dermatol 1990;122:Suppl 36:57–69.
58. Mason J. Renal side effects of cyclosporin A. Br J Dermatol 1990;122:Suppl 36:71–77.
59. Mason J, Moore LC. Indirect assessment of renal dysfunction in patients taking cyclosporin A for autoimmune diseases. Br J Dermatol 1990;122: Suppl 36:79–84.
60. Mihatsch MJ, Thiel G, Ryffel B. Renal side–effects of cyclosporin A with special reference to autoimmune diseases. Br J Dermatol 1990;122:Suppl 36:101–115.
61. Mihatsch MJ, Wolff K. Consensus conference on cyclosporin A for psoriasis, February 1992. Br J Dermatol 1992;126:621–623.
62. Stoof TJ, Korstanje MJ, Bilo HJ, Starink TM, Hulsmans RF, Donker AJ.

Does fish oil protect renal function in cyclosporin-treated psoriasis patients? J Intern Med 1989;226;6:437–441.

63. Raman, G, Feehally, J, Coates, R, Elliott, H, Griffin, P, Olubodun, J, Wilkinson, R. Renal effects of amlodipine in normotensive renal transplant recipients. Nephrol Dial Transplant 1999;14:384–388.

64. Raman GV, Campbell SK, Farrer A, Albano JD, Cook J. Modifying effects of amlodipine on cyclosporin A-induced changes in renal function in patients with psoriasis. J Hypertens Suppl 1998;16:S39–S41.

65. Koo JYM, Lee CS, Maloney JE. Cyclosporine and related drugs. In: Wolverton SE, ed. Comprehensive Dermatologic Drug Therapy. Philadelphia: WB Saunders, 2001:205–229.

66. Zachariae H, Hansen HE, Kragballe K, Olsen S. Morphologic renal changes during cyclosporine treatment of psoriasis. J Am Acad Dermatol 1992;26:415–419.

67. Young EW, Ellis CN, Messana JM, Johnson KJ, Leichtman AB, Mihatsch MJ, Hamilton TA, Grossier DS, Fradin MS, Voorhees JJ. A prospective study of renal structure and function in psoriasis patients treated with cyclosporin. Kidney Int 1994;46:1216–1222.

68. Marcil I, Stern RS. Squamous-cell cancer of the skin in patients given PUVA and ciclosporin: nested cohort crossover study. Lancet 2001;358:1042–1045.

69. Kirby B, Owen CM, Blewitt RW, Yates VM. Cutaneous T-cell lymphoma developing in a patient on cyclosporin therapy. J Am Acad Dermatol 2002; 47:S165–S167.

70. Zackheim HS, Koo J, LeBoit PE, McCalmont TH, Bowman PH, Kashani-Sabet M, Jones C, Zehnder J. Psoriasiform mycosis fungoides with fatal outcome after treatment with cyclosporine. J Am Acad Dermatol 2002;47:155–157.

71. Gupta AK, Cooper KD, Ellis CN, Nickoloff BJ, Hanson CA, Brown MD, Voorhees JJ. Lymphocytic infiltrates of the skin in association with cyclosporine therapy. J Am Acad Dermatol 1990;23:1137–1141.

72. Mockli G, Kabra PM, Kurtz TW. Laboratory monitoring of cyclosporine levels: guidelines for the dermatologist. J Am Acad Dermatol 1990;23:1275–1279.

73. Feutren G, Friend D, Timonen P, Barnes A, Laburte C. Predictive value of cyclosporin A level for efficacy or renal dysfunction in psoriasis. Br J Dermatol 1990;122:Suppl 36:85–93.

74. Ieiri I, Nakayama J, Murakami H, Hori Y, Higuchi S. Evaluation of the therapeutic range of whole blood cyclosporin concentration in the treatment of psoriasis. Int J Clin Pharmacol Ther 1996;34:106–111.

75. Kokelj F, Torsello P, Plozzer C. Calcipotriol improves the efficacy of cyclosporine in the treatment of psoriasis vulgaris. J Eur Acad Dermatol Venereol 1998;10:143–146.

76. Gottlieb SL, Heftler NS, Gilleaudeau P, Johnson R, Vallat VP, Wolfe J, Gottlieb AB, Krueger JG. Short-contact anthralin treatment augments therapeutic efficacy of cyclosporine in psoriasis: a clinical and pathologic study. J Am Acad Dermatol 1995;33:637–645.

77. Bagot M, Grossman R, Pamphile R, Binderup L, Charue D, Revuz J, Dubertret L. Additive effects of calcipotriol and cyclosporine A: from in vitro experiments to in vivo applications in the treatment of severe psoriasis. Cr Acad Sci III 1994;317:282–286.

78. Grossman RM, Thivolet J, Claudy A, Souteyrand P, Guilhou JJ, Thomas P, Amblard P, Belaich S, de Belilovsky C, de la Brassinne M. A novel therapeutic approach to psoriasis with combination calcipotriol ointment and very low-dose cyclosporine: results of a multicenter placebo-controlled study. J Am Acad Dermatol 1994;31:68–74.

79. Ameen M, Smith HR, Barker JN. Combined mycophenolate mofetil and cyclosporin therapy for severe recalcitrant psoriasis. Clin Exp Dermatol 2001; 26:480–483.

80. Clark CM, Kirby B, Morris AD, Davison S, Zaki I, Emerson R, Saihan EM, Chalmers RJ, Barker JN, Allen BR, Griffiths CE. Combination treatment with methotrexate and cyclosporin for severe recalcitrant psoriasis. Br J Dermatol 1999;141:279–282.

81. Petzelbauer P, Honigsmann H, Langer K, Anegg B, et al. Cyclosporin A in combination with photochemotherapy (PUVA) in the treatment of psoriasis. Br J Dermatol 1990;123:641–647.

82. Ellis CN, Voorhees JJ. Etretinate therapy. J Am Acad Dermatol 1987;16:267–291.

83. Halioua B, Saurat JH. Risk: benefit ratio in the treatment of psoriasis with systemic retinoids. Br J Dermatol 1990;122:Suppl 36:135–150.

84. Korstanje MJ, van de Staak WJ. Combination-therapy cyclosporin-A—etretinate for psoriasis. Clin Exp Dermatol 1990;15:172–173.

85. Movsowitz C, Epstein S, Fallon M, Ismail F, Thomas S. Cyclosporin A in vivo produces severe osteopenia in the rat. Effect of dose and duration of administration. Endocrinology 1988;123:2571–2578.

86. Boubigot B, Moal MC, Cledes J. Bone histology in renal transplant patients receiving cyclosporin. Lancet 1988;1:1048.

87. Gupta AK, Ellis CN, Siegel, MT, Duell EA, Griffiths CEM, Hamilton TA, Nickoloff BJ, Voorhees JJ. Sulfasalazine improves psoriasis: a double-blind analysis. Arch Dermatol 1990;126:487–493.

88. Ellis CN, Reiter KL, Bandekar RR, Fendrick AM. Cost-effectiveness comparison of therapy for psoriasis with a methotrexate-based regimen versus a rotation regimen of modified cyclosporine and methotrexate. J Am Acad Dermatol 2002;46:242–250.

89. Krueger JG. The immunologic basis for the treatment of psoriasis with new biologic agents. J Am Acad Dermatol 2002;46:1–23.

90. Singri P, West DP, Gordon KB. Biologic therapy for psoriasis: the new therapeutic frontier. Arch Dermatol 2002;138:657–663.

91. Ellis CN, Krueger GG, Alefacept Clinical Study Group: Treatment of chronic plaque psoriasis by selective targeting of memory-effector T lymphocytes. N Engl J Med 2001;345:248–255.

92. Jegasothy BV, Ackerman CD, Todo S, Fung JJ, Abu-Elmagd K, Starzl TE. Tacrolimus (FK 506)—a new therapeutic agent for severe recalcitrant psoriasis. Arch Dermatol 1992;128:781–7815.
93. The European FK 506 Multicentre Psoriasis Study Group. Systemic tacrolimus (FK 506) is effective for the treatment of psoriasis in a double-blind, placebo-controlled study. Arch Dermatol 1996;132:419–423.
94. Kaplan MJ, Ellis CN, Bata-Csorgo Z, Kaplan RS, Endres JL, Fox DA: Systemic toxicity following administration of sirolimus (formerly rapamycin) for psoriasis: association of capillary leak syndrome with apoptosis of lesional lymphocytes. Arch Dermatol 1999;135:553–557.
95. Reitamo S, Spuls P, Sassolas B, Lahfa M, Claudy A, Griffiths CE. Efficacy of sirolimus (rapamycin) administered concomitantly with a subtherapeutic dose of cyclosporin in the treatment of severe psoriasis: a randomized controlled trial. Br J Dermatol 2001;145:438–45.
96. Ho VC, Griffiths CEM, Ellis CN, Gupta AK, McCuaig CC, Nickoloff BJ, Cooper KD, Hamilton TA, Voorhees JJ. Intralesional cyclosporine in the treatment of psoriasis. A clinical, immunologic, and pharmacokinetic study. J Am Acad Dermatol 1990;22:94–100.
97. Burns MK, Ellis CN, Eisen D, Duell E, Griffiths CEM, Annesley TM, Hamilton TA, Birnbaum JE, Voorhees JJ. Intralesional cyclosporine for psoriasis: relationship of dose, tissue levels, and efficacy. Arch Dermatol 1992; 128:786–790.
98. Powles AV, Baker BS, McFadden J, et al. Intralesional injection of cyclosporin in psoriasis. Lancet 1988;I:537

8

Combination, Rotational, and Sequential Therapy

Mark Lebwohl
Mount Sinai School of Medicine, New York, New York, U.S.A.

I. ROTATIONAL THERAPY

The concept of rotational therapy was first introduced by Weinstein and White (1). At that time ultraviolet B (UVB) plus tar, psoralen plus UVA (PUVA), methotrexate, and etretinate were the treatments available for severe psoriasis. Weinstein and White advocated using each form of therapy for 1–2 years and then switching to the next form. By rotating these treatments, the cumulative toxicity of each individual form of therapy could be minimized, thus reducing the carcinogenesis of PUVA, the hepatic fibrosis and need for liver biopsies with methotrexate, and the musculoskeletal toxicity of retinoids. As new treatments, such as cyclosporine, were developed, they were added to the rotation, allowing further reductions in cumulative dosage over time.

II. COMBINATION THERAPY

Combination therapy has been used for a long time, but the concept of using low-dosage combinations of different treatments to minimize toxicity and enhance efficacy was formally introduced at a consensus conference chaired by Dr. Alan Menter and funded by the National Psoriasis Foundation in 1994 (2). The concept was to minimize toxicity and enhance efficacy by combining lower dosages of different systemic therapies.

III. SEQUENTIAL THERAPY

The concept of sequential therapy, formally introduced by Dr. John Koo, took advantage of the overlap between combination therapy and rotational therapy. As originally stated, sequential therapy involved three phases: a clearing phase, a transitional phase, and a maintenance phase. As an example, cyclosporine at maximal dosage was used for the clearing phase followed by the addition of acitretin during the transitional phase. Once maximal dosages of acitretin were tolerated, cyclosporine was gradually tapered and acitretin continued for long-term maintenance. Phototherapy with UVB or PUVA was added if additional improvement was needed for maintenance (3).

The benefits of combination, rotational, and sequential therapy rely on the use of lower dosages of therapeutic agents to minimize toxicity. In the case of combination therapy, additive or synergistic effects may result in enhanced efficacy as well. The dangers of additive toxicity or the possibility that one treatment might inactivate another must be considered when combining therapies. Finally, topical therapy and phototherapy may be used in combination therapy, rotational therapy, or sequential therapy with systemic agents or with other topical therapies or phototherapeutic modalities. This chapter will emphasize combinations of systemic therapy, but will review topical therapy and phototherapy as well.

IV. TOPICAL THERAPY IN COMBINATION, ROTATIONAL, AND SEQUENTIAL THERAPY WITH OTHER TOPICAL AGENTS

Topical agents are probably the most common medications used in combination therapy. When combining topical agents with phototherapy or with other topical medications, caution must be used because treatments can inactivate one another or, alternatively, can enhance both the efficacy and toxicity of particular agents. For example, the addition of tars to anthralin regimens was advocated in the early 1980s because tar was noted to reduce the cutaneous irritation caused by anthralin (4–6). However, it was subsequently noted that tar inactivates anthralin and is therefore responsible for the reduced irritation (7). Calcipotriene is likewise a relatively unstable molecule that is easily inactivated by acidic compounds. The addition of salicylic acid to calcipotriene completely inactivates this vitamin D_3 analog on contact (8). Other agents, such as topical hydrocortisone valerate or ammonium lactate, also inactivate calcipotriene over time. Halobetasol propionate cream and ointment, however, were found to be entirely compatible with calcipotriene ointment for up to 2 weeks (8).

Before it was known that calcipotriene and halobetasol ointments are compatible, the agents were used separately morning or evening or on different days in combination and sequential regimens. In one study it was shown that once-daily calcipotriene and once-daily halobetasol ointments were superior to either of the individual agents used twice daily for 2 weeks (9). A sequential regimen was then developed in which the first 2 weeks of calcipotriene and halobetasol ointments were followed by a regimen in which halobetasol ointment was used twice daily on weekends and calcipotriene ointment twice daily on weekdays for 6 months (10). The latter regimen was found to be superior to a traditional weekend pulsed therapy regimen with superpotent steroids only. Tazarotene has likewise been shown to be compatible with numerous topical corticosteroids when applied one on top of the other (11). Regimens combining tazarotene with topical corticosteroids have demonstrated increased efficacy and reduced irritation (12, 13).

V. TOPICAL THERAPY COMBINED WITH PHOTOTHERAPY

The use of topical therapy with phototherapy offers unique advantages and disadvantages. For example, some treatments, such as salicylic acid and tar, block UVB (14). Other medications can be affected by ultraviolet light if applied prior to phototherapy. For example, UVA inactivates calcipotriene (15) and both UVA and UVB inactivate calcitriol (16). Other medications pose unique problems. Tars, which were part of the original Goeckerman regimen, caused a photosensitive reaction known as tar smarts when applied prior to UVA irradiation (17). Two weeks of treatment with tazarotene increases the erythemogenicity of UVB, suggesting that phototherapy doses should be reduced by approximately one-third in patients being treated with tazarotene (18). UVA doses should likewise be reduced by 1 or 2 J in patients treated with tazarotene and PUVA, or the tazarotene may make the patients more prone to burning.

The combination of tazarotene and UVB has been shown to result in greater improvement than with UVB and vehicle or UVB alone (19). Tazarotene has also been shown to improve the response to narrowband UVB, as has calcipotriene (20). Another study failed to show a beneficial effect with the addition of calcipotriene to narrow-band UVB (21).

The effect of calcipotriene on a broadband UVB phototherapy regimen has also been questioned. In a bilateral comparison controlled trial, UVB plus calcipotriene was slightly, but statistically significantly, more effective than UVB with vehicle (22). At least two other publications support the increased efficacy of UVB when calcipotriene is added (23, 24), but a third study showed that UVB added to a calcipotriene regimen was no more effective than the calcipotriene alone (25). It has been shown that calcipotriene used in combination with twice-weekly UVB phototherapy is as effective as three times weekly UVB phototherapy (26).

In a bilateral comparison study in which PUVA on one side of the body was compared to PUVA and calcipotriene ointment on the other side, the side treated with both therapies cleared more quickly with lower UVA dosages than the side treated with PUVA alone, supporting a role for calcipotriene in reducing cumulative doses and photocarcinogenesis of PUVA (27). Tazarotene has likewise been used in combination with PUVA (28) but, as noted above, UVA doses should be lowered by 1 or 2 J/cm^2 when tazarotene is added to a PUVA regimen (18).

A leading controversy in the combination of topical agents with phototherapy relates to the concomitant use of topical corticosteroids with UVB and PUVA. One study examined patients treated with UVB phototherapy three times a week. Approximately half the patients applied potent topical corticosteroids twice daily until clear and the other half applied control medication. Although there was a trend toward slightly more rapid clearing in the patients treated with topical corticosteroids, the differences were not significant, nor did those patients require fewer treatments or lower dosages of UVB to achieve clearing. However, those patients had a longer average duration of remission (29). In contrast, a study by Horwitz et al. showed that patients treated with a modified Goeckerman regimen and hydrocortisone valerate cream relapsed after 5.9 weeks compared to 17.9 weeks for patients treated with the modified Goeckerman regimen alone, suggesting that topical corticosteroids shorten the duration of remission (30). Other studies have confirmed the absence of beneficial effects when topical corticosteroids are added to UVB phototherapy regimens (31, 32). In contrast, topical corticosteroids may have a beneficial role when used with PUVA. Patients' disease appears to clear with fewer treatments and lower UVA dosage when corticosteroids are added to a PUVA regimen (33–35).

VI. PHOTOTHERAPY AND SYSTEMIC AGENTS

The addition of systemic therapy to a phototherapy regimen has numerous benefits. Most important is that the number of phototherapy visits can be reduced by addition of systemic therapy, thus minimizing the dose related photodamage and carcinogenicity of treatment such as PUVA (36). Although a number publications have suggested that broadband UVB phototherapy is not carcinogenic (37, 38), addition of systemic therapy to UVB phototherapy allows more rapid and more effective clearing than monotherapy with UVB, as well as faster clearing with lower UVB doses and less photodamage. Conversely, the total dosages and toxicities of systemic agents can be minimized by combining phototherapy with those agents in combination, rotational, or sequential regimens. Combination therapy involves the use of lower dosages of UVB (or, for PUVA, of UVA) with lower dosages of systemic agents. These are described in detail below. In rotational therapy, patients are given rest periods off systemic therapy or off phototherapy, thus minimizing total cumulative dosages of either treatment. In sequential therapy, clearing is initiated with powerful systemic agents such as cyclosporine or methotrexate. In a transition phase, phototherapy is gradually added and the systemic agents gradually tapered until phototherapy is used as monotherapy for maintenance.

A.   Retinoids and Phototherapy

Both etretinate and its active metabolite acitretin have been studied in conjunction with phototherapy. In high dosages retinoids are associated with numerous mucocutaneous side effects including hair loss, cheilitis, thinning of nail plates, development of pyogenic granulomas, and dry or sticky skin. Systemic toxicities include hyperlipidema and bony changes, such as osteophyte formation and osteoporosis, as well as calcification of ligaments and tendons, which have been described with long-term use.

When combining retinoids with UVB phototherapy, lower dosages from 10 to 25 mg daily, can be used, minimizing mucocutaneous side effects and reducing long-term cumulative dosages. Several studies have examined the combination of acitretin or etretinate with broadband UVB (39, 40). All studies have shown that the addition of low-dosage retinoids allows a marked reduction in UVB exposure and much more effective clearing. In current practice, acitretin in dosages of 10–25 mg daily is started 1–2 weeks before initiating UVB phototherapy (Table 1). Starting dosages of UVB and increments should be reduced by one-third to one-half to avoid burning. If retinoids are added in the middle of a course of UVB phototherapy, UVB dosages should be reduced by 50%. Retinoids thin the stratum corneum, allowing more penetration by UVB and thus increasing the erythemogenicity of UVB. Thinning of the stratum corneum occurs over 1 week, so the increased susceptibility to burning may not be apparent until several days after oral retinoids are started.

As with broadband UVB, retinoids increase the efficacy of narrow-band UVB (41). Again, acitretin dosages of 10–25 mg are started 1–2 weeks before initiating phototherapy and narrow-band UVB doses are reduced by one-third to one-half. Retinoids likewise increase the efficacy of PUVA and the combination of retinoids and PUVA is among the most powerful psoriasis treatments available. Published studies have demonstrated faster clearing with lower dosages of UVA (42). When used with PUVA, retinoids have the

Table 1 Combination Therapy: Acitretin and UVB or PUVA

Start acitretin 10-25mg/day.

After 1–2 weeks, add UVB 10-50 mJ/cm^2 or oxsoralen + UVA ½–3J/ cm^2 according to skin type.

Daily acitretin should be continued and phototherapy administered three times per week with incremental (10-30 mJ/cm^2 UVB or ¼ - 2 J/cm^2) UVA.

added advantage of suppressing the development of skin cancers at least while patients are receiving retinoid therapy.

In women of childbearing potential, isotretinoin has been shown to be effective in combination with UVB or PUVA (43). Although isotretinoin is teratogenic, the period of risk is only 1 month after treatment, compared to much longer periods of teratogenicity with acitretin or etretinate.

B. Methotrexate and Phototherapy

A combination of methotrexate and broadband UVB phototherapy has been used for many years for the treatment of psoriasis (44). In one study, three weekly doses of methotrexate 15 mg were given before starting UVB phototherapy. Standard dosages of UVB were used and methotrexate was continued for several more weeks until complete clearing, at which point the methotrexate was discontinued and the patient maintained with UVB. The total dosage of methotrexate used in this regimen is usually under 200 mg for an entire course. One side effect of methotrexate that might be of concern, radiation recall, is rarely seen. This side effect has been reported when using a number of chemotherapy agents after radiation or ultraviolet-induced burns. Affected patients develop erythema and burning in previously burned sites even though they are no longer exposed to ultraviolet light or radiation. Methotrexate can be used with narrow-band UVB in regimens similar to its use with broadband UVB.

The combination of methotrexate and PUVA is somewhat controversial. Both treatments have been used successfully, allowing lower dosages of methotrexate and of UVA with faster and more effective clearing (45). However, there is some evidence that patients treated with methotrexate have a higher risk of squamous cell carcinoma when treated with PUVA (46).

C. Cyclosporine and Phototherapy

The development of squamous cell carcinoma in patients treated with cyclosporine for the prevention of organ transplant rejection is well known (47).

That has led to great concern about the combination of phototherapy with cyclosporine, particularly when considering PUVA. The risk of developing squamous cell carcinoma after treatment with PUVA has been described above (36). The development of squamous cell carcinomas after initiating cyclosporine therapy in patients treated with excessive amounts of PUVA is well described (48). There is less concern when treating UVB-treated patients with cyclosporine since numerous studies have shown low skin cancer risks with broadband UVB (37, 38). Nevertheless, most have avoided using phototherapy with cyclosporine. Some have advocated calming down severe flaring psoriasis with cyclosporine and then tapering the cyclosporine dosage once PUVA is initiated (49).

D. Combinations of Biological Agents with Phototherapy

Although experience with biological agents in combination with phototherapy for psoriasis is limited, these agents appear to be safer than cyclosporine with respect to development of malignancies. One paper documents the development of squamous cell carcinomas in seven patients after treatment with etanercept (50). However, extensive safety data, including postmarketing information on more than 100,000 treated patients, does not show an increase in squamous cell carcinomas or in other immunosuppression-related malignancies such as lymphomas. An increase in squamous cell carcinomas or lymphoproliferative diseases has not been documented in patients treated with infliximab, etanercept, alefacept, or efalizumab, although experience with the latter two drugs is limited. In all likelihood, combination therapy with broadband ultraviolet B and narrow-band UVB will be performed with the biological agents, and in some patients PUVA may be combined with those agents.

VII. SYSTEMIC THERAPY

For patients responsive to conventional psoriasis therapy, the combination of systemic agents offers a way to reduce dosages and toxicities of those agents while maintaining improvement in psoriasis. For patients with the most refractory disease, the combination of systemic agents offers the most effective way of clearing their skin, but must be cautiously used since some combinations can be dangerous. The toxicity of each of the components of a combination regimen must be considered. Nevertheless, combinations of systemic agents for the treatment of psoriasis can be used safely.

Topical therapy and phototherapy can be added to any of the systemic combinations as long as the information presented above on interactions between systemic agents and phototherapy is considered. Specifically, the combination of PUVA and cyclosporine may predispose to squamous cell carcinomas and is therefore avoided by many clinicians. Some also hesitate to combine UVB with cyclosporine because of any potential for additive carcinogenicity even though that has not been demonstrated. When combining retinoids with ultraviolet light, lower ultraviolet dosages must likewise be used as described above.

The role of systemic therapy and rotational therapy has already been described above, and the concept of sequential therapy can be applied to combinations of systemic agents as well. The goal with combination systemic therapy would be to clear patients' skin and then gradually reduce the most dangerous drugs in the combination regimen so that patients can ultimately be maintained with the safest components of the combination. In some instances, remissions may be obtained, allowing drug holidays during which therapy is not required. For patients with responsive disease, PUVA, alefacept, and infliximab offer the longest remissions, but patients with the most difficult disease may not necessarily achieve complete clearing or long periods of clearing.

For purposes of safety, systemic drugs can be classified according to their major toxicities (Table 2). To minimize toxicity while maximizing efficacy, attempts should be made to avoid combinations of drugs whose toxicities might be additive or synergistic. For example, methotrexate and hydroxyurea both affect the bone marrow. Although these two agents have been used together (51), additive bone marrow toxicity is the main obstacle to their concomitant use. In general, physicians should avoid combining agents that each individually cause bone marrow toxicity when treating psoriasis. On the occasions when those combinations must be overlapped, both the dosages and duration of overlap should be minimized. Table 2 includes acute, life-threatening toxicities such as bone marrow suppression or immunosuppression. Drugs such as sulfasalazine that do not have any of these toxicities can be safely added to most of the therapies listed. The combination of sulfasalazine and methotrexate, for example, has been used safely (52).

Table 2 By Dividing Drugs According to Their Major Acute Toxicities, Combinations Can Be Selected that Avoid Overlapping Toxicities

Bone marrow suppression	Immunosuppression	Other
Methotrexate	Cylosporine	Acitretin
Hydroxyurea	Mycophenolate mofetil	Sulfasalazine
6-Thioguanine	Biologicals	

Side effects other than those listed in Table 2, such as hepatotoxicity, can occur and warrant additional monitoring. For example, etretinate has been used safely and effectively in combination with methotrexate for the treatment of erythrodermic and pustular psoriasis (53–55). Because of the potential for additive hepatotoxicity, liver function tests should be checked 1 week after using the two medications together for the first time and at least monthly thereafter. Because etretinate may raise plasma concentrations of methotrexate (56), a complete blood count (CBC) and platelet count should be obtained 1 week after combining the two treatments and should be repeated at least monthly (Table 3).

Retinoids are among the safest agents we have for the treatment of psoriasis and have been combined not only with medications that affect the bone marrow but also with medications that may be immunosuppressive. In fact, retinoids such as acitretin may suppress the development of squamous cell carcinomas that occur as a result of immunosuppressive therapies such as cyclosporine (57). Monotherapy with retinoids is not as effective as cyclosporine or methotrexate and, as a consequence, attempts to taper patients off of cyclosporine onto acitretin are not always successful (58). The combination of retinoids with cyclosporine has been used safely, but that combination is not always effective (59). It should be recognized, however, that published cases of retinoids used in conjunction with cyclosporine usually document patients whose psoriasis is severe and refractory to conventional therapy. Nevertheless, this combination may be useful in selected patients. Because retinoids and cyclosporine can both cause hyperlipidemia, serum lipids should be monitored at baseline, every 2 weeks after using the combination for the first month, and at least monthly thereafter.

The combination of agents that are immunosuppressive with agents that affect the bone marrow is particularly effective. It should be recognized that agents affecting the bone marrow are also immunosuppressive, so physicians must be particularly vigilant about the possibility that opportunistic infections might arise.

The combination of methotrexate and cyclosporine was one of the first to be used. Because methotrexate is hepatotoxic and cyclosporine is metabolized in the liver, and because cyclosporine is nephrotoxic and methotrexate is excreted through the kidneys, this combination was first thought to be unsafe (60). Rheumatologists subsequently showed that combination therapy with cyclosporine and methotrexate was more effective in the treatment of rheumatoid arthritis than methotrexate (61). Cyclosporine in dosages of 2.5–5 mg/kg daily, with a mean dosage of 2.97 mg/kg per day, was added to the maximal tolerated dosage of methotrexate to achieve dramatic improvements in rheumatoid arthritis. Cyclosporine and methotrexate were also effectively combined to treat severe psoriatic arthritis

Table 3 Blood monitoring recommendations when combining systemic therapies[a]

Combination therapy	Monitoring modifications
Mtx + acitretin	Liver function tests: Baseline, 1 weeks, at least monthly for 3 months, then every 3 months if normal CBC + platelets: Baseline, 1 week, and at least monthly Lipids: Baseline, 1–2 weeks, monthly for 3 months, every 3 months, if stable
Acitretin + cylosporine	Lipids: Baseline, 2 week intervals first month, monthly until stable for several months. Then every 3 months Chem screen including: BUN, creatinine, Mg#, LFTs, uric acid: Baseline, 2 weeks, 4 weeks, and monthly thereafter
Mtx + cyclosporine	CBC platelets: Baseline, repeat every 1–2 weeks first month, then monthly Chem screen including LFTs, lipids, BUN, creatinine, Mg#, uric acid: Baseline, repeat every 1-2 weeks first month, then monthly
Biologics + Mtx	In addition to mtx monitoring obtain baseline PPD and chest x-ray if PPD is positive. Alefacept may require monitoring of lymphocytes.
Cyclosporine + mycophenolate mofetil	CBC + differential + platelets: Baseline, every 1-2 weeks first month, at least monthly thereafter. Chem screen including LFTs, lipids, BUN, creatinine, Mg#, uric acid: every 2 weeks first month and monthly thereafter

Mtx, methotrexate; BUN, blood urea nitrogen; Mg#, Magnesium; LFTs, liver function tests; PPD, purified protein derivative.
[a] Liver biopsy monitoring + pregnancy monitoring recommendations are not changed.

(62). Finally, methotrexate and cyclosporine were combined in 19 patients with severe recalcitrant psoriasis. Nine of the patients were taking methotrexate and 10 were taking cyclosporine at maximal dosages before starting combination therapy. Both psoriasis and psoriatic arthritis improved. With long-term therapy (a mean of 193.2 weeks), six patients showed that elevations of serum creatinine that improved with reduction in the dosage of cyclosporine. In three patients, however, impaired renal function did not normalize (63).

When combining methotrexate and cyclosporine, maximal dosages can be used but are seldom necessary. Maximal tolerated dosages of methotrexate (15–30 mg/week) have been combined with cyclosporine dosages as high as 5 mg/kg administered in two equal divided daily doses. However, dosages of methotrexate or cyclosporine can be reduced rapidly when the two agents are used together. When cyclosporine is added, reduction of the weekly methotrexate dosage by as much as 2.5 mg/week has been accomplished without flare of psoriasis. When methotrexate is added to cyclosporine, the cyclosporine dosage can either be tapered or abruptly discontinued if necessary without a flare of psoriasis.

In addition to the potential for added immunosuppression, close attention must be paid to liver function tests, blood urea nitrogen (BUN), creatinine, CBC, and platelet counts when combining methotrexate and cyclosporine. Low-dosage cyclosporine has also been used effectively with hydroxyurea for the treatment of severe psoriasis (64).

Biological agents are being introduced for the treatment of psoriasis. Specifically, alefacept, efalizumab, etanercept and infliximab, are all likely to be approved for the treatment of psoriasis. Infliximab and etanercept are already available for the treatment of Crohn's disease and rheumatoid arthritis. For rheumatoid arthritis, they are administered along with methotrexate. There have been no additive toxicities as far as the bone marrow is concerned, but the combined regimens may result in immunosuppression.

Etanercept is administered in dosages of 25 mg subcutaneously twice per week. It requires no additional monitoring; when added to methotrexate, the same monitoring ordinarily performed for patients on methotrexate should be continued (65–67).

Infliximab is administered by slow intravenous (IV) infusion. Initial trials of infliximab for the treatment of psoriasis have examined dosages of 5 mg/kg given at baseline and weeks 2 and 6 (68). The combination of infliximab with methotrexate has been used for rheumatoid arthritis (69) and more recently for severe recalcitrant psoriasis (70).

In all likelihood all of the biological agents will be used in combination with drugs such as methotrexate for at least some patients. However, caution should be used because of the potential for additive immunosuppression. There have been numerous anecdotes of opportunistic infections in patients treated with infliximab and etanercept. Because of the emergence of latent tuberculosis (71) purified protein derivative (PPD) testing should be considered in these patients and chest x-ray obtained when the PPD is positive.

Questions will undoubtedly be raised about the possibility of combining cyclosporine with the new biological agents. Again, concern about additive immunosuppression must be raised. Nevertheless, cyclosporine has been combined with other immunosuppressive agents such as mycophenolate mofetil. The latter combination has been used for years to prevent organ transplant rejection. In a published study, seven of nine patients whose psoriasis had failed to clear with cyclosporine alone or were unable to tolerate higher dosages of cyclosporine, experienced improvement when mycophenolate mofetil was added to their regimen. The maximum dosage of mycophenolate mofetil was 3 g daily and the mean dosage of cyclosporine was 2.5 mg/kg daily (72).

Addition of mycophenolate mofetil to a cyclosporine regimen does not necessitate any modification in cyclosporine dosage, although patients may be able to reduce their cyclosporine dosages gradually. Attempts to switch patients from cyclosporine to mycophenolate mofetil in cases of severe psoriasis are only occasionally successful: mycophenolate mofetil monotherapy is not nearly as effective as cyclosporine, although it is safer when considering cyclosporine's nephrotoxicity. In one study, eight patients treated with long-term cyclosporine were changed to mycophenolate mofetil. Five of the patients experienced significant exacerbations of their psoriasis, while three patients had only mild recurrences of psoriasis. All six patients who had impaired renal function as a result of the cyclosporine therapy experienced improvement in renal function following the change to mycophenolate mofetil (73).

In summary, the availability of so many psoriasis treatments offers many options for our patients. By utilizing combinations, by rotating from one treatment to another, and by applying the principles of sequential therapy, we should be able to improve the outcomes for our patients while reducing the toxicities of psoriasis therapies.

REFERENCES

1. Weinstein GD, White GM. An approach to the treatment of moderate to severe psoriasis with rotational therapy. J Am Acad Dermatol 1993;28(3):454–459.
2. Menter MA, See JA, Amend WJ, Ellis CN, Krueger GG, Lebwohl M, Morison WL, Prystowsky JH, Roenigk HH Jr, Shupack JL, Silverman AK, Weinstein GD, Yocum DE, Zanolli MD. Proceedings of the Psoriasis Combination and Rotation Therapy Conference. Deer Valley, Utah, Oct. 7–9, 1994. J Am Acad Dermatol. 1996;34(2 Pt 1):315–21.
3. Koo J. Systemic sequential therapy of psoriasis: a new paradigm for improved therapeutic results. J Am Acad Dermatol. 1999;41(3 Pt 2):S25–8.
4. Schulze HJ, Steigleder GK. [Experiences in half-side treatment with tar additive to cignolin-salicylic-acid-white-vaseline therapy of psoriasis vulgaris] Z Hautkr. 1984;9(10):654–6.

5. Schulze HJ, Steigleder GK, Pullmann H, Bloedhorn H. [The effect of a tar admixture to dithranol-salicylic-acid-white-petrolatum therapy on the cytokinetics of psoriasis] Z Hautkr. 1984;59(5):288–90, 295–7.

6. Steigleder GK, Schulze HJ. [A new Cologne therapy scheme—addition of tar to cignoline-salicylic acid-white vaseline therapy in psoriasis vulgaris] Z Hautkr. 1984;59(3):188, 191-2.

7. Muller R, Naumann E, Detmar M, Orfanos CE. [Stability of cignolin (dithranol) in ointments containing tar with and without the addition of salicylic acid. Oxidation to danthron and dithranol dimer] Hautarzt. 1987; 38(2):107–11.

8. Patel B, Siskin S, Krazmien R, Lebwohl M. Compatibility of calcipotriene with other topical medications. J Am Acad Dermatol. 1998;38(6 Pt 1):1010–1.

9. Lebwohl M, Siskin SB, Epinette W, Breneman D, Funicella T, Kalb R, Moore J. A multicenter trial of calcipotriene ointment and halobetasol ointment compared with either agent alone for the treatment of psoriasis. J Am Acad Dermatol. 1996;35(2 Pt 1):268–9.

10. Lebwohl M, Yoles A, Lombardi K, Lou W. Calcipotriene ointment and halobetasol ointment in the long-term treatment of psoriasis: effects on the duration of improvement. J Am Acad Dermatol. 1998;39(3):447–50.

11. Hecker D, Worsley J, Yueh G, Lebwohl M. In vitro compatibility of tazarotene with other topical treatments of psoriasis. J Am Acad Dermatol. 2000;42(6): 1008–11.

12. Lebwohl M, Lombardi K, Tan MH. Duration of improvement in psoriasis after treatment with tazarotene 0.1% gel plus clobetasol propionate 0.05% ointment: comparison of maintenance treatments. Int J Dermatol. 2001;40(1): 64–6.

13. Lebwohl MG, Breneman DL, Goffe BS, Grossman JR, Ling MR, Milbauer J, Pincus SH, Sibbald RG, Swinyer LJ, Weinstein GD, Lew-Kaya DA, Lue JC, Gibson JR, Sefton J. Tazarotene 0.1% gel plus corticosteroid cream in the treatment of plaque psoriasis. J Am Acad Dermatol. 1998;39(4 Pt 1):590–6.

14. Lebwohl M, Martinez J, Weber P, DeLuca R. Effects of topical preparations on the erythemogenicity of UVB: implications forpsoriasis phototherapy. J Am Acad Dermatol. 1995;32(3):469–71.

15. Lebwohl M, Hecker D, Martinez J, Sapadin A, Patel B. Interactions between calcipotriene and ultraviolet light. J Am Acad Dermatol. 1997;37(1):93–5.

16. Lebwohl M, Quijije J, Gilliard J, Rollin T, Watts O. Interactions between ultraviolet light and topical calcitriol (submitted).

17. Diette KM, Gange RW, Stern RS, Arndt KA, Parrish JA. Coal tar phototoxicity: characteristics of the smarting reaction. J Invest Dermatol. 1985;84(4):268–71.

18. Hecker D, Worsley J, Yueh G, Kuroda K, Lebwohl M. Interactions between tazarotene and ultraviolet light. J Am Acad Dermatol. 1999;41(6):927–30.

19. Koo JY, Lowe NJ, Lew-Kaya DA, Vasilopoulos AI, Lue JC, Sefton J, Gibson JR. Tazarotene plus UVB phototherapy in the treatment of psoriasis. J Am Acad Dermatol. 2000 Nov;43(5 Pt 1):821–8.

20. Schiener R, Behrens-Williams SC, Pillekamp H, Kaskel P, Peter RU, Kerscher M. Calcipotriol vs. tazarotene as combination therapy with narrowband ultraviolet B(311 nm): efficacy in patients with severe psoriasis. Br J Dermatol. 2000;143(6):1275–8.

21. Brands S, Brakman M, Bos JD, de Rie MA. No additional effect of calcipotriol ointment on low-dose narrow-band UVB phototherapy in psoriasis. J Am Acad Dermatol. 1999;41(6):991–5.

22. Hecker D, Lebwohl M. Topical calcipotriene in combination with UVB phototherapy for psoriasis. Int J Dermatol. 1997;36(4):302–3.

23. Molin L. Topical calcipotriol combined with phototherapy for psoriasis. The results of two randomized trials and a review of the literature. Calcipotriol-UVB Study Group Dermatology. 1999;198(4):375–81.

24. Kokelj F, Lavaroni G, Guadagnini A. UVB versus UVB plus calcipotriol (MC 903) therapy for psoriasis vulgaris. Acta Derm Venereol. 1995;75(5):386–7.

25. Kragballe K. Combination of topical calcipotriol (MC 903) and UVB radiation for psoriasis vulgaris. Dermatologica. 1990;181(3):211–4.

26. Ramsay CA, Schwartz BE, Lowson D, Papp K, Bolduc A, Gilbert M. Calcipotriol cream combined with twice weekly broad-band UVB phototherapy: a safe, effective and UVB-sparing antipsoriatic combination treatment. The Canadian Calcipotriol and UVB Study Group. Dermatology. 2000;200(1):17–24.

27. Speight EL, Farr PM. Calcipotriol improves the response of psoriasis to PUVA. Br J Dermatol. 1994;130(1):79–82.

28. Behrens S, Grundmann-Kollmann M, Peter RU, Kerscher M. Combination treatment of psoriasis with photochemotherapy and tazarotene gel, a receptor-selective topical retinoid. Br J Dermatol. 1999;141(1):177.

29. Dover JS, McEvoy MT, Rosen CF, Arndt KA, Stern RS. Are topical corticosteroids useful in phototherapy for psoriasis? J Am Acad Dermatol. 1989; 20(5 Pt 1):748–54.

30. Horwitz SN, Johnson RA, Sefton J, Frost P. Addition of a topically applied corticosteroid to a modified Goeckerman regimen for treatment of psoriasis: effect on duration of remission. J Am Acad Dermatol. 1985;13(5 Pt 1):784–91.

31. Petrozzi JW. Topical steroids and UV radiation in psoriasis. Arch Dermatol. 1983;119(3):207–10.

32. LeVine MJ, Parrish JA. The effect of topical fluocinonide ointment on phototherapy of psoriasis. J Invest Dermatol. 1982;78(2):157–9.

33. Hanke CW, Steck WD, Roenigk HH Jr. Combination therapy for psoriasis. Psoralens plus long-wave ultraviolet radiation with betamethasone valerate. Arch Dermatol. 1979;115(9):1074–7.

34. Schmoll M, Henseler T, Christophers E. Evaluation of PUVA, topical corticosteroids and the combination of both in the treatment of psoriasis. Br J Dermatol. 1978;99(6):693–702.

35. Gould PW, Wilson L. Psoriasis treated with clobetasol propionate and photochemotherapy. Br J Dermatol. 1978;98(2):133–6.

36. Stern RS, Laird N, Melski J, Parrish JA, Fitzpatrick TB, Bleich HL. Cutaneous

squamous-cell carcinoma in patients treated with PUVA. N Engl J Med. 1984; 310(18):1156–61.

37. Larko O, Swanbeck G. Is UVB treatment of psoriasis safe? A study of extensively UVB-treated psoriasis patients compared with a matched control group. Acta Derm Venereol. 1982;62(6):507–12.

38. Pittelkow MR, Perry HO, Muller SA, Maughan WZ, O'Brien PC. Skin cancer in patients with psoriasis treated with coal tar. A 25-year follow-up study. Arch Dermatol. 1981;117(8):465–8.

39. Ruzicka T, Sommerburg C, Braun-Falco O, Koster W, Lengen W, Lensing W, Letzel H, Meigel WN, Paul E, Przybilla B, et al. Efficiency of acitretin in combination with UV-B in the treatment of severe psoriasis. Arch Dermatol. 1990;126(4):482–6.

40. Orfanos CE, Steigleder GK, Pullmann H, Bloch PH. Oral retinoid and UVB radiation: a new, alternative treatment for psoriasis on an out-patient basis. Acta Derm Venereol. 1979;59(3):241–4.

41. Halasz CL. Narrowband UVB phototherapy for psoriasis: results with fixed increments by skintype (as opposed to percentage increments). Photodermatol Photoimmunol Photomed. 1999;15(2):81–4.

42. Tanew A, Guggenbichler A, Honigsmann H, Geiger JM, Fritsch P. Photochemotherapy for severe psoriasis without or in combination with acitretin: a randomized, double-blind comparison study. J Am Acad Dermatol. 1991;25(4): 682–4.

43. Anstey A, Hawk JL. Isotretinoin-PUVA in women with psoriasis. Br J Dermatol. 1997;136(5):798–9.

44. Paul BS, Momtaz K, Stern RS, Arndt KA, Parrish JA. Combined methotrexate–ultraviolet B therapy in the treatment of psoriasis. J Am Acad Dermatol. 1982;7(6):758–62.

45. Morison WL, Momtaz K, Parrish JA, Fitzpatrick TB. Combined methotrexate-PUVA therapy in the treatment of psoriasis. J Am Acad Dermatol. 1982; 6(1):46–51.

46. Stern RS, Laird N. The carcinogenic risk of treatments for severe psoriasis. Photochemotherapy follow-up study. Cancer. 1994 Jun 1;73(11):2759–64.

47. Frezza EE, Fung JJ, van Thiel DH. Non-lymphoid cancer after liver transplantation. Hepatogastroenterology. 1997;44(16):1172–81.

48. Marcil I, Stern RS. Squamous-cell cancer of the skin in patients given PUVA and ciclosporin: nested cohort crossover study. Lancet. 2001;358(9287):1042–5.

49. Korstanje MJ, Hulsmans RF. Combination therapy cyclosporin A—PUVA in psoriasis. Acta Derm Venereol. 1990;70(1);89–90.

50. Smith KJ, Skelton HG. Rapid onset of cutaneous squamous cell carcinoma in patients with rheumatoid arthritis after starting tumor necrosis factor alpha receptor IgG1-Fc fusion complex therapy. J Am Acad Dermatol. 2001;45(6): 953–6.

51. Sauer GC. Combined methotrexate and hydroxyurea therapy for psoriasis. Arch Dermatol. 1973;107(3):369–70.

52. Islam MN, Alam MN, Haq SA, Moyenuzzaman M, Patwary MI, Rahman

MH. Efficacy of sulphasalazine plus methotrexate in rheumatoid arthritis. Bangladesh Med Res Counc Bull. 2000;26(1):1–7.

53. Allegue Rodriguez F, Sendagorta Gomendio E, Freire Murgueytio P, Moreno Izquierdo R, Ledo Pozueta A. [Treatment of erythrodermic and pustulous psoriasis with a combination of methotrexate and etretinate] Med Cutan Ibero Lat Am. 1988;16(1):43–9.

54. Rosenbaum MM, Roenigk HH Jr. Treatment of generalized pustular psoriasis with etretinate (Ro 10-9359) and methotrexate. J Am Acad Dermatol. 1984; 10(2 Pt 2):357–61.

55. Tuyp E, MacKie RM. Combination therapy for psoriasis with methotrexate and etretinate. J Am Acad Dermatol. 1986;14(1):70–3.

56. Larsen FG, Nielsen-Kudsk F, Jakobsen P, Schroder H, Kragballe K. Interaction of etretinate with methotrexate pharmacokinetics in psoriatic patients. J Clin Pharmacol. 1990;30(9):802–7.

57. van de Kerkhof PC, de Rooij MJ. Multiple squamous cell carcinomas in a psoriatic patient following high-dose photochemotherapy and cyclosporin treatment: response to long-term acitretin maintenance. Br J Dermatol. 1997; 136(2):275–8.

58. Salomon D, Mesheit J, Masgrau-Peya E, Feldmann R, Saurat JH. Acitretin does not prevent psoriasis relapse related to cyclosporin A tapering. Br J Dermatol. 1994;130(2):257–8.

59. Kuijpers AL, van Dooren-Greebe JV, van de Kerkhof PC. Failure of combination therapy with acitretin and cyclosporin A in 3 patients with erythrodermic psoriasis. Dermatology. 1997;194(l):88–90.

60. Korstanje MJ, van Breda Vriesman CJ, van de Staak WJ. Cyclosporine and methotrexate: a dangerous combination. J Am Acad Dermatol. 1990;3(2 Pt 1): 320–1.

61. Tugwell P, Pincus T, Yocum D, Stein M, Gluck O, Kraag G, McKendry R, Tesser J, Baker P, Wells G. Combination therapy with cyclosporine and methotrexate in severe rheumatoid arthritis. The Methotrexate–Cyclosporine Combination Study Group. N Engl J Med. 1995;333(3):137–41.

62. Mazzanti G, Coloni L, De Sabbata G, Paladini G. Methotrexate and cyclosporin combined therapy in severe psoriatic arthritis. A pilot study. Acta Derm Venereol Suppl (Stockh). 1994;186:116–7.

63. Clark CM, Kirby B, Morris AD, Davison S, Zaki I, Emerson R, Saihan EM, Chalmers RJ, Barker JN, Allen BR, Griffiths CE. Combination treatment with methotrexate and cyclosporin for severe recalcitrant psoriasis. Br J Dermatol. 1999;141(2):279–82.

64. Kirby B, Harrison PV. Combination low-dose cyclosporin (Neoral) and hydroxyurea for severe recalcitrant psoriasis. Br J Dermatol. 1999;140(1):186–7.

65. Cutolo M. Etanercept improves rheumatoid arthritis partially responsive to methotrexate. Clin Exp Rheumatol. 2001;19(6):626–7.

66. Bankhurst AD. Etanercept and methotrexate combination therapy. Clin Exp Rheumatol. 1999;17(6 Suppl 18):S69–72.

67. Weinblatt ME, Kremer JM, Bankhurst AD, Bulpitt KJ, Fleischmann RM, Fox

RI, Jackson CG, Lange M, Burge DJ. A trial of etanercept, a recombinant tumor necrosis factor receptor: Fc fusion protein, in patients with rheumatoid arthritis receiving methotrexate. N Engl J Med. 1999;340(4):253–9.

68. Chaudhari U, Romano P, Mulcahy LD, Dooley LT, Baker DG, Gottlieb AB. Efficacy and safety of infliximab monotherapy for plaque-type psoriasis: a randomised trial. Lancet. 2001;357(9271):1842–7.

69. Maini R, St Clair EW, Breedveld F, Furst D, Kalden J, Weisman M, Smolen J, Emery P, Harriman G, Feldmann M, Lipsky P. Infliximab (chimeric anti-tumour necrosis factor alpha monoclonal antibody)versus placebo in rheumatoid arthritis patients receiving concomitant methotrexate: a randomised phase III trial. ATTRACT Study Group. Lancet. 1999;354(9194):1932–9.

70. Kirby B, Marsland AM, Carmichael AJ, Griffiths CE. Successful treatment of severe recalcitrant psoriasis with combination infliximab and methotrexate. Clin Exp Dermatol. 2001;26(1):27–9.

71. Keane J, Gershon S, Wise RP, Mirabile-Levens E, Kasznica J, Schwieterman WD, Siegel JN, Braun MM. Tuberculosis associated with infliximab, a tumor necrosis factor alpha-neutralizing agent. N Engl J Med. 2001;345(15):1098–104.

72. Ameen M, Smith HR, Barker JN. Combined mycophenolate mofetil and cyclosporin therapy for severe recalcitrant psoriasis. Clin Exp Dermatol. 2001; 26(6);480–3.

73. Davison SC, Morris-Jones R, Powles AV, Fry L. Change of treatment from cyclosporin to mycophenolate mofetil in severe psoriasis. Br J Dermatol. 2000; 143(2):405–7.

9

Pediatric Psoriasis

Peggy Lin and Amy S. Paller
Children's Memorial Hospital and Northwestern University Feinberg School of Medicine, Chicago, Illinois, U.S.A.

Psoriasis is one of several papulosquamous diseases that represent 10% of all cutaneous disorders seen in a busy pediatric dermatology clinic (1). Psoriasis itself accounts for 4% of all dermatoses seen in patients under the age of 16 years (2). In childhood, psoriasis may vary from a life-threatening neonatal pustular or exfoliative dermatosis to an entity of almost subclinical impact.

I. EPIDEMIOLOGY

Thirty-one to 45% of adults with psoriasis had the onset of disease during the first 2 decades of life (3–5). To some extent, the incidence estimates have been hampered by the unclear definitions of childhood psoriasis, particularly the question of whether psoriatic diaper rash is true psoriasis (see below). In the childhood population, there is a slight female preponderance with a female/ male ratio of 1.13:1 (6) to 1.25:1 (3). As in the adult populations, white children develop psoriasis more commonly than African-American children, who in turn develop it more commonly than Native Americans or Asians (7). Although Farber and Nall noted that 2% of all patients with psoriasis had the initial onset of disease by 2 years of age (4), a recent survey of 1262 Australian children with psoriasis, including diaper region psoriasis, found that 16% of the patients were less than 1 year of age and 27% were under 2 years (6). Neonatal and congenital onsets of psoriasis have been reported.

The origin of psoriasis appears to be multifactorial, with both genetic and environmental factors playing major roles. A positive family history of psoriasis has been found in up to 70% of pediatric patients, regardless of

197

inclusion of psoriatic diaper rash (3, 6, 8), and twins with psoriasis have been reported. Swanbeck et al. investigated the first-degree relatives of more than 3000 patients with psoriasis and showed a lifetime risk of inheriting psoriasis if no parent, one parent, and two parents had psoriasis of 4%, 28%, and 65%, respectively (9). Human leukocyte antigen (HLA) types Cw6 and DR7 are linked to early-onset psoriasis (under 40 years of age) (10). Tiilikainen et al. noted the prevalence of HLA-Cw6 in 72.7% of patients with the guttate form of psoriasis and 45.9% of patients overall with the medium to large plaque form (vs. 7.4% of the general population of Finland) (11).

II. MANIFESTATIONS OF PEDIATRIC PSORIASIS

In general, the diagnosis of psoriasis in children is based on clinical features. Biopsy confirmation is rarely necessary, and should be avoided unless critical to the diagnosis, such as in pustular psoriasis. Psoriasis may take on several presentations in the pediatric population. Most common is the medium to large plaque type (34–84%) (5, 6, 8, 12). The knees are the most common body location of plaques (4). The plaques are usually smaller and the scale finer and softer in children than in adults. In dark-skinned children, the scale may be so subtle that the lesions appear to be areas of hypopigmentation, with the scale only obvious when the lesions are scratched. The appearance of psoriatic lesions after skin injury (Koebner phenomenon) has been described in 50% of pediatric patients, in contrast to 39% of adults (3). Although lesions may be pruritic in 80% of children, the itchiness tends to be mild (3).

The small plaque of guttate (or teardrop-shaped) psoriasis is the presentation in 6.4–44% of patients, depending on the survey (5, 6) and whether diaper area psoriasis is included. The 1–3 mm guttate lesions are most commonly distributed on the trunk and proximal extremities (Fig. 1). The association of the guttate form with recent streptococcal infection (usually 1–3 weeks earlier), particularly of the throat or perianal area, is well known (5, 13). In a questionnaire study of 5600 patients, 17% of patients 9 years of age and under and 32% of patients between 10 and 19 years of age reported a recent throat infection as an initial trigger of their psoriasis (4). The incidence of guttate psoriasis in a given population may reflect the frequency and form of streptococcal infection.

Morris et al. have proposed that psoriatic diaper rash (Fig. 2) and psoriatic diaper rash with dissemination be considered psoriasis or at least precursors to psoriasis in some children. In their recent series, 13% of children presented with psoriatic diaper rash with dissemination and 4% with localized psoriatic diaper rash (6). The major difficulty with this classification lies in differentiating it from infantile seborrheic dermatitis. The sharp definition of

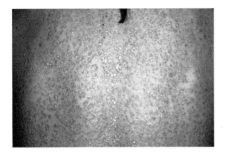

Figure 1 The small guttate plaques of psoriasis, most common on the trunk, are frequently the presenting feature of pediatric psoriasis, especially following streptococcal infection. (Refer to the color insert.)

plaques, brightly erythematous coloration, shininess, and larger and drier scale of plaques of psoriasis help to differentiate it from seborrheic dermatitis (14–19). The frequency of diaper area psoriasis in infants likely reflects the Koebner phenomenon, triggered by the trauma from exposure to stool and urine. The diagnosis should be based strictly on clinical grounds, since biopsy of lesions at this age is usually inappropriate. Because scale is often absent in the moist diaper area, the diagnosis may be obscured. Psoriatic diaper rash with dissemination is the most common form of psoriasis in infancy. Several of these infants have later shown other forms of psoriasis (6). Psoriasis may also involve the groin area in older children. In young girls, psoriasis is the diagnosis of 17% of prepubertal girls presenting with a vulvar region complaint (20). However, diaper area genital involvement more commonly persists into childhood and adolescence in boys. Lesions may present as well-

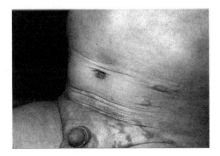

Figure 2 Diaper area psoriasis shows brightly erythematous, well-demarcated plaques. (Refer to the color insert.)

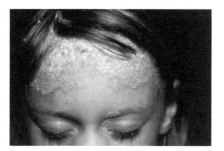

Figure 3   Facial psoriasis is more common in children than in adults. (Refer to the color insert.)

demarcated, red, nonscaling, symmetrical plaques involving the vulva, perineum, and often the natal cleft, but never the vagina.

Facial involvement has been described more commonly in children than in adults (Fig. 3). A rash on the face is the sole manifestation in 4–5% of patients (6, 21), although 38–46% have facial involvement in addition to involvement elsewhere (5, 6, 22). Psoriatic lesions tend to be more clearly demarcated than patches of atopic dermatitis, are less itchy, and commonly have an annular configuration. Involvement of the periorbital area is particularly common, although distribution in the nasolabial folds and perioral area is also not uncommon. Lesions may range in intensity from subtle to florid. In a recent series, facial involvement was noted in 98% of children with psoriatic diaper rash with dissemination (6).

Psoriasis of the scalp is the most common presenting feature for many children—in several studies it is the site of onset for 40–60% of patients prior to 20 years of age (22, 23). Scalp psoriasis is usually characterized by discrete patches of erythema with overlying scale, but many authors consider pityriasis amiantacea (tinea amiantacea) to be a form of psoriasis or a precursor to it. The classic sign of pityriasis amiantacea is the micalike scale adherent to the hair and large plates of scale attached to the scalp (Fig. 4). Typical psoriatic plaques of the scalp or elsewhere are not seen at onset. Focal hair loss and secondary infection may be associated. Pityriasis amiantacea usually begins during the teenage years and occasionally progresses to clear psoriasis (2.5–15% of patients after a mean of 6–8 years) (24, 25). Localized scalp psoriasis may also occur at the nape of the neck in young children overlying a salmon patch.

Several of the cutaneous variants of psoriasis seen in adults occur rarely in children. These include pustular, acropustular, erythrodermic, linear (26), and follicular forms. Geographic tongue may also represent a form of psoriasis in children. Pustular psoriasis has been described in

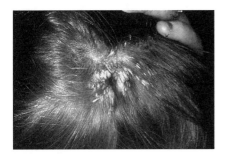

Figure 4 Pityriasis amiantacea is characterized by patches of erythema and micalike scale adherent to the hair and scalp. (Refer to the color insert.)

more than 300 children. Five clinical patterns of sterile pustules have been noted: generalized or von Zumbusch form, annular, exanthematic, localized, and a mixed variant with features of both the generalized and annular patterns. Of these, the annular form is the most common in children (60% of the pustular psoriasis in children) (27, 28), with a mean age of onset being 6 years of age. Pustular psoriasis has been described as early as the first week of life (28, 29). Diagnosis should be confirmed by biopsy, which shows spongiotic pustules and Munro's abscesses in addition to the classic parakeratosis and elongated ridges of psoriasis. Associated fever, malaise, and anorexia may be severe. All forms can have a recurrent course over years to decades, although the episodes are usually less severe in the annular and mixed forms than in the generalized form. Lytic bone lesions may be associated (29, 30). In contrast to the occurrence of pustular psoriasis after a history of psoriasis vulgaris in adults, the occurrence of pustular psoriasis in a child is not uncommonly the presenting sign of psoriasis. The erythrodermic form is quite rare. It is characterized by erythema involving more than 90% of the total body surface and with less scaling than in the plaque type of psoriasis. Patients with erythrodermic or extensive pustular psoriasis usually require hospitalization, and courses are not uncommonly complicated by bacterial septicemia (28).

Approximately 5% of pediatric patients show an eczema/psoriasis overlap (6). These patients may either have both typical plaques of psoriasis and features of eczema, or may show scaling erythematous patches with features intermediate between eczema and psoriasis. Most children with the latter initially show typical nummular dermatitis. Almost all patients with the overlap have a family history of both atopic disease and psoriasis.

Nail psoriasis occurs in up to 40% of patients with psoriasis under 18 years of age (Fig. 5) (5, 22, 31). Although these are more common during the

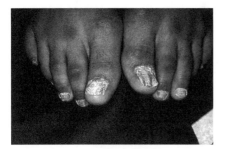

Figure 5   Nail psoriasis is more common in adolescents than in young children, and is characterized by nail pitting, discoloration, onycholysis, and/or subungual hyperkeratosis. (Refer to the color insert.)

second decade of life than the first (32), Farber and Jacobs found nail changes in 79% of patients with infantile psoriasis (33). Nail pitting has also been observed at birth in a neonate who developed diaper area psoriasis at 2 weeks of age (31). The nail changes seen in children are similar to those in adults. Most common is nail pitting, caused by tiny psoriatic lesions of the nail matrix. Discoloration, onycholysis (separation of the distal and lateral nail plate edges), and subungual hyperkeratosis (lifting of the nail plate with nail thickening) are also commonly seen in children with nail involvement. Secondary bacterial, candidal, or occasionally dermatophyte infections occur with increased frequency.

The only noncutaneous features of childhood psoriasis are psoriatic arthritis and psoriatic uveitis. Although rare in children, several large series of juvenile psoriatic arthritis have been reported (34–38). In the past, the diagnosis of psoriatic arthritis was difficult to make without the presence of skin lesions. However, researchers have now established criteria for making the diagnosis, even without the cutaneous changes of psoriasis. These so-called Vancouver Criteria include nail pitting, dactylitis, a psoriasis-like rash, and a family history of psoriasis (34). Definite juvenile psoriatic arthritis is defined as having three of the four criteria; if two of the four are present, the diagnosis is probable. Rheumatoid factor is always negative, but antinuclear antibody (ANA) is positive in 50–63% of affected patients (34, 38), especially in affected girls with more severe disease (35). Psoriatic arthritis is considered a relatively common form of chronic arthropathy that differs clinically, genetically, and serologically from both juvenile ankylosing spondylitis and juvenile rheumatoid arthritis (38). A female predominance has been correlated with earlier age of onset of the arthritis (38). Up to 50% of patients with psoriatic arthritis have a family history of psoriasis. Most patients have involvement of a single joint/pauciarthritis at onset, most commonly the knee, but the pauciarticular involvement progresses to asymmetrical polyarthritis in 64% of patients (34). Either the skin disease or arthritis may develop initially, and in most patients, flares of joint and skin disease are not correlated. Psoriatic uveitis, an asymmetrical anterior uveitis, is found in 14–17% of children with juvenile psoriatic arthritis (34, 38). The outcome of the joint disease does not correlate with either the presence of a positive ANA or uveitis. Although human leukocyte antigen (HLA) B27 was found in 53% of children with definite psoriatic arthritis and a positive family history, but in only 5% without a family history of psoriasis (35), no such association has been described in other studies, in contrast to the documented relationship in adults with psoriatic arthritis (38, 39).

III. IMPORTANT HISTORICAL INFORMATION

Evaluation of the pediatric patient always takes longer than that of the adult patient, because of the time needed to gain the trust of a child and establish rapport. In taking the history of a pediatric patient with a scaly inflammatory disease suspected to be psoriasis, there are several useful questions:

1. Is there a family history of psoriasis?
2. Is the eruption periodic?
3. Do new lesions appear in areas where he or she has been bruised, scratched, burned, or otherwise traumatized?
4. Is there a family history of arthritis?
5. What time of year did the eruption begin? (Psoriasis onset is more common in fall or winter than in summer.)
6. Is there a specific time of year when the eruption gets better? Is there a benefit from sunlight?
7. Has there been a recent or chronic history of sore throat or streptococcal infection?

IV. PSYCHOSOCIAL ASPECTS

Psoriasis inflicts an emotional toll on affected children and their families. The highly visible disorder has an impact on one's self-esteem, psychosocial development, and ability to function socially (40). As with any visible and chronic skin disorder, the embarrassment and effect on social relationships can affect patients and families differently, based on the individual's personality and sensitivity to the opinions of others. However, teenagers and older children need to become well educated about psoriasis in order to face the

Table 1 Tips for Teens and Older Children

Become educated about psoriasis

Develop responses to questions about the psoriasis and practice them; make sure to
impart that psoriasis is not contagious or self-inflicted but a medical condition

Be open about the disorder—don't try to hide it; however, you may choose to
wear long sleeves, for example, to make coping in public easier

Use your therapy as directed, but seek guidance from your physician if the results
are not satisfactory

Check out the National Psoriasis Foundation's Web site: message boards, live chat,
and pen pal programs. Request one of the free booklets for kids, youth, teens.
Become a member and receive regular mailings with columns and information
just for kids

Seek support on a personal level with your doctor, other adults and peers; discuss
your feelings; remember that real friends want to know about psoriasis and
want to help

Expect some negative experiences, but have the resolve to get past them

Acknowledge that confusion and anger are normal reactions; seek help if you feel sad
or depressed

Focus on positive experiences—with family, friends, hobbies, travel, sports; there is
more to life than the skin condition

Decide to be happy and have fun—and then do it; you are in control,
not your psoriasis

---

disorder healthily (Table 1). In addition, parents of children with psoriasis
need to become involved in their child's psoriasis to encourage healthy
psychosocial development and effective therapy (Table 2). The National
Psoriasis Foundation (NPF) has a youth program specifically designed for
children and teenagers, their parents, and caregivers. It includes educational
booklets, web site activities, and other information that encourages dealing
with the psoriasis through education and emotional support (www.psoriasis.
org). The NPF also has a special column in its member newsletter dedicated to
kids and teens.

V. DISORDERS THAT RESEMBLE PSORIASIS

Psoriasis in children or adolescents with guttate psoriasis may be confused
with pityriasis rosea or parapsoriasis (including parapsoriasis lichenoides et
varioliformis acuta and parapsoriasis lichenoides chronica). Pityriasis rubra
pilaris is the hardest to differentiate, especially when involving largely the
palms, soles, elbows, and knees. The follicular accentuation, focal areas of
sparing, and sometimes more salmon coloration of pityriasis rubra pilaris can

Table 2 Tips for Parents

Learn about psoriasis; if you are educated, you can teach others

Explain to the child that the more people understand psoriasis, the better; encourage your child to practice telling you about the psoriasis as if you were a friend or teacher; make sure that the child can impart that the psoriasis is not self-inflicted or contagious, but a medical condition of skin cells that grow too fast associated with inflammation

Listen to your child and try to elicit feelings about the psoriasis and how it affects him or her; always acknowledge the feelings and that having psoriasis is not easy; encourage your child to ask for support

Help the child find friends with whom he or she can identify, who can see beyond the psoriasis

Dealing with psoriasis in a child can be time-consuming, but recognize the potential impact on the entire family; spend equal time with other children and encourage their involvement in care of the disorder

Find the right doctor who can educate, be supportive, and provide optimal care for this chronic disorder

Set up a "treatment center" in the home and show the commitment to the treatment regimen that sets the example for your child in developing future responsibility

Use games when applying treatments so that the interaction becomes pleasant and the kids are engaged in the treatment

As the child gets older, encourage him or her to share in the responsibility of therapy and making appropriate choices; responsibility fosters independence and a sense of control over the condition; by the age of 6–7 years, most children can participate in the application of moisturizers or topical medications

Always be positive and hopeful, since your attitude affects your child and sets the example

Contact the National Psoriasis Foundation and get current information, support from other parents, and many resources to help your child, including Web activities, pen pals, message boards, story books and more. Call (800) 723-9166 or visit www.psoriasis.org

---

help to differentiate the conditions clinically; biopsy sections of pityriasis rubra pilaris may show perifollicular inflammation. In addition, widespread chronic eczematous dermatosis, lichen planus, drug eruption, or widespread dermatophytosis may also be confused with psoriasis (Table 3). When scaling plaques of psoriasis affect the sun-exposed areas of the face, they must be differentiated from lesions of discoid lupus erythematosus; nasolabial and periauricular involvement in the affected adolescent patient may resemble seborrheic dermatitis. Diaper area psoriasis is often confused with candidal diaper dermatitis with or without an id reaction, seborrheic dermatitis, or irritant contact dermatitis. Scalp psoriasis may be mistaken for tinea capitis

Table 3 Disorders to Be Differentiated from Psoriasis in Children

Parapsoriasis (e.g., parapsoriasis lichenoides et varioliformis acuta
  and parapsoriasis lichenoides chronica)
Pityriasis rubra pilaris
Pityriasis rosea
Lichen planus
Dermatophytosis
Diaper area
Irritant dermatitis
Candidal dermatitis
Nail
Onychomycosis
Trachyonychia
Scalp
Tinea capitis
Seborrheic dermatitis
Chronic dermatosis
Other: drug eruption, pityriasis rubra pilaris, secondary syphilis,
  T-cell lymphoma (adolescent)
Hand/feet: dermatitis (atopic, dyshidrotic), contact dermatitis, severe
  tinea pedis

or, if more widespread, severe seborrheic dermatitis. The differential diagnosis of psoriasis of the nail includes nail changes after trauma, onychomycosis, and lichen planus, the latter being the least common in a child. Pustular
psoriasis may be misdiagnosed as infection (impetigo, staphylococcal folliculitis or staphylococcal scalded skin syndrome, candidal pustulosis, or
widespread herpes simplex infection) or, when exfoliative, as toxic epidermal
necrolysis. Erythrodermic psoriasis may be confused with extensive pityriasis
rubra pilaris and ichthyotic disorders, particularly congenital ichthyosiform
erythroderma and erythrokeratodermia variabilis.

VI. THERAPY

Education is a key component of the therapy of psoriasis. Patients and
parents must understand the chronicity of the disorder and the tendency for
spontaneous remissions, particularly in the pediatric population (3). In
addition, the concept of the Koebner phenomenon or isomorphic response
(that injury to skin may exacerbate psoriasis) should be imparted (Table 4).
Other trigger factors should also be considered, including infection (especially

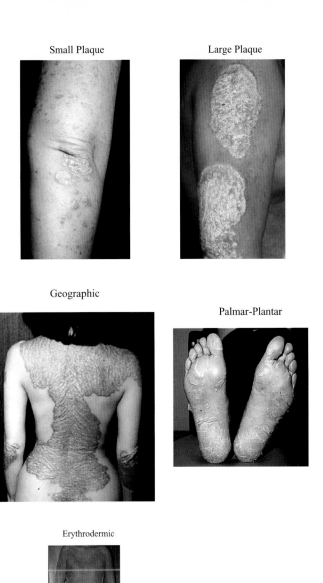

Figure 1.1 Morphological variants of psoriasis: Is this one disease?

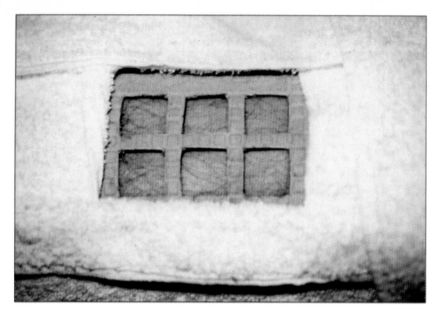

Figure 3.1 In conducting formal MED testing, a different amount of UVB radiation is applied sequentially to each opening in the template, which is made of an opaque material such as a thick piece of cardboard. The increment of UVB exposure used is usually 15 or 30 s when a UVB box with fluorescent lights is utilized.

Figure 3.2 The result of MED testing on the body.

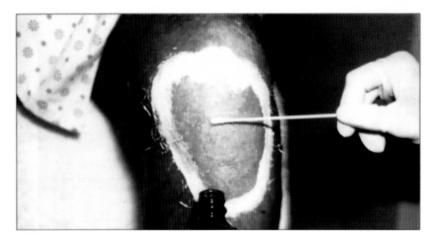

Figure 3.7 The application of topical "paint" PUVA therapy to selected, resistant psoriatic plaques is shown. Zinc oxide paste is sometimes used to prevent inadvertent application of 0.1% Oxsoralen solution to the noninvolved skin.

A   B

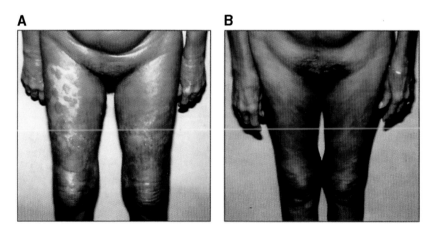

Figure 3.8 Erythrodermic patient with psoriasis and intense leg edema before (A) and after (B) short-term cyclosporine followed by long-term UVB phototherapy. This therapeutic regimen makes use of the powerful anti-inflammatory property of cyclosporine while minimizing the risk of systemic effects, which may be associated with long-term use of cyclosporine.

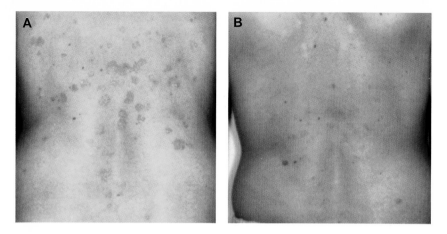

Figure 6.2   Patient with recalcitrant plaque-type psoriasis (A) before and (B) after treatment with 25 mg acitretin each day plus etanercept 25 mg twice a week subcutaneously for 8 weeks.

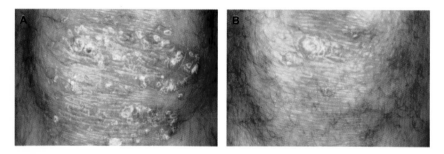

Figure 6.3   Patient with plaque-type psoriasis (A) before and (B) after treatment with oral tazarotene 4.2 mg each day for 12 weeks.

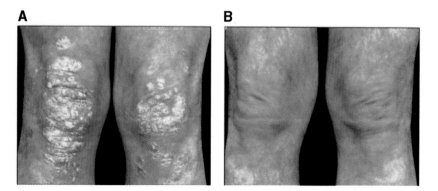

Figure 7.1   A typical optimal response to cyclosporine therapy for psoriasis. (A) Pretherapy. (B) After 8 weeks of cyclosporine, 3 mg/kg/day.

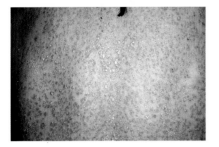

Figure 9.1 The small guttate plaques of psoriasis, most common on the trunk, are frequently the presenting feature of pediatric psoriasis, especially following streptococcal infection.

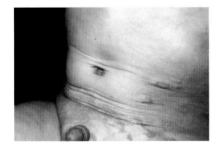

Figure 9.2 Diaper area psoriasis shows brightly erythematous, well-demarcated plaques.

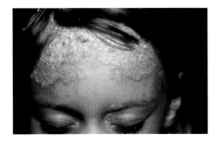

Figure 9.3 Facial psoriasis is more common in children than in adults.

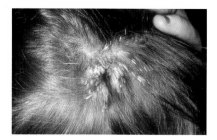

Figure 9.4 Pityriasis amiantacea is characterized by patches of erythema and micalike scale adherent to the hair and scalp.

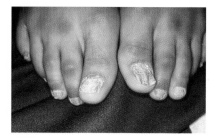

Figure 9.5 Nail psoriasis is more common in adolescents than in young children, and is characterized by nail pitting, discoloration, onycholysis, and/or subungual hyperkeratosis.

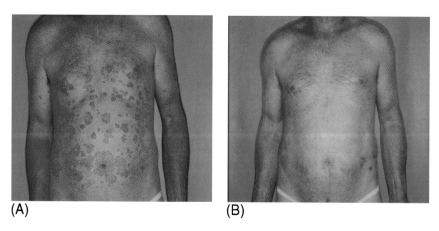

(A)   (B)

Figure 14.6 Photographic record of infliximab therapy.

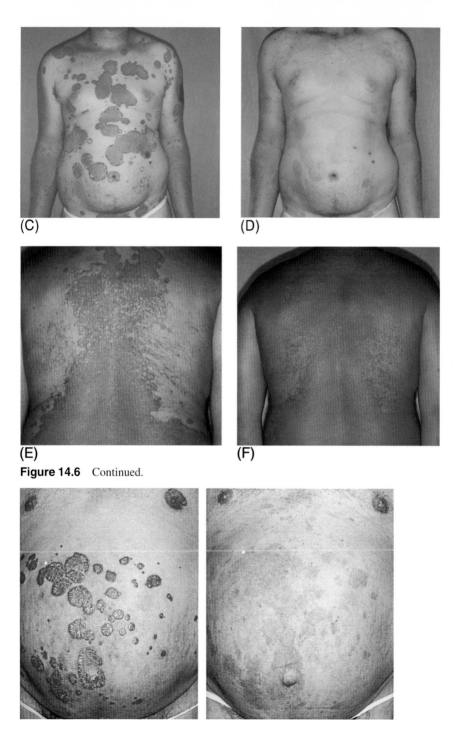

Figure 14.6 Continued.

Figure 15.9 Representative patient responses.

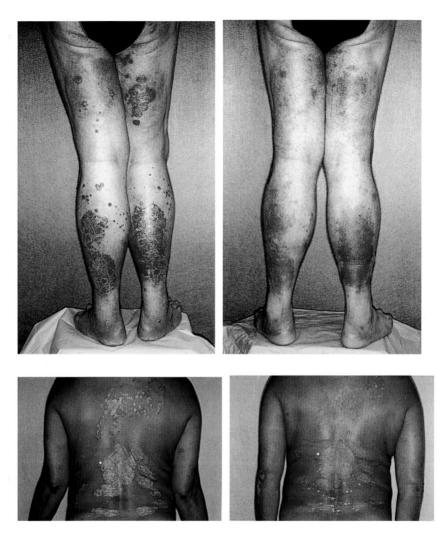

Figure 15.9 Continued.

Table 4 Prevention of Psoriasis in Pediatric Patients

Location	Intervention
Face	Avoid overexposure to ultraviolet light and irritating soaps
Creases and folds	Avoid irritating underarm deodorants
Genital and perianal regions	Avoid irritation from accumulation of feces and urine and from tight garments
Hands and feet	Avoid contact with irritating soaps or other substances
	Avoid tight shoes and accumulation of moisture, including sweat, on the feet
Scalp	Avoid vigorous combing, picking, or scratching of the scalp
Nails	Avoid long fingernails or toenails, trauma to nails in play situations, or wearing tight shoes

streptococcal) and medications (e.g., systemic steroids, lithium, antimalarials, and beta blockers). Above all, therapy should be conservative as appropriate for the type and severity of the psoriasis, and parents must realize the potential side effects of prescribed therapy.

A. Topical Therapy

The most commonly used topical therapies in children include topical corticosteroids, calcipotriene, tar preparations, and anthralin (short-contact therapy). Emollients are used as adjunctive agents to decrease the associated scaling and dryness, but should not replace medications when inflammation is present.

In plaque-stage psoriasis, the mainstay of treatment remains corticosteroid preparations (Table 5). Most commonly, application up to twice daily of class II–IV midpotency topical steroids is most useful for lesions on the trunk and extremities. Use of halogenated steroids, however, should be avoided in the diaper area, intertriginous areas, and on the face. Topical steroid options for these sensitive areas should never be stronger than nonhalogenated low- to medium-strength preparations, such as hydrocortisone acetate preparations (1.0–2.5%), desonide, and aclometasone dipropionate, hydrocortisone butyrate, or prednicarbate. Topical calcipotriene and tacrolimus ointment are steroid-sparing alternatives (see below).

Once the acute lesions are under control, treatment can be tapered to lower-potency steroids and/or emollients. If individual thick plaques fail to respond, higher-potency topical steroid preparations can be used, but should be limited to no longer than 2 week continuing courses. As in adults, weekend therapy with class I steroids can be used in adolescents with severe

Table 5 Treatment of Psoriasis in Children

	Use in children	Potential side effects
Topical preparations		
Emollients	Useful in mild disease; adjunct	None
Topical steroids	Firstline therapy: all types of psoriasis	Tachyphylaxis
		Local side effects: atrophy, striae
		Systemic side effects: impaired growth, adrenal suppression, cataracts
Tar/anthralin	Thicker plaques; short contact anthralin	Irritation, staining
Calcipotriene	Limited plaques	Irritation
Tazarotene gel	Limited plaques	Irritation
Tacrolimus	Face, intertriginous areas	Burning with first applications
Phototherapy		
Ultraviolet B	Widespread plaques	Cost, inconvenience, premature aging, skin cancer
Psoralens–UVA	Rarely indicated	As for UVB; cataracts with systemic psoralens
Systemic therapy		
Methotrexate	Recalcitrant extensive plaques, erythrodermic, pustular psoriasis, psoriasic arthritis	Bone marrow and hepatotoxicity
Cyclosporine	Recalcitrant severe psoriasis	Renal and hepatic toxicity, hypertrichosis, immunosuppression, UVB-induced skin cancer
Acetretin	Especially for pustular psoriatis	Cheilitis, hyperlipidemia, musculoskeletal pain, hair loss, skin fragility, bone toxicity if used long-term

disease, but their use must be monitored carefully (41). It should be noted that the preadolescent/adolescent population is particularly at risk for developing striae from the use of the superpotent steroids. Use of keratolytic agents to enhance penetration, such as 6% salicylic acid compounded into steroid ointment or at a separate time (e.g., Keralyt gel), occlusion, or steroid-impregnated tapes are alternative treatments for more hyperkeratotic, resistant lesions. Selected resistant lesions may respond to the use of intralesional triamcinolone (diluted to 3–5 mg/ml). Intralesional injections are rarely used in pediatric patients because of the associated discomfort. However, the availability of topical anesthetic creams (e.g., EMLA or Elamax) may prove helpful in diminishing the discomfort of injections, especially in younger children.

B. Tar and Anthralin Preparations

Tar preparations, especially when used in association with daily incremental outdoor ultraviolet light, are a time-honored and effective adjunct to the topical treatment of psoriasis. Tar (in the form of 1–10% crude coal tar or liquor carbonis detergens) can be compounded into preparations or used alone: either at bedtime and left on overnight or applied for 30 mins before ultraviolet light exposure (Goeckerman regimen). Tar may also be administered in the form of a tar bath. Tar preparations, however, stain skin and clothing, and have an odor that is often objectionable to children and adolescents.

Anthralin preparations provide an alternative to tar treatment. Short-contact anthralin therapy (SCAT) led to remission in 81% of children with plaque psoriasis, treated for 30 mins with up to 1% anthralin cream (42). SCAT can be applied in the form of a 1% anthralin cream (Micanol, Psoriatec), a microencapsulated form that results in marked reduction in discoloration of skin or clothing (43, 44). This medication is formulated in a temperature-sensitive vehicle that releases the active medication at the skin surface temperature; the medication must be washed out with cold water to avoid release of the anthralin from vehicle during washing (41). Short-contact anthralin application should start with 5 min applications of the 1% anthralin (the only concentration currently available commercially), and can be increased in duration every other day as tolerated and needed for efficacy, limiting the duration of application to no more than 1 h. If the 1% anthralin causes too much irritation, it can be diluted. Bland emollient or protective paste can be applied on the normal skin surrounding the area of psoriasis to minimize the risk of irritation of noninvolved skin. Contact with face, eyes, and mucous membranes should be avoided. Triethanolamine, marketed as CuraStain, markedly reduces the minimal staining and irritation of anthralin when sprayed on skin or fabrics before and after cleaning.

C. Vitamin D₃ Derivatives

Calcipotriene, an analog of vitamin D_3, has been formulated as a 0.005% ointment that is most effective when combined with topical steroids, but serves as a steroid-sparing agent and has been efficacious in children as monotherapy as well (45, 46). However, care must be taken to ensure compatibility of the calcipotriene ointment and the topical steroid. For example, calcipotriene can be mixed directly with halobetasol ointment for so-called weekend therapy, but is destabilized by hydrocortisone valerate ointment or ammonium lactate lotion, and is completely inactivated by salicylic acid. Calcipotriene is best applied twice daily, but the onset of action is slow (maximal response is 6–8 weeks). Calcipotriene is also available as a solution for scalp psoriasis and a cream that is slightly less effective than the ointment, but is devoid of the propylene glycol present in the ointment and solution forms. Irritant dermatitis, particularly on the face and intertriginous areas, occurs in up to 20% of patients.

D. Tazarotene

The topical retinoid tazarotene gel is available in 0.05% and 0.1% strengths, and can serve as a steroid-sparing agent. Because it is quite irritating as monotherapy, tazarotene is best applied once a day in combination with a medium to potent topical steroid, applied at another time during the day. Even with the combination therapy, use of tazarotene may not be tolerated in children.

E. Tacrolimus 0.1% Ointment

Tacrolimus ointment has recently become available for the treatment of atopic dermatitis in adults and children. A calcineurin inhibitor, tacrolimus blocks the release of inflammatory cytokines by a mechanism that differs from that of topical corticosteroids. It is devoid of the potential local side effects of corticosteroids, particularly atrophy and ocular effects. Although not found to be useful in double-blind trials in adults, our experience and that of others anecdotally is that twice-daily application of tacrolimus ointment 0.1% ointment is effective in the majority of children for facial and intertriginous psoriatic plaques. It often leads to improvement in plaques elsewhere, since the psoriatic plaques in children tend to be thinner than those of adults.

F. Ultraviolet Light

When psoriasis involves more than 15–20% body surface area or involves the palms and soles, and is recalcitrant to topical therapy, children may need and respond to artificial ultraviolet B (UVB) light (290–320 nm), preferably narrow-band UVB (312 nm) (47, 48). The narrow-band UVB has a higher ratio of therapeutic to toxic wavelengths (49). The UVB is best initiated in a light box at a dermatology office as outpatient therapy. Once patients and parents know how to increase the dosages of UV light gradually, judge the effects of the daily treatment, and practice preventive eye care, home light box therapy can be initiated. Home light boxes are ultimately less invasive to the activities of a family and more cost-effective than treatment administered away from home. In general, ultraviolet light therapy is started at 70–75% of the minimal erythema dose and increased by about 10–20% with each treatment, as tolerated. A minimum of three treatments per week is required to clear psoriasis. Although rarely used in young children, phototherapy may be administered to young children who are accompanied by parents in the light unit. Tricks such as use of a radio or CD player with earphones can be used to distract the child during treatment. Acutely, UVB therapy is associated with skin darkening, a chance of skin burning, and, not infrequently, with early pruritus. Although data are lacking on children with psoriasis, recurrent exposure to UVB increases the long-term risk of skin cancer and premature aging. Psoralens and ultraviolet A (PUVA) light are used rarely in children because of the ocular toxicity, generalized photosensitivity, and the risk of later development of cutaneous carcinomas (50). If PUVA is used for severe psoriasis, 8-methoxypsoralen (0.6 mg/kg) is administered, with ultraviolet light dosages similar to those of adults. UVB tends to be less effective in children with skin type IV–VI due to their greater skin pigmentation, although PUVA may be effective. Protective eyewear and clothing as appropriate must be worn by patients receiving ultraviolet light treatments.

VII. TOPICAL SCALP AND NAIL CARE

A. Scalp

Psoriatic scalp lesions are a frustrating and sometimes recalcitrant component of psoriasis. Several techniques and forms of medication are available. Topical corticosteroids may be applied in the form of oils, solutions, or foams. For example, a fluocinolone in peanut oil solution (DermaSmoothe-FS) under shower cap occlusion can be applied for a few hours to overnight to the wet, affected scalp, followed by shampooing with a tar-containing or steroid-containing shampoo. As an alternative, a phenol and saline (P & S) solution with a shower cap for occlusion can be applied overnight. In the morning, one can wash with a keratolytic and/or tar shampoo and gentle massage, followed by application of a steroid solution. Recently, foam preparations of betamethasone valerate and clobetasol have become available to allow delivery of steroids without greasiness.

B. Nails

Psoriatic nail lesions can be difficult to treat, because of the failure of topical agents to penetrate the nail plate. Instillation of steroid preparations into the subproximal nail fold area can be successful, but nightly application of flurandrenolide-impregnated tape to the base of the nail for approximately 6 months yields better results and is not painful, in contrast to steroid injections. Parents must understand that response to therapy is measured in terms of months and that there is no instant gratification. For adolescents, the use of PUVA in a hand/foot box has proven effective in many patients. Methotrexate or other systemic therapies are the most effective means of treatment, but rarely indicated in the pediatric population and never for isolated nail changes. The development of nail psoriasis can be partially prevented by hydration of nails before trimming, keeping nails trimmed, avoidance of manipulation of the cuticles, and wearing shoes that fit properly.

VIII. SYSTEMIC THERAPY

Although most moderate and moderate-to-severe psoriasis will respond to treatment with topical steroids, tar and ultraviolet light, and/or anthralin, in some instances additional therapies may be necessary, particularly for more severe plaque-type, erythrodermic, and pustular forms of psoriasis. In general, systemic corticosteroids should be avoided. Although occasionally effective, they are often ineffective or lead to worsening of psoriasis; furthermore, corticosteroid withdrawal tends to precipitate flares, particularly of pustular psoriasis. Before considering more toxic therapy, some practitioners will prescribe a course of antistreptococcal antibiotics, especially for guttate psoriasis. The association of group A beta-hemolytic streptococci and psoriasis has been well established, and probably relates to M-protein super- antigen expression by the streptococcal organism. These superantigens bypass normal immunological pathways and stimulate the activation of T lymphocytes that are key to the development of psoriasis. Patients with guttate or a significant flare of plaque-type psoriasis without an obvious sore throat or history of recent streptococcal infection may be carriers for strep- tococcal organisms that can be grown by culture. Although the results of therapy are controversial (51, 52), treatment is indicated if culture demonstrates streptococcal infection of the pharynx. Culture should also be performed if the perianal area shows erythema because of the demonstrated relation between perianal streptococcal cellulitis in children and psoriasis (53). Penicillin, erythromycin, and amoxicillin are most commonly used and administered for 4 weeks; one should consider the addition of rifampin if a carrier state is suspected. Other uncontrolled studies have suggested that tonsillectomy is superior to antibiotic administration in the clearance of psoriasis in children (54, 55).

A. Methotrexate

Methotrexate is indicated for severe unresponsive psoriasis, exfoliative erythrodermas, pustular psoriasis, and psoriatic arthritis. Its mechanisms combine antimitotic, antichemotactic, and anti-inflammatory activities. Methotrexate treatment in children is similar to that in adults (56, 57). After appropriate screening tests, oral methotrexate is initiated at a test dosage of 2.5 mg, then up to 20 mg/week is given, depending on weight. Concurrent administration of folic acid 1–5 mg/day ameliorates the risk of nausea, mucosal ulcerations, and macrocytic anemia (58). Screening tests and complications are the same as for adults, with the most common side effects being nausea, fatigue, headaches, and anorexia. The most significant is bone marrow suppression. Liver function should be monitored by blood testing; liver biopsy is unnecessary in children, and hepatic toxicity is rare. During childhood, live vaccines such as measles, mumps, and rubella (MMR) and poliovirus vaccines may not be given to a child taking weekly methotrexate (in the latter case, a killed polio vaccine can be substituted.) Long-term oncogenic risks in children taking methotrexate are of concern but have not been clearly delineated. An option for those who cannot tolerate oral methotrexate is weekly intramuscular or intravenous methotrexate. Clearing is generally seen within 3–6 weeks after initiation of treatment. Once clearing is achieved, the methotrexate dosage should be gradually lowered (for example, 2.5 mg/month) during the subsequent months until a maintenance level is achieved.

B. Retinoids

In general, retinoids tend to be less effective than methotrexate or cyclosporine for treating plaque-type psoriasis, but can be quite effective for pustular psoriasis that does not respond to more conservative therapy, including compresses and topical corticosteroids, and for exfoliative erythrodermas (59, 60). Acitretin normalizes epidermal differentiation and has an anti-inflammatory effect. The usual regimen is 0.5–1.0 mg/kg/day, although the dosage can be titrated, depending on patient response and laboratory results (56). Complications related to acetretin therapy in children are the same as for adults, but the risk of skeletal toxicity (premature epiphyseal closure and hyperostosis), although rare, must be monitored by radiographic evaluations during infancy, childhood, and puberty (60, 61, 62). Screening tests otherwise are the same as for adults (56). As with adults, practitioners should be concerned about teratogenic effects in young women. Isotretinoin may be an alternative retinoid for adolescent girls with pustular psoriasis because of its much more rapid clearance, but it is not generally as effective as acetretin.

C. Cyclosporine

Cyclosporine has been used in young patients with severe unresponsive psoriasis, exfoliative erythrodermas, or pustular psoriasis (56, 63). Its mechanism of action involves inhibition of cytokine statement by T lymphocytes. It has been used for children in regimens that include up to 5 mg/kg/day in oral doses during a 3–4 month period followed by gradual downward titration and discontinuance. The complications of this medicine in children are the same as in adults, particularly hypertension and renal and hepatic toxicity; however, concerns about potential leukemias, lymphomas, cutaneous carcinomas, and other oncogenic risks are heightened with childhood use. Live vaccines (e.g., MMR and poliovirus) cannot be used in patients receiving cyclosporine therapy.

D. Therapy for Psoriatic Arthritis

Most patients with psoriatic arthritis require only nonsteroidal anti-inflammatory drugs, maintenance of joint position, functional splinting, and physiotherapy. Intra-articular corticosteroid injections, oral corticosteroids, intramuscular gold, sulfasalazine, hydroxychloroquine, and methotrexate have also been used as medical therapy for more recalcitrant cases. Occasionally arthroscopic synovectomy or joint replacement is required.

IX. EXPERIMENTAL THERAPIES

Experiments with biological therapies are an exciting and growing field. Currently, adult clinical trials involving biological agents fall into three classes (antibodies, fusion proteins, and recombinant cytokines) (64) and include efalizumab, alefacept, infliximab, etanercept, and interleukins 10 and 11. Etanercept is now approved by the Food and Drug Administration (FDA) for adults with psoriatic arthritis. These therapies have not been studied in children with psoriasis to date, although the tumor necrosis factor-α inhibitor infliximab has been tested in children with Crohn's disease and etanercept is FDA-approved for juvenile rheumatoid arthritis in children 4 years of age and older.

X. CONCLUSIONS

The treatment of psoriasis in children involves a conventional therapeutic regimen of emollients, steroids, calcipotriene, tars, keratolytics, antibiotics, and/or antihistamines. On the other hand, severe unresponsive psoriasis, exfoliative erythrodermas, and pustular psoriasis may require ultraviolet light therapy or treatment with systemic agents, methotrexate, acetretin, or cyclosporine. The use of mycophenolate mofetil and the new biological agents in pediatric patients with severe disease deserves investigation.

REFERENCES

1. Schachner L, Ling MS, Press S. A statistical analysis of a pediatric dermatology clinic. Pediatr Dermatol 1983;1:157–164.
2. Beylot C, Puissant A, Bioulac P, Saurat JH, Pringuet R, Doutre MS. Particular clinical features of psoriasis in infants and children. Acta Derm Venereol Suppl (Stockh). 1979;87:95–7.
3. Raychaudhuri SP, Gross J. A comparative study of pediatric onset psoriasis with adult onset psoriasis. Pediatr Dermatol. 2000;17:174–8.
4. Farber EM, Nall ML. The natural history of psoriasis in 5600 patients. Dermatologica. 1974;109:207–11.
5. Nyfors A, Lemholt K. Psoriasis in children. A short review and a survey of 245 cases. Br J Dermatol. 1975;92:437–42.
6. Morris A, Rogers M, Fischer G, et al. Childhood psoriasis: a clinical review of 1262 cases. Pediatr Dermatol. 2001;18:188–98.
7. Kinney JA. Psoriasis in the American black. In: Farber EM, Cox AJ, eds. Psoriasis: Proceedings of the International Symposium. Stanford University. Stanford, CA: Stanford University Press, 1971:49.
8. Al-Fouzan AS, Nanda A. A survey of childhood psoriasis in Kuwait. Pediatr Dermatol. 1994;116–9.
9. Swanbeck G, Inerot A, Martinsson T, Enerback C, Enlund F, Samuelsson L, Yhr M, Wahlstrom J. Genetic counseling in psoriasis: empirical data on psoriasis among first-degree relatives of 3095 psoriatic probands. Br J Dermatol. 1997 Dec;137:939–42.
10. Henseler T. The genetics of psoriasis. J Am Acad Dermatol. 1997;37:S1–11.

11. Tiilikainen A, Lassus A, Karvonen J, et at. Psoriasis and HLA-Cw6. Br J Dermatol.1980;192:179–84.
12. Menter MA, Whiting DA, McWilliams J. Resistant childhood psoriasis: an analysis of patients seen in a day-care center. Pediatr Dermatol. 1984;2:8–12.
13. Patrizi A, Costa AM, Fiorillio L, et al. Perianal streptococcal dermatitis associated with guttate psoriasis and/or balanoposthitis. Pediatr Dermatol. 1994;11:168.
14. Andersen S, La C, Thomsen K. Psoriasiform napkin dermatitis. Br J Dermatol. 1971;84:316–9.
15. Neville EA, Finn OA. Psoriasiform napkin dermatitis—a follow up study. Br J Dermatol. 1975;92:279–85.
16. Rasmussen HB, Hagdrup JI, Schmidt H. Psoriasiform napkin dermatitis. Acta Dermatol Venereol (Stockh). 1986;66:534–6.
17. Thomsen K. Seborrhoeic dermatitis and napkin dermatitis. Acta Dermatol Venereol (Stockh). 1981; 95:40–2.
18. Menni S, Piccino R, Baietta S, Ciuffreda A, Scotti L. Infantile seborrheic dermatitis: seven year follow-up and some prognostic criteria. Pediatr Dermatol. 1989; 6:13–5.
19. Rattet J, Headley J, Barr R. Diaper dermatitis with psoriasiform id eruption. Int J Dermatol. 1981; 20:122–5.
20. Fischer G, Rogers M. Vulvar disease n children: a clinical audit of 130 cases. Pediatr Dermatol. 2000; 17:1–6.
21. Farber EM. Facial psoriasis. Cutis. 1992; 50:25–8.
22. Nanda A, Kaur S, Kaur I, Kumar B. Childhood psoriasis: an epidemiologic survey of 112 patients. Pediatr Dermatol. 1990; 7:19–21.
23. Farber EM, Nall L. Natural history and treatment of scalp psoriasis. Cutis. 1992; 174.
24. Hersle K, Lindholm A, Mobacken H, Sandberg L. Relationship of pityriasis amiantacea to psoriasis: a follow-up study. Dermatologica. 1979; 159:245–50.
25. Hansted B, Lindskov R. Pityriasis amiantacea and psoriasis. Dermatologica. 1983; 166:314–5.
26. Atherton DJ, Kahan M, Russell-Jones R. Naevoid psoriasis. Br J Dermatol.1989; 120:837–41.
27. Liao PB, Rubinson R, Howard R, Sanchez G, Frieden IJ. Annular pustular psoriasis—most common form of pusular psoriasis in children: report of three cases and review of the literature. Pediatr Dermatol. 2002; 19:19–25.
28. Zelickson BD, Muller SA. Generalized pustular psoriasis in childhood. J Am Acad Dermatol. 1991; 24:186–94.
29. Ivker RA, Grin-Jorgensen CM, Vega VK, Hoss DM, Grant-Kels JM. Infantile generalized pustular psoriasis associated with lytic lesions of the bone. Pediatr Dermatol. 1993; 10:277–82.
30. Prose NS, Fahrner LJ, Miller CR, Layfield L. Pustular psoriasis with chronic recurrent multifocal osteomyelitis and spontaneous fractures. J Am Acad Dermatol. 1994; 31(2 Pt 2):376–9.
31. Farber EM, Nall L. Nail psoriasis. Cutis.1992; 50:174–8.

32. Barth JH, Dawber RPR. Diseases of nails in children. Pediatr Dermatol. 1987; 4:275–90.
33. Farber EM, Jacobs AH. Infantile psoriasis. Am J Dis Child. 1977; 131:1266–9.
34. Southwood TR, Petty RE, Malleson PN, Delgado EA, Hunt DWC, Wood B, Schroeder M-L. Psoriatic arthritis is children. Arthritis Rheum. 1989; 32:1007–1013.
35. Shore A, Ansell BM. Juvenile psoriatic arthritis: an analysis of 60 cases. J Pediatr.1982; 100:529–35.
36. Perlman SG. Psoriatic arthritis in children. Pediatr Dermatol. 1984; 1:283–7.
37. Hafner R, Michels H. Psoriatic arthritis in children. Curr Opin Rheumatol. 1996; 8:467–72.
38. Robertson DM, Cabral DA, Malleson PN, Petty RE. Juvenile psoriatic arthritis: followup and evaluation of diagnostic criteria. J Rheumatol 1996; 23:166–70.
39. Hamilton ML, Gladman DD, Shore A, Laxer R, Silverman ED. Juvenile psoriatic arthritis and HLA arthritis. Ann Rheum Dis. 1990; 49:694–7.
40. Leary MR, Rapp SR, Herbst KC, Exum ML, Feldman SR. Interpersonal concerns and psychological difficulties of psoriasis patients: effects of disease severity and fear of negative evaluation. Health Psychol. 1998; 17:530–6.
41. Lebwohl M, Ali S. Treatment of psoriasis. Part 1. Topical therapy and phototherapy. J Am Acad Dermatol. 2001; 45:487–98.
42. Zvulonov A, Anisfeld A, Metzker A. Efficacy of short-contact therapy with dithranol in childhood psoriasis. Int J Dermatol. 1994; 38;808–10.
43. Lowe NJ, Ashton RE, Koudsi H, Verschoore M, Schaefer H. Anthralin for psoriasis: short-contact anthralin therapy compared with topical steroid and conventional anthralin. J Am Acad Dermatol. 1984; 10:69–72.
44. Harris DR. Old wine in new bottles: the revival of anthralin. Cutis. 1998; 62:201–3.
45. Darley CR, Cunliffe WJ, Green CM, Hutchinson PE, Klabers MR, Downes N. Safety and efficacy of calcipotriol ointment (Dovonex) in treating children with psoriasis vulgaris. Br J Dermatol. 1996; 135:390–3.
46. Oranje AP, Marcoux D, Svensson A, Prendiville J, Krafchik B, O'Toole J, et al. Topical calcipotriol in childhood psoriasis. J Am Acad Dermatol. 1997; 36:203–8.
47. Tay Y, Morelli JG, Weston WL. Experience with UVB phototherapy in children. Pediatr Dermatol. 1996; 13:406–9.
48. Atherton DJ, Cohen BL, Knobler E, Garzon M, Morelli JG, Tay Y, et al. Phototherapy for children. Pediatr Dermatol. 1996; 13:415–26.
49. Barbagallo J, Spann CT, Tutrone WD, Weinberg JM. Narrowband UVB phototherapy for the treatment of psoriasis: a review and update. Cutis. 2001; 68:345–7.
50. Stern RS, Nichols KT, and the PUVA Follow-up Study. Therapy with orally administered methoxsalen and ultraviolet A radiation during childhood increases the risk of basal cell carcinoma. J Pediatr. 1996; 129:915–7.
51. Owens CM, Chalmers RJG, O'Sullivan T, Griffiths CRM. Antistreptococcal

interventions for guttate and chronic plaque psoriasis (Cochrane Review). In: The Cochrane Library, Issue 1, 2002. Oxford, OK: Update Software.

52. Vincent F, Ross JB, Dalton M, Wort AJ. A therapeutic trial of the use of penicillin V or erythromycin with or without rifampin in the treatment of psoriasis. J Am Acad Dermatol. 1992; 26:458–61.

53. Honig PJ. Guttate psoriasis associated with perianal streptococcal disease. J Pediatr. 1988; 113:1037–9.

54. Hone SW, Donnelly MJ, Powell F, Blayney AW. Clearance of recalcitrant psoriasis after tonsillectomy. Clin Otolaryngol Allied Sci 1996; 21:546–7.

55. Nyfors A, Rasmussen PA, Lemholt K, Eriksen B. Improvement of recalcitrant psoriasis vulgaris after tonsillectomy. J Laryngol Otol. 1976; 90:789–94.

56. Lebwohl M, Ali S. Treatment of psoriasis. Part 2. Systemic therapies. J Am Acad Dermatol. 2001; 45:649–61.

57. Bright RD. Methotrexate in the treatment of psoriasis. Cutis. 1999; 64:332–4.

58. Duhra P. Treatment of gastrointestinal symptoms associated with methotrexate therapy for psoriasis. J Am Acad Dermatol. 1993; 288:466–9.

59. Shelnitz LS, Esterly NB, Honig PJ. Etretinate therapy for generalized pustular psoriasis in children. Arch Dermatol. 1987; 123:230–3.

60. Orfanos CE. Treatment of psoriasis with retinoids: present status. Cutis. 1999; 64:347–53.

61. Lacour M, Mehta-Nikhar B, Atherton DJ, Harper JI. An appraisal of acetretin therapy in children with inherited disorders of keratinization. Br J Dermatol. 1996; 134:1023–9.

62. Halkier-Sorensen L, Laurberg G, Andresen J. Bone changes in children on long-term treatment with etretinate. J Am Acad Dermatol. 1987; 16:999–1006.

63. Sebnem Kilic S, Hacimustafaoglu M, Celebi S, Karadeniz A, Ildirim I. Low dose cyclosporin A treatment: generalized pustular psoriasis. Pediatr Dermatol. 2001; 18:246–8.

64. Krueger JG. The immunologic basis for the treatment of psoriasis with new biologic agents. J Am Acad Dermatol.2002; 46:1–23.

10
Psoriatic Arthritis

Dafna D. Gladman
University of Toronto, Toronto Western Research Institute, and Toronto Western Hospital, Toronto, Ontario, Canada

I. EPIDEMIOLOGICAL EVIDENCE

The occurrence of arthritis in patients with psoriasis has been recognized since the 19th century. However, psoriatic arthritis (PsA) was identified as a distinct entity primarily as a consequence of the efforts of the late Professor Verna Wright of Leeds, England, and his colleague Dr. John Moll of Sheffield, England (1). Epidemiological studies have noted that among patients with psoriasis, arthritis occurs in a higher prevalence than in the general population (2). Whereas the frequency of arthritis in the general population is estimated to be 3–5%, among patients with psoriasis 7–42% have been identified as having PsA. Likewise, psoriasis occurs in a higher frequency among patients with arthritis (7%) than among the general population (1–3%). Although there are individuals who disagree with the identification of PsA as a distinct entity (3), it is now widely accepted that there is a specific form of arthritis associated with psoriasis (4).

II. CLINICAL DEFINITION

Based on their observations, Moll and Wright defined psoriatic arthritis as an inflammatory arthritis associated with psoriasis, usually seronegative for rheumatoid factor. Inflammatory-type arthritis presents with pain, swelling, and stiffness in the affected joints. The pain and stiffness are usually worse with rest and are improved with activity, and patients complain of morning stiffness usually greater than 45 min in duration. Any of the peripheral joints may be affected. The larger the number of joints affected, the more likely it is to be in a symmetrical distribution. In addition to the peripheral joint disease, inflammation of the sacroiliac and apophyseal joint of the spine also occur in almost half the patients with PsA. About 40% of patients with PsA carry the human leukocyte antigen (HLA)-B*27 allele.

Because of the presence of the spondyloarthropathy in 40–50% of the patients, the usual absence of rheumatoid factor, and the association with HLA-B*27, PsA has been classified among the seronegative, HLA-B*27-associated spondyloarthropathies.

III. CLINICAL PATTERNS

Moll and Wright described five clinical patterns of the disease: distal arthritis, involving primarily the distal interphalangeal joints of the hands and feet; oligoarthritis, in which four or fewer joints were affected often in an asymmetrical distribution; polyarthritis, in which five or more joints are affected, often indistinguishable from rheumatoid arthritis; arthritis mutilans, which is a destructive form of arthritis; and a spondyloarthropathy with inflammation in the spine and sacroiliac joints (1).

Since the observations of Moll and Wright, several cohorts of patients with psoriatic arthritis have been described, and it has become clear that there was no consensus as to the frequency of the specific patterns. Moreover, while these patterns may be defined at presentation, they tend to change over time, as more joints accrue in some patients and some joints settle in others. As the disease progresses there is often an increasing number of joints involved and the disease becomes more symmetrical (5, 6). The variation of the clinical patterns with time, as well as the fact that psoriatic arthritis is generally less tender than rheumatoid arthritis (RA), have made it difficult to create widely accepted classification criteria for the disease.

IV. EXTRA-ARTICULAR MANIFESTATIONS

In addition to the psoriasis and nail lesions, patients with PsA have other extra-articular manifestations that help to identify the correct diagnosis. These include iritis, mucous membrane lesions, urethritis, bowel symptoms, and aortic dilatation. These features are common to the other spondyloarthropathies (Table 1).

Table 1 Comparison of PsA and Other Arthropathies

Features		PsA	RA	OA	Arthritic condition AS	ReA	IBD	Gout
Gender distribution		Equal	F > M	Equal	M > F	M > F	M > F	M > F
Age at onset (years)		35–45	20–50	> 50	20–30	20–30	30–40	> 30
Peripheral joints		Common	Common	Common	Uncommon	Common	Common	Common
Distal joints		Common	Rare	Common	Uncommon	Uncommon	Uncommon	Common
Distribution		Asymmetrical	Symmetrical	Symmetrical	Asymmetrical	Asymmetrical	Asymmetrical	Asymmetrical
Red hot joints		Yes	No	No	No	Yes	No	Yes
Dactylitis		Yes	No	No	NO	Yes	No	No
Back involvement (%)		40–50	Rare	Common	100	100	30	Rare
Nodules		No	Common	No	No	No	No	Tophi
Psoriasis		Yes	No	No	No	No	No	No
Nail lesions		Yes	No	No	No	Yes	No	No
Enthesitis		Yes	No	No	Yes	Yes	Yes	No

V. DIFFERENTIATING BETWEEN PSORIATIC ARTHRITIS AND OTHER ARTHROPATHIES

Despite the variation in disease presentation, there are distinct features of PsA that differentiate it from rheumatoid arthritis (RA), osteoarthritis (OA), and other spondyloarthropathies (SpA) (Table 1).

A. Features that Differentiate PsA from RA

PsA commonly affects the distal interphalangeal (DIP) joints, which are uncommonly affected in RA. PsA tends to be asymmetrical compared to RA, and the joints tend to be affected in a ray distribution: all the joints of a single digit are involved but the same digit on the opposite limb is spared. This contrasts with the symmetrical distribution of RA, in which the same joints on both hands or feet are affected. The affected joints in PsA tend to have a purplish discoloration compared to RA. The degree of tenderness in patients with PsA is less than that of RA (7). Almost half the patients with PsA may have a spondyloarthropathy, which is distinctly uncommon in RA. Enthesitis, the inflammation at tendon insertion into bone, is uncommon in RA but is a classic feature of PsA. Dactylitis, the inflammation and swelling of a whole digit, is also a distinct feature of PsA and does not occur in RA. The extra-articular manifestations of PsA are also different from those of RA. Psoriasis in a patient presenting with joint symptoms should certainly alert the physician to the presence of PsA. Nail lesions are thought to be specific differentiating features. In a study comparing patients with PsA to patients with uncomplicated psoriasis, nail involvement was the only clinical feature that was significantly different, occurring in 87% of patients with PsA and 40% of patients with psoriasis (8). Other specific extra-articular features of PsA include iritis, urethritis, aortic root dilatation, and at times gut involvement. On the other hand, the presence of rheumatoid nodules is an exclusion criterion for the diagnosis of PsA, since it occurs only in patients with RA. Patients with RA tend to have conjunctivitis, lung nodules or interstitial lung disease, pericarditis or myocarditis, and compression neuropathies or mononeuritis multiplex. Skin involvement in RA is usually in the form of nail fold infarcts or periungual erythema, or the leg ulcers that are typical of Felty's syndrome. It should be noted that the co-occurrence of RA and psoriasis is possible. Since psoriasis occurs in 1–3% of the population, and RA occurs in close to 1% of the population, the likelihood of a coexistence of the two conditions in the same patient may reach 1:10,000. The features noted above should help identify whether the patient has PsA or psoriasis with RA.

   The changes in joint distribution described clinically may also be noted in the assessment of radiographs from patients with PsA compared to RA.

While joint erosions occur in both PsA and RA (9), the radiological changes specific to PsA include extensive joint lysis with pencil-in-cup change, as well as ankylosis (Fig. 1). In addition, periosteal reaction is a feature of PsA not seen in patients with RA. The presence of sacroiliitis and syndesmophytes is also typical for PsA and does not occur in RA.

B. Features that Differentiate PsA from OA

The DIP joints are classically affected in patients with OA. OA is the most common rheumatic disease, therefore its association with psoriasis is expected. DIP involvement in OA usually presents with pain, which is usually noninflammatory in nature (not associated with prolonged morning stiffness and aggravated by activity rather than rest), whereas the DIP involvement in PsA patients is typically inflammatory. Moreover, on physical examination OA presents with bony overgrowth that is recognized clinically as Heberden's nodes, whereas in PsA the DIP are often swollen on palpation. Radiographs further help to differentiate the two conditions: the erosions seen in PsA are

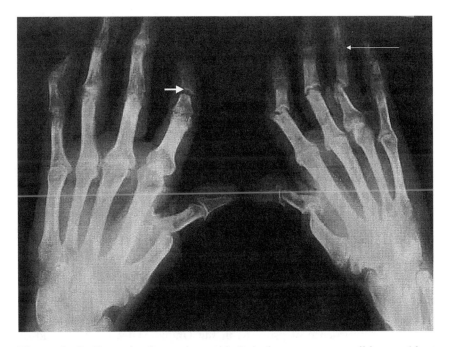

Figure 1 Radiograph of a patient with PsA demonstrates pencil-in-cup (short arrow) and ankylosing (long arrow) features.

marginal as opposed to the cartilage changes seen in OA. In the spine, OA presents with degenerative disc and apophyseal joint disease, and with traction osteophytes, compared with the syndesmophytes seen in PsA. Sacroiliitis is not a feature of OA. The back disease in OA is of the mechanical type as opposed to the inflammatory features of back involvement in PsA.

C. Features that Differentiate PsA from Other Spondyloarthropathies

The spondyloarthropathy of PsA can be differentiated from that of other spondyloarthropathies, particularly ankylosing spondylitis (AS), by the presence of the peripheral arthritis, the asymmetrical nature of the syndesmophytes, as well as the sacroiliac involvement. In addition, the spondyloarthropathy of PsA tends to be less symptomatic than that of AS (10). However, as a member of the seronegative HLA-B27 spondyloarthropathy group, PsA shares many of the extra-articular features with other conditions in the group, including AS, reactive arthritis, and the arthritis of inflammatory bowel disease.

D. Features that Differentiate PsA from Crystal-Induced Arthritis

Another condition than needs to be differentiated from PsA is crystal-induced arthritis, particularly gout. Gout presents as an acute monoarthritis with a red hot swollen toe (podagra) or a swollen knee or ankle. These are joints commonly involved in PsA. Since patients with psoriasis may have an increased uric acid concentration in their plasma, they are often misdiagnosed as having gout. It is important to aspirate the joint and look for crystals to ascertain the diagnosis. If there are no uric acid crystals in the fluid, it is most likely the acute onset of PsA. This is another reason why patients with psoriasis who present to their dermatologist with joint complaints should be referred to a rheumatologist.

VI. PREVALENCE AMONG PATIENTS WITH PSORIASIS

The exact prevalence of PsA in the general population is unknown. Estimates reported in the literature vary from 0.1% in the Mayo Clinic to 1.4% in the Faroe Islands. A recent survey by the National Psoriasis Foundation estimated a prevalence of psoriasis in the United States of 2.1%, and of psoriatic arthritis at 0.5% (11). The reported prevalence of PsA among patients with psoriasis has been variable from 7 to 42%. The value of 7%

was reported from a hospital study including only patients with polyarthritis in Sweden in 1948, and the higher value was from an outpatient facility in South Africa. The difficulty in getting accurate information arises from the lack of widely accepted classification criteria, and from the fact that patients with PsA do not complain of as much pain and therefore their disease may be unnoticed until they have clear deformities. Moreover, even rheumatologists do not always make the correct diagnosis (12). A recent study performed at the University of Toronto identified 30% of patients with psoriasis as having psoriatic arthritis (13).

As will be noted later, correct and early diagnosis is crucial for appropriate therapy for patients with PsA. Therefore, it is important for dermatologists to identify patients with psoriasis who have any joint complaints and refer them to a rheumatologist, and it is important for a rheumatologist to look for skin and nail changes in patients with inflammatory arthritis and refer the patient to a dermatologist for the correct diagnosis of the skin lesion.

VII. JOINT ASSESSMENT OF PATIENTS WITH PsA

While the dermatologist is not expected to perform a joint assessment, it is important that the dermatologist asks the patient about the presence of joint symptoms including joint pain, joint stiffness, or swelling, and identifies the presence of joint changes during the skin examination. From a rheumatologist's perspective, a detailed history looking for extra-articular features suggesting another condition is important. It is also important to note whether the patient has extra-articular features of PsA, which include iritis and mucous membrane lesions. The joint assessment should include an evaluation of the number of actively inflamed and damaged joints (14), assessment of function by the grip strength, and assessment of back involvement. Evaluation of so-called sausage digits or dactylitis and attention to the sites of tendon insertion into bones (entheses) such as the Achilles tendon, or the plantar fascia is important. In addition to the clinical evaluation, a laboratory assessment is usually performed including a test for rheumatoid factor and antinuclear factor. These are usually done to rule out other rheumatological disorders such as systemic lupus erythematosus, (which may present with a psoriasiform rash and arthritis), and rheumatoid arthritis (which may coexist with psoriasis). Radiographs are then requested to help make the correct diagnosis and to evaluate the extent of the arthritis. Since the pain is not as much of an issue for patients with PsA, they may have joint destruction that has gone unnoticed. Moreover, the only way to determine the presence of the spondyloarthropathy is through radiological assessment (15).

The assessment of skin disease should be performed by a dermatologist. Preferably, a psoriasis area severity index score (PASI) should be determined and followed.

VIII. RELATIONSHIP BETWEEN SKIN AND JOINTS IN PSORIATIC ARTHRITIS

The relationship between skin and joint manifestations in PsA is not uniform. Although many dermatologists believe that patients with severe psoriasis are those who developed arthritis, this is not necessarily the case. Two studies that found a high prevalence of PsA among patients with psoriasis were performed on inpatients, who presumably had severe psoriasis, but the higher frequency of PsA was noted among outpatients. Moreover, in each of the large reported series about 15% of patients have arthritis that precedes the diagnosis of psoriasis. While it is possible that the diagnosis of psoriasis was missed because patients were not undressed or questioned about the condition, it certainly suggests that the psoriasis was not extensive. Recent studies support the notion that there is no direct relationship between the severity of skin and joint manifestations. In a cross-sectional study, no relationship between skin and joint severity was found (16). In two longitudinal studies there was no statistical association between the severity of skin and joint manifestations, although it was noted that in patients who presented with skin and joints simultaneously there tended to be a relation between skin and joint manifestations (17).

IX. PROGNOSIS

Several studies reported in the past 20 years document that the prognosis of PsA is more serious than previously thought. About 20% of patients with PsA may develop a destructive form of arthritis than can be devastating to them and their families (5). These patients have more than five totally damaged joints and consequently they have a reduced quality of life and function. Moreover, it has been demonstrated that patients with PsA are at an increased risk of death compared to the general population (18). While the causes of death are similar to those noted in the general population, the predictive factors for mortality include active and severe disease at presentation, which are similar to those predictive of progressive joint damage (19, 20). It has therefore been suggested that early diagnosis and aggressive therapy may prevent these adverse outcomes in patients with PsA. Not all patients with PsA fare poorly. Some 18% of patients sustained periods of remission lasting an average of 2.5 years (21). Male patients, and those with a smaller number of affected joints at presentation, are more likely to achieve periods of remission.

X. MANAGEMENT

Despite the fact that there is no direct relationship between the skin and joint manifestations in PsA, the two components of the disease require consideration when planning patients' management. The management plan begins with educating the patient that the condition is chronic, inflammatory in nature, and that consistent therapy is required. Patients should also be instructed to maintain a healthy lifestyle, as many patients with PsA have risk factors for coronary artery disease (22). In this chapter only the treatment of the joint disease will be considered. Specific therapy is tailored to individual patients (23).

A. Nonsteroidal Anti-Inflammatory Drugs

When the joint disease is mild, nonsteroidal anti-inflammatory drugs (NSAIDs) are used. NSAIDs provide analgesia and anti-inflammatory activity. In many patients NSAIDs are sufficient to control the inflammatory joint disease. There are many preparations, and none is considered superior to the others. The new COX-2-selective inhibitors may be less harmful to the gastrointestinal tract, but they are not superior to the traditional NSAIDs in terms of anti-inflammatory activity. It should be noted that, on occasion, NSAIDs have caused an exacerbation of the psoriasis, which is why patients need to be evaluated by both a dermatologist and a rheumatologist (24).

B. Slow-Acting Antirheumatic Drugs

Patients who continue to demonstrate persistent inflammatory activity or who have erosive disease detected on radiographs usually deserve treatment with slow-acting antirheumatic drugs (SAARDs). However, NSAIDs remain important therapy in patients with severe PsA. The majority of patients require NSAIDs even while taking other medications. Studies have shown that patients who present with five or more swollen joints on their first visit are at increased risk of disease progression (25). Therefore patients with significant joint disease should be treated aggressively early on, even if their skin disease is mild.

SAARDs or disease-modifying antirheumatic drugs (DMARDs) typically take several weeks to months to reach therapeutic effect. The latter definition has been replaced with the former, since none of the drugs to date have actually demonstrated the ability to modify the disease process. None of the drugs was developed specifically for PsA. The majority of these drugs were borrowed from the treatment of RA. Initially, medications such as antimalarials, gold, and penicillamine were used. More recently sulfasalazine, methotrexate, and cyclosporine A have been introduced (23, 26).

1. Antimalarials

Both chloroquine and hydroxychloroquine have been used for the treatment of PsA. While there have been several anecdotal reports that these drugs aggravate psoriasis, this concern has not been confirmed in case-controlled studies (27). However, there has not been a randomized controlled trial of antimalarials in the treatment of PsA.

2. Gold

Gold has been used for the treatment of PsA since a study in 1978 demonstrated its effect (28). An oral preparation was tested but showed very minimal improvement over placebo (29). A comparison of intramuscular to oral gold in PsA demonstrated superiority of the former (30). While gold may work for some patients with PsA, it has not provided protection from progression of joint disease (31). Moreover, with skin rash being one of the major side effects, its differentiation from psoriasis is difficult.

3. Penicillamine

Penicillamine has been studied in a controlled trial in patients with PsA. While it did provide some benefit, its slow action and multiple side effects have precluded it from routine use in the treatment of PsA (23, 26).

4. Sulfasalazine

Three double-blind controlled studies of sulfasalazine support its role in the treatment of PsA (32–34). However, the therapeutic effect noted has been modest at best. One of the difficulties encountered in clinical trials of PsA is the lack of established criteria for improvement. Investigators have used the response criteria for RA, which are defined as a 20% improvement in actively inflamed joint count, effusion count, the Health Assessment Questionnaire, and a reduction in either erythrocyte sedimentation rate (ESR) or C-reactive protein (CRP). However, patients with PsA do not always have an elevated ESR, and if it is elevated, it is difficult to discern whether it is due to skin or joint disease. Clegg and colleagues (34) defined improvement as a 30% improvement in the absence of deterioration (a worsening of 30%) in two of the following four items: actively inflamed joint count, swollen joint count, patient global assessment, and physician global assessment. At least one of the two had to be an objective joint assessment. Using these criteria these investigators enrolled 220 patients in a double-blind randomized placebo-controlled trial of sulfasalazine in PsA (34). They demonstrated a very small difference: 54% improvement in the active treatment group compared to 45% in the placebo group. Although this was statistically significant at the $p < 0.05$ level, it does not seem to be a clinically important difference (34).

In a clinical setting, many patients were unable to tolerate sulfasalazine, with a withdrawal rate of 44%, and the drug did not provide long-term protection from disease progression (35).

5. Methotrexate

Methotrexate has been considered the drug of choice for the treatment of PsA since 1964, because it works for both skin and joint manifestations of the disease (36, 37). A meta-analysis of therapies used in PsA demonstrated that parenteral methotrexate and sulfasalazine were the only drugs effective for PsA, but noted that the effect was modest. Methotrexate has also not been found to be helpful in preventing progression of joint destruction (38). Methotrexate may be give orally, intramuscularly, or subcutaneously. Patients can self-administer parenteral methotrexate (39). Both patients and physicians are reluctant to use methotrexate because of its potential liver toxicity, hair loss, predisposition to infection, and the fact that it is unsafe for use during pregnancy.

6. Cyclosporine A

Cyclosporine A has also been used to treat patients with PsA. There are no published placebo-controlled trials of cyclosporin A in PsA, but a randomized controlled trial comparing cyclosporin to methotrexate demonstrated both to be effective for the treatment of PsA (40). A study comparing cyclosporin A to sulfasalazine demonstrated that the former was more effective for the peripheral arthritis (41). Cyclosporine is less well tolerated than methotrexate, with many patients discontinuing it because of hypertension and renal toxicity (42).

C. Other Medications that May Control Skin and Joint Disease in PsA

If both skin and joint manifestations of PsA are severe, a common approach is taken. Systemic medications are likely required, and medications that treat both skin and joint disease are preferred. These include, in addition to methotrexate and cyclosporine A, retinoids (43) and psoralen/ultraviolet A (PUVA) (44). These latter medications have demonstrated efficacy in the treatment of psoriasis, but there effect in PsA has not been impressive. Moreover, these medications are toxic and physicians have been reluctant to use them.

XI. NEW THERAPIES BASED ON PATHOGENESIS

Based on new insights into the pathogenesis of PsA, the new millenium has provided a new era of therapy for PsA. Although the exact causes and pathogenesis of PSA are unknown, genetic, environmental, and immunological factors are considered important contributors.

A. Genetic Factors

It is well recognized that a family history of psoriatic or PsA may be obtained from some 40% of patients. A family investigation performed in 1973 identified a strong familial predisposition (45), with 5.5% if the relatives of patients with PsA having PsA compared to its estimated prevalence in the UK population of 0.1%. Thus the risk ($\lambda 1$) for PsA among first-degree family members using current methodology is 55 (46). Further genome scans identified a number of genetic regions associated with psoriasis (47). The HLA locus on chromosome 6p has been identified as a strong susceptibility locus (7) and HLA antigens have been associated with disease progression (48). Other genes within the major histocompatibility complex (MHC) have also been associated with PsA. These include the MHC class I-related chain (MIC) A (49) and tumor necrosis factor (TNF), genes (50). However, with regard to therapy, at the present time it is unlikely that we can change the genetic make-up of a patient in an attempt to modify their disease.

B. Environmental Factors

Environmental factors thought to contribute to the susceptibility of PsA include trauma and infection (51). These also are not modifiable by specific therapy.

C. Immunological Factors

Immunological abnormalities have been suspected in patients with PsA because of the inflammatory nature of the joint and skin lesions (52). The role of T cells has been clearly recognized (53). In particular, a clonal expansion of CD8 + cells has been identified (54). T-cell antigen-receptor beta-chain variable-gene repertoires in skin and synovium are similar, suggesting that there may be a common antigen triggering the disease. T-cell activation may lead to the increased levels of cytokines noted in the synovial tissues in patients with PsA (55). In particular, the increased TNF levels have been important therapeutically (56). Since levels of TNF are elevated, and there appears to be a specific polymorphism for the TNF promoter gene among patients with PsA, it is likely that TNF plays an important role in the pathogenesis of the disease.

XII. NEW BIOLOGICAL AGENTS

Based on similar pathogenic considerations, several agents have been tried in the treatment of RA as well as in psoriasis. These include anti-TNF agents, anti-CD4 agents, anti-CD11, and CTLA4-Ig.

A. Anti-TNF Agents

In the past few years several anti-TNF agents have been developed and proven effective in the treatment of RA. Etanercept (Enbrel) is a human dimeric fusion protein consisting of the extracellular portion of two TNF receptors (p75) connected to the Fc portion of human immunoglobulin G1 (IgG1). Two double-blind controlled trials have now been completed in PsA (57, 58). The first included 60 patients from a single center: half were randomized to etanercept while the others received placebo. Within each group half the patients took methotrexate while the remainder received etanercept as monotherapy. Response in joint disease was determined at 3 months by both the American College of Rheumatology (ACR) 20 response (which is borrowed from rheumatoid arthritis studies) and the PsA Response Criteria (PsARC, which were modified from criteria developed for PsA by Clegg et al. (34). Response in skin disease was determined by a reduction in the PASI score as well as target lesion assessment. There was a remarkable improvement in both joint and skin manifestations, with only injection site reactions being a major untoward effect. An extension of this study in which patients originally treated with etanercept were continued on it, while those initially taking placebo were given the active drug, demonstrated a similar degree of improvement (59). The magnitude of improvement (73% of the patients) noted in these studies is unparalleled in the literature.

The second study was a phase 3 multicenter trial including 205 patients, which was similar in design to the first trial (58). This trial also demonstrated remarkable improvement in both joint and skin manifestations of PsA. Enbrel has now been approved for treatment of patients with PsA.

Infliximab is a chimeric monoclonal antibody, composed of human constant and murine variable regions, that binds specifically to human TNF. It has also been used effectively for the treatment of RA and is currently approved for that indication. There is one randomized controlled trial of infliximab in patients with severe psoriasis (60). There are a few uncontrolled trials of infliximab in patients with PsA. A multicenter trial has recently been completed but the results are not available. Several other anti-TNF agents have been used for the treatment of RA, but have yet to be tested in the treatment of PsA.

B. Other Biologicals

Several other medications have been used for the treatment of psoriasis, including CTLA-4Ig and anti-CD11 antibody, but these have not been tested in the treatment of PsA. The disappointing fact is that none of the medications work for all patients, suggesting that the pathogenesis is indeed multifactorial, and that perhaps combination therapy may be required for some patients.

C. Who Should Be Treated with New Therapies?

While the new medications provide new hope for patients with psoriatic arthritis, they are very expensive. In addition, their role as so-called disease modifying drugs in psoriatic arthritis remains to be demonstrated. Although at present the anti-TNF agents appear safe, with the major side effects being injection site reactions and allergic reactions, as well as infections, their long-term adverse event profile is unknown. Thus, while dermatologists tend to consider methotrexate toxicity prohibitive, it is not clear that the new medications are indeed better. However, if these drugs are proven to modify the course of psoriatic arthritis by preventing joint damage, providing better control of the psoriasis, and achieving better quality of life for the patients, then it would be important to include them early in the management plan. It would be advantageous if we had markers for disease expression that would allow us to identify those patients who require these drugs, so that we can avoid putting patients with mild disease at risk. Initial studies suggest that patients with HLA-B*27 in the presence of HLA-DRB1*07, patients with HLA-B*39, and patients with HLA-DQB1*03 in the absence of HLA-DRB1*07 are predictive of progression in clinical damage, while HLA-B*22 is protective (48). Studies are currently underway to address this issue further.

D. Management of Psoriatic Arthritis Requires Team Effort

The best way for patients with psoriatic arthritis to be managed is through a team effort including the rheumatologist and dermatologist. Such collaborative effort exists in our Psoriatic Arthritis Program at the University of Toronto. All our patients are reviewed by their dermatologists at regular intervals, and communication with them allows us to use appropriate therapies.

XIII. SUMMARY

Over the past 2 decades PsA has been recognized as a more severe form of arthritis than initially described. The course and prognosis of the disease suggest that early diagnosis and more aggressive treatment are important. While several clinical and HLA markers for disease progression have been identified, further work in this area is required. Therefore, it is important for dermatologists to recognize the features of the arthritis, and it is important for rheumatologists to look for evidence of psoriasis in patients with arthritis. The management of patients with PsA is best performed with team effort so that both aspects of the disease are dealt with. There are new and exciting treatments that should be available to these patients.

REFERENCES

1. Wright V, Moll JMH, eds. Seronegative Polyarthritis. Amsterdam: North Holland Publishing Company, 1976: 169–223.
2. O'Neill T, Silman A. Psoriatic arthritis. Historical background and epidemiology. Baillières Clin Rheumatol 1994; 8:245–261.
3. Cats A. Psoriasis and arthritis. Cutis 1990; 46:323–329.
4. Gladman DD. Psoriatic arthritis. Baillières Clin Rheumatol 1995; 9:319–329.
5. Gladman DD. The natural history of psoriatic arthritis. Baillières Clin Rheumatol 1994;8:379–394.
6. Helliwell PS, Hetthen J, Sokoll K, Green M, Marchesoni A, Lubrano E, et al. Joint symmetry in early and late rheumatoid and psoriatic arthritis: comparison with a mathematical model. Arthritis Rheum 2000; 43:865–871.
7. Buskila D, Langevitz P, Gladman DD, Urowitz S, Smythe H. Patients with rheumatoid arthritis are more tender than those with psoriatic arthritis. J Rheumatol 1992; 19:1115–1119.
8. Gladman DD, Anhorn KB, Schachter RK, Mervart H. HLA antigens in psoriatic arthritis. J Rheumatol 1986;13:586–592.

9. Rahman P, Gladman DD, Cook RJ, Zhou Y, Young G, Salonen D. Radiological assessment in psoriatic arthritis. Br J Rheumatol 1998, 37:760–765.
10. Gladman DD. Clinical aspects of spondyloarthropathies. Am J Med Sci 1998; 316:234–238.
11. http://www.psoriasis.org/npfsurveyfactsheet.htm
12. Gorter S, van der Heijde DM, van Der LS, et al. Psoriatic arthritis: performance of rheumatologists in daily practice. Ann Rheum Dis 2002, 61:219–224.
13. Brockbank JE, Schentag C, Rosen C, Gladman DD: Psoriatic arthritis (PsA) is common among patients with psoriasis and family medical clinic attendees. Arthritis Rheum 2001;44(suppl 9):S94.
14. Gladman DD, Farewell VT, Buskila D, Goodman R, Hamilton L, Langevitz P, et al. Reliability of measurements of active and damaged joints in psoriatic arthritis. J Rheumatol 1990; 17:62–64.
15. Khan M, Gladman D, Schentag C. Clinical and radiological changes during psoriatic arthritis disease progression: working toward classification criteria. J Rheumatol 2002;29:1569.
16. Cohen MR, Reda DJ, Clegg DO. Baseline relationships between psoriasis and psoriatic arthritis: analysis of 221 patients with active psoriatic arthritis. Department of Veterans Affairs Cooperative Study Group on Seronegative Spondyloarthropathies. J Rheumatol 1999; 26:1752–1756.
17. Elkayam O, Ophir J, Yaron M, Caspi D. Psoriatic arthritis: interrelationships between skin and joint manifestations related to onset, course and distribution. Clin Rheumatol 2000;19:301–305.
18. Wong K, Gladman DD, Husted J, Long J, Farewell VT. Mortality studies in psoriatic arthritis. Results from a single centre. I. Risk and causes of death. Arthritis Rheum 1997;40:1868–1872.
19. Gladman DD, Farewell VT, Husted J, Wong K: Mortality studies in psoriatic arthritis. Results from a single centre. II. Prognostic indicators for mortality. Arthritis Rheum 1998;41:1103–1110.
20. Gladman DD, Farewell VT. Progression in psoriatic arthritis: role of time varying clinical indicators. J Rheumatol 1999; 26:2409–2413.
21. Gladman DD, Ng Tung Hing E, Schentag CT, Cook R: Remission in psoriatic arthritis. J Rheumatol 2001;28:1045–1048.
22. Bruce IN, Schentag C, Gladman DD. Hyperuricemia in psoriatic arthritis (PsA) does not reflect the extent of skin involvement. J Clin Rheumatol 2000; 6:6–9.
23. Gladman DD, Brockbank J. Psoriatic arthritis. Exp Opin Invest Drugs 2000; 9:1511–1522.
24. Griffiths CE. Therapy for psoriatic arthritis: sometimes a conflict for psoriasis. Br J Rheumatol 1997; 36:409–410.
25. Gladman DD, Farewell VT, Nadeau C. Clinical indicators of progression in psoriatic arthritis (PSA): multivariate relative risk model. J Rheumatol 1995; 22:675–679.
26. Jones G, Crotty M, Brooks P. Interventions for psoriatic arthritis. Cochrane Database Syst Rev 2000;CD000212.

27. Gladman DD, Blake R, Brubacher B, Farewell VT: Chloroquine therapy in psoriatic arthritis. J Rheumatol 1992;19:1724–1726.
28. Dowart BB, Gall EP, Schumacher HR, Krauser RE. Chrysotherapy in psoriatic arthritis: efficacy and toxicity compared to rheumatoid arthritis. Arthritis Rheum 1978; 21:513–515.
29. Carrett S, Calin A. Evaluation of auranofin in psoriatic arthritis: a double blind placebo controlled trial. Arthritis Rheum 1989;32:158–165.
30. Palit J, Hill J, Capell HA, et al. A multicentre double-blind comparison of auranofin, intramuscular gold thiomalate and placebo in patients with psoriatic arthritis. Br J Rheumatol 1990; 29:280–283.
31. Mader R, Gladman DD, Long J, Gough J, Farewell VT. Does injectable gold retard radiologic evidence of joint damage in psoriatic arthritis? Clin Invest Med 1995;18:139–143.
32. Gupta AK, Grober JS, Hamilton TA, Ellis CN, Siegel MT, Voorhees JJ, et al. Sulfasalazine therapy for psoriatic arthritis: a double blind, placebo controlled trial. J Rheumatol 1995; 22:894–898.
33. Dougados M, vam der LS, Leirisalo-Repo M, Huitfeldt B, Juhlin R, Veys E, et al. Sulfasalazine in the treatment of spondylarthropathy. A randomized, multicenter, double-blind, placebo-controlled study. Arthritis Rheum 1995; 38:618–627.
34. Clegg DO, Reda DJ, Mejias E, Cannon GW, Weisman MH, Taylor T, et al. Comparison of sulfasalazine and placebo in the treatment of psoriatic arthritis. A Department of Veterans Affairs Cooperative Study. Arthritis Rheum 1996; 39:2013–2020.
35. Rahman P, Gladman DD, Zhou Y, Cook RJ. The use of sulfasalazine in psoriatic arthritis: a clinic experience. J Rheumatol 1998;25:1957–61.
36. Black RL, O'Brien WM, Van Scott EJ, Auerbach R, Eisen AZ, Bunim JJ. Methotrexate therapy in psoriatic arthritis. Double blind study on 21 patients. JAMA, 1964; 189:743–747.
37. Chang DJ. A survey of drug effectiveness and treatment choices in psoriatic arthritis. Arthritis Rheum. 1999; 42(Suppl 9):S372.
38. Abu-Shakra M, Gladman DD, Thorne JC, Long J, Gough J, Farewell VT. Longterm methotrexate therapy in psoriatic arthritis: clinical and radiologic outcome. J Rheumatol 1995;22:241–245.
39. Arthur AB, Klinkhoff AV, Teufel A. Safety of self-injection of gold and methotrexate. J Rheumatol 1999; 26:302–305.
40. Spadaro A, Riccieri V, Sili-Scavalli A, Sensi F, Taccari E, Zoppini A. Comparison of cyclosporin A and methotrexate in the treatment of psoriatic arthritis: a one-year prospective study. Clin Exp Rheumatol 1995; 13:589–593.
41. Salvarani C, Macchioni P, Olivieri I, Marchesoni A, Cutolo M, Ferraccioli G, et al. A comparison of cyclosporine, sulfasalazine, and symptomatic therapy in the treatment of psoriatic arthritis. J Rheumatol 2001; 28:2274–2282.
42. Spadaro A, Taccari E, Mohtadi B, Riccieri V, Sensi F, Zoppini A. Life-table analysis of cyclosporin A treatment in psoriatic arthritis: comparison with

other disease-modifying antirheumatic drugs. Clin Exp Rheumatol 1997; 15:609–614.

43. Klinkhoff AV, Gertner E, Chalmers A, Gladman DD, Stewart WD, Schachter DG, Schachter RK. Pilot study of etretinate in psoriatic arthritis. J Rheumatol 1989; 16:789–791.

44. Perlman SG, Gerber LH, Roberts M, et al. Photochemotherapy and psoriatic arthritis. A prospective study. Ann Intern Med 1979; 91: 717–722.

45. Moll JM, Wright V. Familial occurrence of PsA. Ann Rheum Dis 1973; 32:181–201.

46. Risch N. Linkage strategies for genetically complex traits. 1. Multilocus model. Am J Hum Genet 1990; 46:222–228.

47. Elder JT, Nair RP, Henseler T, Jenisch S, Stuart P, Chia N, Chritophers E, Voorhees JJ. The genetics of psoriasis 2001. The odyssey continues. Arch Dermatol 2001; 137:1447–1454.

48. Gladman DD, Farewell VT, Kopciuk K, Cook RJ. HLA antigens and progression in psoriatic arthritis. J Rheumatol 1998; 25;730–733.

49. Gonzalez S, Martinez-Borra J, Lopez-Vazquez A, Garcia-Fernandez S, Torre-Alonso JC, Lopez-Larrea C. MICA rather than MICB, TNFA, or HLA-DRBI is associated with susceptibility to psoriatic arthritis. J Rheumatol 2002; 29:973–978.

50. Hohler T, Grossmann S, Stradmann-Bellinghausen B, Kaluza W, Reuss E, de Vlam K, Veys E, Marker-Hermann E. Differential association of poly-morphisms in the TNFα region with psoriatic arthritis but not psoriasis. Ann Rheum Dis 2002; 61:213–218.

51. Abu-Shakra M, Gladman DD. Aetiopathogenesis of psoriatic arthritis. Rheumatol Rev 1994; 3:1–7.

52. Gladman DD. Toward unravelling the mystery of psoriatic arthritis. Editorial. Arthritis Rheum 1993; 36:881–884.

53. Hohler T. Marker-Hermann E. Psoriatic arthritis: clinical aspects, genetics, and the role of T cells. Curr Opin Rheumatol 2001; 13:273–279.

54. Costello P, Bresnihan B, O'Farrell C, Fitzgerald O. Predominance of CD8+ T lymphocytes in Psoriatic Arthritis. J Rheumatol 1999; 26:1117–1124.

55. Ritchlin C, Haas-Smith SA, Hicks D, Cappuccio J, Osterland CK, Looney RJ. Patterns of cytokine production in psoriatic synovium. J Rheumatol 1998; 25:1544–1552.

56. Partsch G, Wagner E, Leeb BF, Dunky A, Steiner G, Smolen JS. Upregulation of cytokine receptors sTNF-R55, sTNF-R75, and sIL-2R in psoriatic arthritis synovial fluid. J Rheumatol. 1998; 25:105–110.

57. Mease PJ, Goffe BS, Metz J, Vanderstoep A, Finck B, Burge DJ. Etanercept in the treatment of psoriatic arthritis and psoriasis: a randomised trial. Lancet. 2000; 356:385–390.

58. Mease P, Kivitz A, Burch F, Siegel E, Cohen S, Burge D. Improvement in disease activity in patients with psoriatic arthritis receiving etanercept (ENBREL): results of a phase 3 multicenter clinical trial. Arthritis Rheum. 2001; 44(suppl):S90.

59. Mease PJ, Goffe BS, Metz J, VanderStroep A, Burge DJ. ENBREL® (etanercept) in patients with psoriatic arthritis and psoriasis. Arthritis Rheum 2001; 43(suppl 9):S403.

60. Chaudhari U, Romano P, Mulcahy LD, Dooley LT, Baker DG, Gottlieb AB. Efficacy and safety of infliximab monotherapy for plaque-type psoriasis: a randomised trial. Lancet. 2001; 357:1842–1847.

11

Immunobiologicals for Psoriasis: Using Targeted Immunotherapies as Pathogenic Probes in Psoriasis

Alice B. Gottlieb
University of Medicine and Dentistry of New Jersey–Robert Wood Johnson Medical School, New Brunswick, New Jersey, U.S.A.

I. TARGETED IMMUNOBIOLOGICS

Biotechnology-created immunobiologicals targeted immunotherapies that offer hope for safe and effective long-term management of moderate to severe psoriasis vulgaris (Table 1). These treatments are here now: Etanercept (Enbrel) is approved by the Food and Drug Administration (FDA) for treatment of psoriatic arthritis with or without methotrexate. Alefacept (Amevive) is recommended for approval, by the FDA Dermatology Advisory Panel, as monotherapy for moderate to severe psoriasis vulgaris. Infliximab (Remicade), etanercept, and efalizumab (Raptiva) are in relatively advanced stages of development as monotherapies for moderate to severe psoriasis. Targeted immunobiologicals have also been invaluable therapeutic probes into the pathogenesis of psoriasis. The studies summarized in this article demonstrate the power of clinical research not only to improve patient care but also to produce good science.

II. ACTIVATED TYPE 1 T CELLS SECRETING TYPE 1 CYTOKINES

Psoriasis vulgaris is a chronic, inflammatory, papulosquamous dermatosis characterized by cellular immune activation, keratinocyte hyperproliferation,

Table 1 Targeted Immunosuppression Strategies Used as Pathogenic Probes in Psoriasis

Strategy	Drug	Target	References
Cytokines			
Inhibit T1 cytokines	Infliximab, Etanercept	TNF-α	11, 58, 63, 64
Monoclonal antibodies	Anti-IL-8 (no longer in development for psoriasis	IL-8	Reviewed in 11
Immune deviation	IL-10 (no longer in development for psoriasis), IL-11 IL-4	Alter the cytokine balance	44, 45, 81
Inhibit T-cell activation			
	Alefacept, Siplizumab	CD2-LFA-3	36, 82
	Anti-CD11a (Efalizumab)	LFA-1-ICAM-1	1, 41, 43
	Anti-CD80 (IDEC 114)	CD28-CD80	83
	CTLA4Ig (no longer in development for psoriasis)	CTLA4-CD80, CD86	25, 84
	Anti-CD25 (Daclizumab)	IL-2 Receptor	85
	Denileukin difitox	IL-2 Receptor	6, 17
Inhibit T-cell trafficking	Anti-CD11a (Efalizumab)	LFA-1-ICAM-1	See above

and abnormal differentiation. The inflammatory response in psoriatic plaques is initiated in part by activated T cells and dendritic cells in the epidermis and dermis (1–6).

Cytokine-producing T cells can be classified into type 1 (T1) T cells, which make interleukin (IL)-2, γ-interferon, and tumor necrosis factor alpha (TNFα); and type 2 (T2) T cells, which make IL-4, IL-5, IL-6, IL-9, IL-10, and IL-13 (Table 2). T1-type T cells predominate in plaques and release a number of inflammatory cytokines including TNFα (7). TNFα, γ-interferon, IL-6, IL-8, and other inflammatory cytokines are elevated in psoriatic lesions but not in the normal skin of psoriatic patients (8–10). TNFα increases the synthesis of proinflammatory cytokines such as IL-1, IL-6, and IL-8 and activates nuclear transcription factors such as NFκB (7, 11–14). NFκB plays a crucial role in inflammation and is a nuclear transcription heterodimer

Table 2 Immunological Terminology

Term	Explanation
T1 (type 1) T cells (86)	Mediate cellular immune responses Make IL-2, γ-interferon, TNF-α Stimulate IgG1 and IgG3 secretion
T2 (type 2) T cells	Mediate effective humoral immunity Make IL-4, IL-5, IL-6, IL-9, IL-10, IL-13 Stimulate IgE and IgG4 secretion Support mast cell and eosinophil growth
NFκB (nuclear transcription factor-κB) (12)	Promotes mRNA transcription of TNF-α, IL-1β, IL-2 IL-6, granulocyte–macrophage CSF, granulocyte CSF, macrophage CSF, IL-8, macrophage inhibitory protein 1α, inducible nitric oxide synthase, inductible cyclooxygenase-2, ICAM-1, VCAM-1, E-selectin, IL-2 receptor (α chain), and the T-cell receptor β chain

consisting of p50 and p65 components. This heterodimer is complexed to its inhibitory protein, IκB. While complexed to IκB, NFκB resides in the cytoplasm. Upon degradation of IκB, the P50,p65 heterodimeric NFκB translocates to the nucleus where it is a nuclear transcription factor for a number of proteins of immunological importance including TNFα, IL-1β, IL-2, IL-6, granulocyte–macrophage colony-stimulating factor (CSF), granulocyte CSF, macrophage CSF, IL-8, macrophage inhibitory protein 1α, inducible nitric oxide synthase, inducible cyclooxygenase-2 intracellular adhesion molecule (ICAM-1), vascular cell adhesion molecule 1 (VCAM-1), E-selectin, IL-2 receptor (α chain), and the T-cell receptor β chain. Nuclear translocation of NFκB, stimulated by degradation of IκB, is stimulated by TNF-α, IL-1β, IL-17, phorbol esters, oxidants, ultraviolet irradiation, various viruses, lipopolysaccharides (LPS), antigen, T-cell mitogens, and antiCD-3 monoclonal antibodies (12).

III. EXPERIMENTAL THERAPIES

Experimental treatment of patients with moderate to severe psoriasis with biologics has successfully targeted:

1. T-cell activation
2. Memory T cells

3. T-cell migration into skin
4. Cytokines (e.g., TNFα)
5. Induction of immune deviation from type 1 to type 2 cytokine predominance in plaques

These five therapeutic strategies can reverse clinical and histological pathology in psoriatic plaques. Murine severe combined immunodeficiency (SCID) models of psoriasis confirm the key role of T cells (CD4+ and CD8+) in both the initiation and maintenance of psoriatic plaques, and suggest a potential role for natural killer (NK) cells in the pathogenesis of psoriasis (15, 16).

IV. ROLE OF ACTIVATED T CELLS IN PSORIASIS

Denileukin diftitox (Ontak) is a fusion protein of IL-2 and diphtheria toxin protein fragments that specifically kills activated T cells. It has no biological activity in vitro against growth factor-stimulated keratinocytes. As a single agent, denileukin diftitox treatment cleared psoriasis clinically and histologically (6, 17). This observation definitively demonstrated that activated T cells were pivotal in maintaining psoriatic plaques and not that T lymphocytes were merely secondarily activated by keratinocytes.

Plaque T cells are more activated (i.e., demonstrate higher IL-2 receptor expression and other markers of T-cell activation) than circulating T cells from patients with psoriasis (5, 7). This observation suggests localized activation of T cells. Activated plaque Langerhans cells are detected by their surface membrane phenotype (increased major histocompatibility complex [MHC], CD40, ICAM-1, CD80, and CD86), increased cytokine production (increased IL-12), and increased potency in stimulating autologous peripheral blood T cells to proliferate (18–24). In addition, two recent papers have shown that Langerhans cells in psoriatic lesions are CD83+ and DC-LAMP+, which establishes that these cells are fully mature dendritic cells. Cells that have matured are considered to have both migratory behavior to lymph nodes and optimal T-cell-stimulating activity (25, 26).

In general, T cells require two signals in order to be activated (Fig. 1). The first signal is provided by antigen bound to class I or II MHC on antigen- presenting cells (e.g., Langerhans cells), interacting with surface membrane T-cell receptors. However, in the absence of a second activating signal, the interaction of antigen with the T-cell receptor fails to activate the T lymphocyte. The second signal can be supplied by a number of pairs of surface molecules (e.g., LFA-1-ICAM-1, CD2-LFA3, and CD80,86-CD28-CTLA4) (27–29). Recent studies suggest that LFA-1–ICAM-1 interactions may be

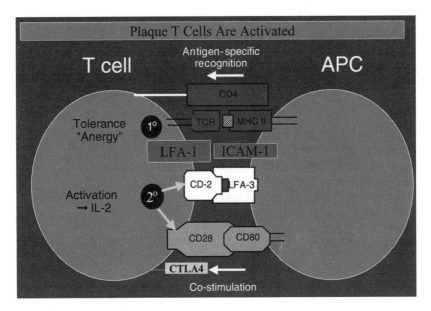

Figure 1 Plaque T cells are activated.

more important in anchoring the immunological synapse between T cells and antigen-presenting cells than in actually providing a second activating signal to T cells (30, 31).

V. ROLE OF T-CELL COSTIMULATION

A. CD80,CD86-CD28, CTLA4 Costimulation in Psoriasis

B7.1 (CD80) and B7.2 (CD86) are membrane proteins expressed primarily on activated antigen-presenting cells (APCs) and on a subset of activated T cells in psoriatic plaques. The interaction of CD28 with CD80, CD86 delivers a second signal, leading to T-cell activation (Fig. 1). After T-cell activation, CTLA-4 is upregulated on the T-cell surface. The interaction of CTLA-4 with CD80,CD86 leads to deactivation of the T cell and suppression of the immune response.

Soluble CTLA4lg inhibits T-cell activation by binding to CD80 and CD86 on antigen-presenting cells. Forty-three patients with moderate to severe plaque-type psoriasis received four intravenous infusions of CTLA4lg. Forty-six percent of all patients experienced 50% or more improvement in physician's global assessment (a clinical research tool used to measure disease activity). Clinical improvement was associated with decreased epidermal thickness and numbers of epidermal CD3+ T cells. Activated/mature dendritic cells in psoriasis lesions were reversed by B7-blockade. Hence, the stimulus for continued T-cell activation, as well as the continuing maturation of dendritic cells, may be sustained by B7-CD28 signaling (25).

IDEC 114 is an anti-CD80 monoclonal antibody that binds specifically and with high affinity. A significant finding is that IDEC 114 blocks the interaction of CD80 with CD28 without affecting the interaction of CD80 and CTLA-4 in vitro. Twenty-four patients received single intravenous infusions of IDEC 114 (32). Evidence of clinical and histological activity was demonstrated.

A multiple-dose study of IDEC 114 in patients with psoriasis was conducted next. Thirty-five patients received four intravenous infusions of IDEC 114 over a 3–6 week period, in dosages ranging from 2.5 to 15.0 mg/kg. Clinical improvement was noted in all dosage groups. Histopathological results, including reduced epidermal CD3+ T-cell counts, reduced epidermal thickness, and normalization of keratinocyte differentiation, were generally consistent with clinical outcome. (These data were presented at the American Academy of Dermatology, the Society for Investigative Dermatology, and at the International Psoriasis Symposium, 2001.)

However, with both CTLA4lg and IDEC 114, a minority of patients cleared, suggesting that other T-cell surface proteins and/or other pathogenic molecular pathways are required for T-cell activation in some patients with psoriasis.

B. Role of Memory T Cells in Psoriasis

CD45RO+ (so-called memory effector) T cells predominate in psoriasis lesions. Alefacept (LFA3TIP) is a 115 kD fusion protein that consists of the first extracellular domain of human LFA-3 fused to the hinge C_H2 and C_H3 sequences of human IgG_1. Alefacept binds CD2 on T cells leading to inhibition of T-cell costimulation and a reversible reduction of memory-effector (CD4+CD45RO+, CD8+CD45RO+) T cells in peripheral blood (Fig. 2) (33). In a small study, clinical response correlated with depletion of T cells from the epidermis (29, 30, 34, 35).

A phase II double-blind, placebo-controlled study of 229 patients with moderate to severe psoriasis given 12 weekly intravenous doses of alefacept (0.025, 0.075, 0.150 mg/kg vs. placebo), followed by a 12 week follow-up period, was performed. At 12 weeks, the mean reduction in psoriasis area severity index (PASI) was 38%, 53%, and 53% in the 0.025, 0.075, and 0.150 mg/kg groups, respectively, compared with 21% in the placebo group. Alefacept treatment required approximately 3 months to show dramatic

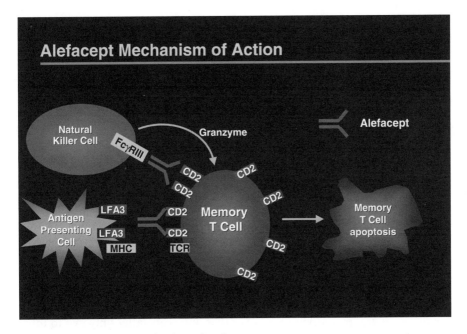

Figure 2 Alefacept mechanism of action.

clinical response. Of the 29 patients whose skin was clear after the 12 week follow up period, the median time until relapse (i.e., patients were no longer clear or almost clear) was 236 days. Early reduction in the number of circulating memory T cells was associated with clinical response. On a population basis, there was a correlation between reduction in the CD45RO+ (memory) T-cell subset early in treatment and clinical improvement, although early reduction in memory T-cell numbers was neither necessary nor sufficient for clinical response (36). The combined data suggest that other T-cell surface proteins and/or other pathogenic molecular pathways are required in some patients with psoriasis.

Phase III trials confirmed and extended the observations made in phase II. Both an intramuscular and intravenous formulation were tested in phase III. After one 12 week course of intramuscular alefacept (15 mg dosed weekly), 33% of patients achieved at least a 75% reduction in PASI. After two 12 week courses of intramuscular alefacept, 43% of patients achieved at least a 75% reduction in PASI (37). Selective reductions in memory-effector (CD45RO+) T cells were related to clinical improvement (38). Alefacept was recently recommended by the FDA's Dermatology Advisory Panel for approval as monotherapy for moderate to severe psoriasis.

VI. ROLE OF ICAM-1-LFA-1

Efalizumab (anti-CD11a, Raptiva) is a non-lymphocyte-depleting, humanized monoclonal antibody against T-cell lymphocyte leukocyte function-associated antigen (LFA-1) that has been studied as monotherapy for patients with moderate to severe plaque psoriasis (1, 39–41). By blocking the interaction between LFA-1 and ICAM-1, efalizumab inhibits T-cell activation and inhibits T-cell migration into skin (1) (Fig. 3).

Two phase III clinical trials, enrolling 1095 subjects, have been completed, partially evaluated, and presented at a number of national and international meetings in 2001. The clinical response to 12 weekly subcutaneous (SC) efalizumab doses was studied. The primary endpoint was achievement of 75% or more improvement in PASI (42). Subjects were randomized to treatment consisting of an initial conditioning dose of 0.7 mg/kg in week 1, followed by 11 weekly doses of either 1.0 mg/kg or 2.0 mg/kg of efalizumab or placebo.

More subjects (29.2%) treated with efalizumab (1 mg/kg) achieved at least 75% PASI improvement than did those receiving placebo (3.4%). Combined results from both trials show that the PASI improvement for both efalizumab groups was improved over that of placebo after only two to four doses (p < 0.005).

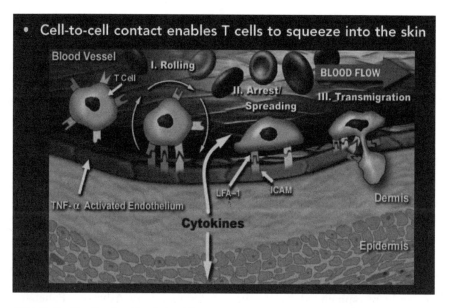

Figure 3 T-cell migration into skin.

Immunohistological studies in phases I and II demonstrated decreased T-cell infiltration in plaques and normalization of keratinocyte differentiation in a minority of patients. Reductions in epidermal T-cell number were accompanied by increases in circulating lymphocytes. Based on these observations, the authors hypothesized that efalizumab inhibits T-cell migration into the skin. CD11a saturation in plaques was necessary but not sufficient for clinical clearance as defined by the primary endpoint above (1, 40, 41, 43).

The combined data suggest that other T-cell surface proteins and/ or other pathogenic molecular pathways are required in some patients with psoriasis.

VII. T1 CYTOKINES PREDOMINATE IN PSORIATIC PLAQUES

A useful way to categorize some the major T-cell cytokines has been to group them into T1 and T2 subclasses (Table 2) (reviewed in (7)). Proinflammatory or T1 cytokines, such as IL-2, TNF-α, lymphotoxin, IL-12, IL-18, and interferon gamma, stimulate cell-mediated immunity and T-cell cytotoxicity. T2 cytokines, such as IL-4, IL-5, IL-6, IL10, and IL-13, stimulate humoral immunity.

Psoriasis is a T1-mediated T-cell disorder. Patients with psoriasis have an increased expression of interferon-gamma over IL-4 in circulating T cells compared with normal volunteers (7, 44). CD3 + T lymphocytes from psoriatic plaque epidermis express increased interferon-gamma compared with IL-4 (7, 44). Pilot, open studies of 1L-10 and IL-11 in the treatment of psoriasis demonstrated decreased T1 cytokine expression and increased T2 cytokine expression in plaques responding to cytokine therapy as compared with baseline plaques (44, 45).

VIII. IMPORTANT ROLE OF TNF-ALPHA IN PSORIASIS AND PSORIATIC ARTHRITIS

The inflammatory response in psoriatic plaques is initiated in part by activated T cells in the epidermis and dermis (reviewed in (46)). T1 T cells predominate in plaques and release a number of inflammatory cytokines, including TNF-α (44). TNF-α, γ-interferon, IL-6, IL-8, and other inflammatory cytokines are elevated in psoriatic lesions but not in the normal skin of psoriatic patients (7–10, 44, 47). TNF-α increases the synthesis of proinflammatory cytokines such as IL-1, IL-6, and IL-8 and activates nuclear transcription factors such as NFκB (48) (Fig. 4).

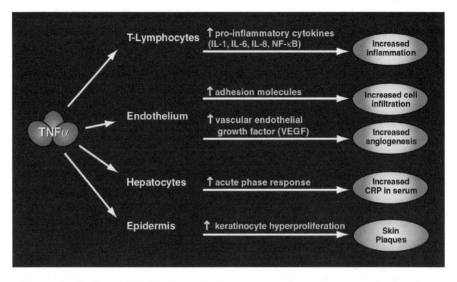

Figure 4 Actions of TNFα in psoriasis.

Psoriasis is an inflammatory, T-cell-mediated disease; however, what causes activation of these T cells is still unknown. After antigen exposure in the skin, Langerhans cells, which are the antigen-presenting cells of the epidermis, must exit the skin and travel to lymph nodes, where presentation of antigen to T cells takes place. TNF-alpha is capable of stimulating Langerhans cells to migrate from the skin to the lymph nodes. Interaction of MHC class I- or II-bound antigen with the T-cell receptor, plus a second activating signal, causes activation of T cells. This leads to T-cell expression of surface membrane proteins (e.g., cutaneous lymphocyte-associated antigen; CLA), allowing them access into the skin. An additional possible method involves E-cadherin, an adhesion molecule in the epidermis that enables Langerhans cell binding to keratinocytes. Expression of E-cadherin potentially retains Langerhans cells in the epidermis, bound to keratinocytes. TNF-α decreases E-cadherin expression (49). A decrease of E-cadherin could facilitate the migration of Langerhans cells from the skin, allowing their travel to lymph nodes and subsequent T-cell activation.

By inducing the synthesis of adhesion molecules on endothelial cells and keratinocytes, TNF-α potentially increases cellular infiltration in skin (50, 51). Leukocyte migration into skin could also be promoted by the induction of vascular endothelial growth factor by TNF-α (52).

TNF-α increases keratinocyte proliferation in vitro (53). TNF-α has been found to increase type I vasoactive intestinal peptide (VIP) receptor mRNA in keratinocytes. Subsequent binding of VIP to its receptor pro-

motes keratinocyte proliferation and stimulates synthesis of proinflammatory cytokines such as IL-6, IL-8, and regulated on activation, normal T-cell
expressed and secreted (RANTES) (54). TNF-α increases plasminogen
activator inhibitor type 2 (PAI-2), a serine proteinase inhibitor, which is
thought to protect cells from apoptosis (55). The prevention of apoptosis
could lead to increased longevity of keratinocytes, and consequently a
thickened epidermis.

TNF-α also increases hepatocyte synthesis of acute-phase reactants
such as C-reactive protein. Thus TNF-α potentially contributes to the clinical
and histological phenotype characteristic of psoriasis.

A. Infliximab

Infliximab is a chimeric IgG1 anti-TNF-α monoclonal antibody that binds to
transmembrane-bound and soluble TNF-α with high specificity, affinity, and
avidity (56). Infliximab neutralizes transmembrane-bound TNF-α on the cells
that synthesize it (e.g., antigen-presenting cells, keratinocytes, mast cells, and
activated T cells) (56). Infliximab acts like a sponge to absorb soluble
circulating TNF-α. Infliximab competes with the TNF receptor for receptor-
bound ligand on target cells (e.g., lymphocytes, antigen-presenting cells,
and keratinocyte). Infliximab has the potential to kill cells bearing surface
TNF-α by both complement-mediated and antibody-dependent, cell-mediated cytotoxicity. Infliximab induces apoptosis of activated lymphocytes in
vitro. Infliximab is not currently indicated for the treatment of psoriasis.
However, it is indicated for the treatment of moderate to severe Crohn's
disease (for the reduction of signs and symptoms and closure of enterocutaneous fistulas) and moderate to severe rheumatoid arthritis (for reduction
of signs and symptoms and inhibition of progression of structural damage)
(56–61).

In psoriasis, the TNF story started with a 57-year-old woman with
recalcitrant, severe psoriasis and Crohn's disease who was treated for
refractory inflammatory bowel disease with a humanized anti-TNF-α monoclonal antibody (infliximab). The patient had a 15 year history of Crohn's
disease with dependence on high-dosage prednisone (up to 60 mg/day), and a
20 year history of moderate to severe psoriasis treated with topical corticosteroids. The patient received a single infusion of infliximab (5 mg/kg).
Dramatic improvement in her psoriasis was demonstrated 2 weeks after the
infusion (58). The PASI values measured at baseline, 2 weeks after Infliximab
infusion, and 4 weeks postinfusion were 34.1, 19.9, and 12.1 respectively. At
16 weeks postinfusion, the patient's PASI had gradually returned to a baseline
value of 34.3. The patient received a second dose of infliximab (5 mg/kg) 16
weeks following first dose. As with the first administration of infliximab, the

patient's psoriasis and Crohn's disease followed a similar course of clinical improvement upon follow-up examinations (58).

Based upon this observation a double blind, placebo-controlled, phase II study of infliximab monotherapy in the treatment of plaque-type psoriasis was executed and recently reported (11). This study was conducted to assess the clinical benefit and safety of infliximab monotherapy in patients with moderate to severe plaque psoriasis. A second aim was to use infliximab as a targeted therapeutic probe to determine the role of TNF-α in the pathogenesis of psoriasis. In this investigator-initiated, double-blind, placebo-controlled, clinical trial, 33 patients with moderate to severe plaque psoriasis were randomized to receive placebo or infliximab 5 or 10 mg/kg infusions at weeks 0, 2, and 6. Patients were assessed at week 10 for the primary endpoint determination, which was the physician's global assessment (PGA). The proportions of responders (good, excellent, or clear rating on PGA) were 9/11 (81.8%) and 10/11 (90.9%) patients in the infliximab 5 and 10 mg/kg groups, respectively, vs. 2/11 (18.2%) patients in the placebo group (p < 0.01 for each infliximab group vs. placebo). Nine of 11 (81.8%) and 8/11 (72.7%) patients had at least 75% improvement in the PASI in the 5 and 10 mg/kg dosing groups, respectively, compared to 2/11 (18.2%) patients in the placebo group (p < 0.05 for each infliximab group vs. placebo). The median time to response was 4 weeks for patients in both infliximab groups. There were no serious adverse events and infliximab was well tolerated. In this controlled trial, patients receiving the anti-TNF-α agent infliximab as monotherapy experienced a high degree of clinical benefit and rapid time to response in the treatment of moderate to severe plaque psoriasis compared to patients who received placebo. These findings strongly suggest that TNF-α plays a pivotal role in the pathogenesis of psoriasis (11).

The pharmacodynamic response to infliximab was next investigated: Immunohistochemical changes were assessed in patients with moderate to severe plaque psoriasis who were treated with infliximab 5 mg/kg, infliximab 10 mg/kg, or placebo, in this double-blind, clinical trial. Immunoperoxidase analysis of lesional (weeks 0, 2, 10) and nonlesional (week 0) biopsies for epidermal CD3+ T cells, epidermal keratin K16 expression, keratinocyte ICAM-1 expression, and epidermal thickness was conducted. Correlation analyses between histological findings and clinical efficacy measures (PASI and PGA) were performed using the Spearman correlation test. Targeted immunotherapy with infliximab resulted in rapid and dramatic decreases in epidermal inflammation and in normalization of keratinocyte differentiation in psoriatic plaques. These changes preceded maximal clinical response and correlated with both PASI and PGA scores (62). The combined clinical and immunohistological data again demonstrate a pivotal role for TNF-α in the pathogenesis of psoriasis and support further clinical development of drugs that target TNF-α.

For the open-label extension portion of the phase II study, the durability of response in patients who were defined as responders in the blinded phase of the study was determined. In this open-label extension, patients with moderate to severe plaque psoriasis received a three-dose induction regimen of infliximab 5 or 10 mg/kg at weeks 0, 2, and 6. During weeks 10–26 patients were evaluated for loss of response (loss of at least half of the improvement in the PASI score achieved at week 10) and retreated with open-label infliximab 5 or 10 mg/kg as needed. Twenty-nine subjects participated in the open-label extension. At week 10, 77% of infliximab-treated patients achieved at least 75% improvement from baseline in the PASI score. Among the 19 patients who continued in the trial through week 26, 58% maintained at least 50% improvement and 48% maintained at least 75% improvement in the PASI score as compared to the baseline score. There were no serious adverse events and infliximab was well tolerated. Thus infliximab is a remittive psoriasis therapy. (These data were presented at the International Psoriasis Symposium and the Society far Investigative Dermatology in 2001 and the American Academy of Dermatology in 2002.)

B. Etanercept

Etanercept is a fusion protein of two TNFα receptor p75 extracellular domains with one IgG1 Fc region and is FDA-approved for the treatment of rheumatoid arthritis and psoriatic arthritis. The American College of Rheumatology criteria for improvement (ACR20) (63) were used to assess clinical response of psoriatic arthritis in phase III studies. In those patients with 3% or greater body surface area involvement with psoriasis, PASI and target lesion assessments were done. Forty-seven percent of patients in both the etanercept and placebo groups were receiving concurrent methotrexate therapy. Twenty percent and 40% of patients were receiving systemic corticosteroids in the etanercept and placebo groups, respectively.

In the phase III study, 205 patients with PsA were enrolled; 101 received etanercept and 104 received placebo. Patients received 25 mg etanercept or placebo twice weekly SC for 24 weeks. Concomitant therapy with methotrexate, oral corticosteroids, and nonsteroidal anti-inflammatory drugs was permitted. The primary arthritis endpoint was the ACR20 at 12 weeks. Psoriasis improvement was measured by target lesion score, and, in a subset of patients with psoriasis involvement $\geq 3\%$ (n = 66 for etanercept; n = 62 for placebo), by the PASI. Arthritis was significantly improved with etanercept treatment. ACR20 was achieved by 59% of the etanercept group and 15% of the placebo group at 12 weeks (p < 0.0001).

Significant improvement in arthritis was maintained with continued etanercept treatment through the end of the study at 24 weeks. ACR70 was achieved in 11% of the etanercept-treated patients vs. 0% of the placebo-treated patients at 12 weeks. Psoriatic target lesions were also significantly improved with etanercept treatment; median improvement at 24 weeks was 33% in etanercept patients and 0% in placebo patients (p < 0.0001). PASI measurements confirm this result. Etanercept was well-tolerated in this patient population (64).

The next study examined the efficacy of etanercept as monotherapy in patients with psoriasis. In a 24-week, multicenter, blinded, randomized study, patients received etanercept 25 mg or placebo by SC injection twice weekly. The primary endpoint was the 75% improvement in PASI at 12 weeks. One hundred twelve patients enrolled in the study. Groups (n = 57 for etanercept; n = 55 for placebo) were well-matched for patient age, psoriasis duration, and disease intensity. The percentage of patients achieving PASI improvement of at least 75% at 12 weeks was significantly higher in the etanercept group than the placebo group (30% vs. 2% respectively; p < 0.0001). Efficacy continued to improve with longer treatment: 56% of etanercept-treated patients and 5% of placebo-treated patients reached PASI improvements of at least 75% at 24 weeks (p < 0.0001). Statistically significant improvements in patient global, physician global, target lesion assessments, and dermatology life quality index (DLQI) confirmed efficacy of etanercept therapy. Etanercept was well tolerated. Numbers of patients reporting adverse events were similar between groups (70% for etanercept, 67% for placebo), as were the rates of adverse events (4.49 per patient year for etanercept, 5.66 per patient year for the placebo group). Etanercept as monotherapy was efficacious, safe, and well-tolerated in the treatment of psoriasis (65).

Taken together, the infliximab and etanercept data point to a key role for TNF-α in the pathogenesis of psoriasis and psoriatic arthritis. The pathogenesis of multiple sclerosis has been frequently grouped with that Crohn's disease and rheumatoid arthritis (RA): all four diseases have been thought to be T1-mediated immune disorders. Recent reports of exacerbation of multiple sclerosis with therapies targeting TNF-α (61, 66), and of β-interferon-induced flares of psoriasis in patients whose multiple sclerosis improved (67), demonstrate that the pathogenesis of multiple sclerosis is different from that of psoriasis, rheumatoid arthritis, and Crohn's disease.

The accumulated data indicate a key role for TNF-α in the pathogenesis of psoriasis and psoriatic arthritis, rheumatoid arthritis, and Crohn's disease. Additionally, both infliximab and etanercept have demonstrated efficacy in the treatment of ankylosing spondylitis, suggesting that this disorder too is at least partially mediated by TNF-α (68, 69). There are case reports and small series of patients with other immune-mediated inflammatory disorders (IMIDs) treated successfully with TNF-targeting immuno-therapies (infliximab). These include uveitis, Sjögren's syndrome, giant cell arteritis, graft vs. host disease, sarcoidosis, hidradenitis suppurativa, and pyoderma gangrenosum (11, 58, 68–80). Thus, rather than considering these disorders as separate and localized to nonoverlapping therapeutic areas, perhaps we should group these IMIDs by common pathogenesis.

IX. CONCLUSION

It is exciting to have so many biologicals in development for the treatment of moderate to severe plaque-type psoriasis. We anxiously await published trials with large numbers of psoriasis patients treated with these targeted immuno-biologicals for prolonged periods of time in order to assess safety risks to patient more accurately. Additionally, we will need data on the combination of targeted immunobiologicals with each other and with current, FDA-approved therapies for psoriasis. However, because no targeted organ toxicity has been demonstrated with any these immunobiologicals to date, we are optimistic that patients will soon have choices among treatments that offer hope for long-term, safe, and effective treatments for this chronic, life-impacting illness. Clinical research with targeted immunotherapeutic probes has also the led the way in determining the pathogenesis of psoriasis and will continue to yield important scientific knowledge.

ACKNOWLEDGMENTS

This work was supported in part by a grant from the David Ju Foundation and by general support to the Clinical Research Center by Merck, Inc.

REFERENCES

1. Gottlieb A, Krueger JG, Bright R, et al. Effects of administration of a single dose of a humanized monoclonal antibody to CD11a on the immunobiology and clinical activity of psoriasis. J Am Acad Dermatol 2000; 42:428–435.
2. Ovigne JM, Baker BS, Brown DW, Powles AV, Fry L. Epidermal CD8+ T cells in chronic plaque psoriasis are Tc1 cells producing heterogeneous levels of interferon-gamma. Exp Dermatol 2001; 10:168–174.
3. Nestle F, Turka L, Nickoloff B. Characterization of dermal dendritic cells in psoriasis. Autostimulation of T lymphocytes and induction of Th1 type cytokines. J Clin Invest 1994; 94:202–209.

4. Jones J, Berth-Jones J, Fletcher A, Hutchinson P. Assessment of epidermal dendritic cell markers and T-lymphocytes in psoriasis. J Pathol 1994; 174:77–82.

5. Gottlieb AB, Lifshitz B, Fu SM, Staiano-Coico L, Wang CY, Carter DM. Expression of HLA-DR molecules by keratinocytes and presence of Langerhans cells in the dermal infiltrate of active psoriatic plaques. J Exp Med 1986; 164:1013–1028.

6. Gottlieb SL, Gilleaudeau P, Johnson R, et al. Response of psoriasis to a lymphocyte-selective toxin (DAB389IL-2) suggests a primary immune, but not keratinocyte, pathogenic basis. Nature Med 1995; 1:442–447.

7. Austin L, Ozawa M, Kikuchi T, Krueger G. Intracellular TNF-alpha, IFN-gamma, and IL-2 identify TC1 and TH1 effector populations in psoriasis vulgaris plaque lymphocytes: single-cell analysis by flow cytometry. J Invest Dermatol 1998; 110:649.

8. Grossman RM, Krueger J, Yourish D, et al. Intedeukin-6 (IL-6) is expressed in high levels in psoriatic skin and stimulates proliferation of cultured human keratinocytes. Proc Natl Acad Sci USA 1989; 86:6367–6371.

9. Sticherling M, Bornscheuer E, Schroder JM, Christophers E. Localization of neutrophil-activating peptide-1/interleukin-8-immunoreactivity in normal and psoriatic skin. J Invest Dermatol 1991; 96:26–30.

10. Livden JK, Nilsen R, Bjerke JR, Matre R. In situ localization of interferons in psoriatic lesions. Arch Dermatol Res 1989; 281:392–397.

11. Chaudhari U, Romano P, Mulcahy LD, Dooley LT, Baker DG, Gottlieb AB. Efficacy and safety of infliximab monotherapy for plaque-type psoriasis: a randomised trial. Lancet 2001; 357:1842–1847.

12. Barnes PJ, Karin M. Nuclear factor-kappaB-A pivotal transcription factor in chronic inflammatory diseases. N Engl J Med 1997; 336:1066–1072.

13. Gomi T, Shiohara T, Munakata T, Imanishi K, Nagashima M. Interleukin 1alpha, Tumor necrosis factor alpha and interferon gamma in psoriasis. Arch Dermatol 1991; 127:827–830.

14. Nickoloff BJ. The immunologic and genetic basis of psoriasis. Arch Dermatol 1999; 135:1104–1110.

15. Nickoloff BJ, Kunkel SL, Burdick M, Strieter RM. Severe combined immunodeficiency mouse and human psoriatic skin chimeras. Validation of a new animal model. Am J Pathol 1995; 146:580–588.

16. Gilhar A, David M, Ullmann Y, Berkutski T, Kalish RS. T-lymphocyte dependence of psoriatic pathology in human psoriatic skin grafted to SCID mice. J Invest Dermatol 1997; 109:283–288.

17. Gottlieb AB, Bacha P, Parker K, Strand V. Use of the interleukin-2 fusion protein, DAB389IL-2, for the treatment of psoriasis. Dermatol Ther 1998; 5:48–63.

18. Horrocks C, Duncan JI, Sewell HF, Ormerod D, Thomson AW. Differential effects of cyclosporine A on Langerhans cell and regulatory T-cell populations in severe psoriasis: an immunohistochemical and flow cytometric analysis. J Autoimmun 1990; 3:559–570.

19. Baker BS, Swain AF, Griffiths CEM, Leonard JN, Fry L, Valdimarsson H. Epidermal T lymphocytes and dendritic cells in chronic plaque psoriasis: the effects of PUVA treatment. Clin Exp Immunol 1985; 61:526–534.

20. Nestle F, Nickoloff B. Dermal dendritic cells are important members of the skin immune system. Adv Exp Mol Biol 1995; 378:111–6.

21. Das P, de Boer O, Visser A, Verhagen C, Bos J, Pals S. Differential expression of ICAM-1, E-selectin and VCAM-1 by endothelial cells in psoriasis and contact dermatitis. Acta Derm Venereol Suppl (Stockh) 1994; 186:21–2.

22. De Boer O, Wakelkamp I, Pals S, Claessen N, Bos J, Das P. Increased expression of adhesion receptors in both lesional and non-lesional psoriatic skin. Arch Dermatol Res 1994; 286:304–11.

23. Ashworth J, Kahan MC, Breathnach SM. PUVA therapy decreases HLA-DR + CDia + Langerhans cells and epidermal cell antigen-presenting capacity in human skin, but flow cytometrically-sorted residual HLA-DR + CDia + Langerhans cells exhibit normal alloantigen-presenting function. Br J Dermatol 1989; 120:329–339.

24. Kimber I, Cumberbatch M, Dearman RJ, Bhushan M, Griffiths CEM. Cytokines and chemokines in the initiation and regulation of epidermal Langerhans cell mobilization. Br J of Dermatol 2000; 142:401–412.

25. Abrams J, Kelley S, Hayes E, et al. Blockade of T lymphocyte costimulation with cytotoxic T lymphocyte-associated antigen 4-immunoglobulin (CTLA4Ig) reverses the cellular pathology of psoriatic plaques, including the activation of keratinocytes, dendritic cells, and endothelial cells. J Exp Med 2000;192:681–94.

26. Dieu-Nosjean M-C, Massacrier, C., Hormey, B., et. al. Macrophage inflammatory protein 3a is expressed at inflamed epithelial surfaces and is the most potent chemokine known in attracting Langerhans cell precursors. J Exp Med 2000; 192:705–717.

27. vanNoesel C, Miedema F, Brouwer M, deRie MA, Aarden LA, vanLier RAW. Regulatory properties of LFA-1 alpha and beta chains in human T-lymphocyte activation. Nature 1988; 333:850–852.

28. June CH, Ledbetter JA, Linsley PS, Thompson CB. Role of the CD28 receptor in T-cell activation. Immunology Today 1990; 11:211–216.

29. Springer TA, Dustin ML, Kashimoto TK, et. al. The lymphocyte function-associated LFA-1, CD2, and LFA-2 molecules: cell adhesion receptors of the immune system. Annu Rev Immunol 1987; 5:223–252.

30. Friedrich M. KS, Henze M., Docke W.D., Sterry W., Asadullah K. Flow cytometric characterization of lesional T cells in psoriasis: intracellular cytokine and surface antigen expression indicates an activated, memory/effector type 1 immunophenotype. Arch Derm Res 2000; 292:59–521.

31. Grakoui A. BSK, Sumen C., et. al. The immunological synapse: A molecular machine controlling T cell activation. Science 1999; 285:221–227.

32. Gottlieb AB, Lebwohl M, Tortoritus MC, Abdulghani AA, Shuey SR, Romano P, Chaudhari U, Allen RS, Lizambri RG. Clinical and histologic response to single-dose treatment of moderate to severe psoriasis with an anti-CD80 monoclonal antibody. J Am Acad Dermatol 2002; 47:692–700.

33. daSilva AJ, Brickelmaier M, Majeau GR, et al. Alefacept, an immuno-modulatory recombinant LFA-3/IgG1 fusion protein, induced CD16 signaling and CD2/CD16-dependent apoptosis of CD2+ cells. J Immunol 2002; 168: 4462–4471.

34. Krueger JG, Gilleaudeau P, Kikuchi T, Lee E. Psoriasis-related subpopulations of memory CD4+ and CD8+ T cells are selectively reduced by Alefacept. J Invest Dermatol 2002; 119:345.

35. Magilavy D. Immunopharmacologic effects of Amevive (LFA3TIP) in chronic plaque psoriasis: selectivity for peripheral memory-effector (CD45RO+) over Naive (CD45RA+) T cells: AMEVIVE Clinical Study Group. Br J Dermatol 1999; 141:990.

36. Ellis CN, Krueger GG, Group ACS. Treatment of chronic plaque psoriasis by selective targeting of memory effector T lymphocytes. N Engl J Med 2001; 345:248–255.

37. Langley RD, Christophers E, Lebwohl M. Efficacy and safety of multiple courses of intramuscular alefacept in patients with chronic plaque psoriasis. J Invest Dermatol 2002; 119:344.

38. Lowe N, Griffiths C, Gottlieb AB. Selective reductions in memory-effector (CD45RO+) T cells by alefacept are related to clinical improvement in psoriasis. J Invest Dermatol 2002; 119:345.

39. Gordon KB, Leonardi C, Tyring S, Gottlieb AB, Walicke P, Dummer W, Papp K. Efalizumab (anti CD11a) is safe and effective in the treatment of psoriasis: pooled reslults of the 12 week first treatment period from 2 phase III trials. J Invest Dermatol 2002; 119:242.

40. Gottlieb AB, Krueger JG, Wittkowski K, Dedrick R, Walicke PA, Garovoy M. Psoriasis as a model for T-cell-mediated disease: Immunobiologic and clinical effects of treatment with multiple doses of efalizumab, an anti-CD11a monoclonal antibody. Arch Dermatol 2002; 138:591–600.

41. Papp K. BR, Krueger J.G., et al. The treatment of moderate to severe psoriasis with a new anti-CD11a monoclonal antibody. J Am Acad Dermatol 2001; 45:665–674.

42. Frederiksson T, Pettersson U. Severe psoriasis oral therapy with a new retinoid. Dermatologica 1978; 157:238–244.

43. Gottlieb AB, Krueger JG, Dedrick R, Walicke PA, Garovoy M, and the HUPS249 Study Group. Psoriasis as a model for T-cell-mediated disease: Immunobiologic and clinical effects of treatment with multiple doses of an anti-CDIIa antibody. Arch Dermatol 2002; 138:591–600.

44. Trepicchio W, Ozawa M, Walters IB, et al. IL-11 is an immune-modulatory cytokine which downregulates IL-12, Type 1 cytokines, and multiple inflamma-tion-associated genes in patients with psoriasis. J Invest Dermatol 1999; 112:598.

45. Asadullah K, Sterry W, Stephanek K, et al. IL-10 is a key cytokine in psoriasis. Proof of principle by IL-10 therapy: a new therapeutic approach. J Clin Invest 1998; 101:783–794.

46. Gottlieb AB. Psoriasis: Immunopathology and immunomodulation. Derm Clinics 2001; 19:649–657.

47. Ettehadi P, Greaves MW, Wallach D, Aderka D, Camp RDR. Elevated tumour necrosis factor-alpha (TNF-alpha)biological activity in psoriatic skin lesions. Clin Exp Immunol 1994; 96:146–151.

48. Choy EHS, Panayi GS. Cytokine pathways and joint inflammation in rheumatoid arthritis. N Engl J Med 2001; 344:907–916.

49. Schwarzenberger K, Udey MC. Contact allergens and epidermal proinflammatory cytokines modulate Langerhans cell E-cadherin expression in situ. J Invest Dermatol 1996; 106:553–558.

50. Norris DA. Cytokine modulation of adhesion molecules in the regulation of immunologic cytotoxicity of epidermal targets. J Invest Dermatol 1990; 95:111S-120S.

51. Griffiths CEM, Voorhees JJ, Nickoloff BJ. Characterization of intercellular adhesion molecule-1 and HLA-DR expression in normal and inflamed skin: modulation by recombinant gamma interferon and tumor necrosis factor. J Am Acad Dermatol 1989; 20:617–629.

52. Sato N, Nariuchi H, Tsuruoka N, et al. Actions of TNF and IFN-gamma on angiogenesis in vitro. J Invest Dermatol 1990; 95:85S-89S.

53. Nickoloff BJ. The cytokine network in psoriasis. Arch Dermatol 1991; 127:871–884.

54. Kakurai M, Fujita N, Murata S, et al. Vasoactive intestinal peptide regulated its receptor expression and functions of human keratinocytes via type I vasoactive intestinal peptide receptors. J Invest Dermatol 2001; 116:743–749.

55. Wang Y, Jensen PJ. Regulation of the level and glycosylation state of plasminogen activator inhibitor type 2 during human keratinocyte differentiation. Differentiation 1998; 63:93–99.

56. Scallon BJ, Moore MA, Trinh H, Knight DM, Ghrayeb J. Chimeric anti-TNF-alpha monoclonal anti-body cA2 binds recombinant transmembrane TNF-alpha and activates immune effector functions. Cytokine 1995; 7:251–259.

57. Maini R, St.Clair EW, Breedveld F, et al. Infliximab (chimeric anti-tumour necrosis factor-alpha monoclonal antibody) versus placebo in rheumatoid arthritis patients receiving concomitant methotrexate: a randomised phase III trial. Lancet 1999; 354:1932–1939.

58. Oh CJ, Das KM, Gottlieb AB. Treatment with anti-tumor necrosis factor-alpha (TNF-alpha) monoclonal antibody dramatically decreases the clinical activity of psoriasis lesions. J Am Acad Dermatol 2000; 42:829–830.

59. Present DH, Rutgeerts P, Targan S, et al. Infliximab for the treatment of fistulas in patients with Crohn's disease. N Engl J Med 1999; 340:1398–1401.

60. Targan SR, Hanauer SB, VanDeventer SJH, et al. A short-term study of chimeric monoclonal antibody cA2 to tumor necrosis factor-alpha for Crohn's disease. N Engl J Med 1997; 337:1029–1035.

61. VanOosten BW, Barkhof F, Truyen L, al. e. Increased MRI activity and immune activation in two multiple sclerosis patients treated with monoclonal anti-tumor necrosis factor antibody CA2. Neurology 1996; 47:1531–1534.

62. Gottlieb AB, Masud S, Ramamurthi R, Abdulghani A, Romano P, Chaudhari U, Dooley LT, Fasanmade AA, Wagner CL. Pharmacodynamic and

pharmacokinetic response to anti-tumor necrosis factor monoclonal antibody (Infliximab) treatment of moderate to severe psoriasis vulgaris. J Am Acad Dermatol 2002; in press.

63. Mease PJ, Goffe BS, Metz J, VanderStoep A, Finck B, Burge DJ. Etanercept in the treatment of psoriatic arthritis and psoriasis: a randomised trial. Lancet 2000; 356:385–390.

64. Mease P, Kivitz A, Burch F, Siegel E, Cohen S, Burge D. Improvement in disease activity in patients with psoriatic arthritis receiving etanercept (Enbrel): Results of a phase 3 multicenter clinical trial. Arthritis Rheum 2001;44:S90.

65. Gottlieb AB, Matheson RT, Lowe NJ, Zitnik RJ. Efficacy of Enbrel in patients with psoriasis. J Invest Dermatol 2002; 119:234.

66. Amason BGW, Lenercept MSSG. TNF neutralization in MS: Results of a randomized, placebo-controlled multicenter study. Neurology 1999; 53:457–465.

67. Webster GF, Knobler RL, Lublin FD, Kramer EM, Hochman LR. Cutaneous ulcerations and pustular psoriasis flare caused by recombinant interferon beta injections in patients with multiple sclerosis. J Am Acad Dermatol 1996; 34:365–367.

68. Braun J, Brandt J, Listing J, et al. Treatment of active ankylosing spondylitis with inflximimab: a randomised controlled multicentre trial. Lancet 2002; 359:1187–1193.

69. Gorman JD, Sack KE, Davis Jr JC. Treatment of ankylosing spondylitis by inhibition of tumor necrosis factor alpha. N Engl J Med 2002; 346: 1349–1356.

70. Braughman RPI, Lower EE. Inflximab for refractory sarcoidosis. Sarcoidosis Vasc. Diffuse Lung Dis 2001; 18:70–74.

71. Botros N, Pickover, L., Das, K.M. Image of the month. Gastroenterology 2000; 118:654.

72. Cambell S, Ghosh S. Infliximab therapy for Crohn's disease in the presence of chronic hepatitis C infection. Eur J Gastroenterol Hepatol 2001; 13:191–192.

73. Couriel DR, Hicks K, Giralt S, Champlin RE. Role of tumor necrosis factor-alpha inhibition with inflximab in cancer therapy and hematopoietic stem cell transplantation. Curr Opin Oncol 2000; 12:582–587.

74. De Clercq E. Perspectives for the chemotherapy of AIDS. Anticancer Res 1987; 7:1023–1038.

75. Fabrizio C, Niccoli L, Salvarani C, Padula A, Olivieri. Treatment of longstanding active giant cell arteritis with infliximab: report of four cases. Arthritis Rheum 2001; 44:2933–2935.

76. Martinez F, Nos P, Benlloch S, Ponce J. Hidradenitis suppurativa and Crohn's disease: response to treatment with infliximab. Inflamm Bowel Dis 2001; 7:323–326.

77. Schothorst AA, Evers LM, Noz KC, Filon R, van Zeeland AA. Pyrimidine dimer induction and repair in cultured human skin keratinocytes or melanocytes after irradiation with monochromatic ultraviolet radiation. J Invest Dermatol 1991; 96:916–920.

78. Smith JR, Levinson RD, Holland GN, et al. Differential effiacy of tumor necrosis factor inhibition in the management of inflammatory eye disease and associated rheumatic disease. Arthritis Care Res 2001;45:252–2557.

79. Steinfeld S, Demols, P., Salmon, I., Kiss, R., Appelboom, T. Infliximab in pateints with primary Sjogren's syndrome: a pilot study. Arthritis Rheum 2001; 44:2371–2375

80. Tan JH, Gordon M, Lebwohl O, George J, Lebwohl MG. Improvement of pyoderma gangrenosum and psoriasis associated with Crohn disease with anti-tumor necrosis factor alpha monoclonal antibody. Arch Dermatol 2001; 137:930-933.

81. Thomas P. IL-4-induced immune deviation as therapy of psoriasis. Arch Dermatol Res 2001; 293:30.

82. Gottlieb AB, Vaishnaw AK. Alefacept (Amevive) does not blunt primary or secondary immune responses. Arthritis Rheum 2001; 44:S91.

83. Gottlieb A, Abdulghani A, Totoritis M, et al. Results of a single-dose, dose-escalating trial of anti-B7.1 monoclonal antibody ((DEC-114) in patients with psoriasis. J Invest Dermatol 2000; 114:840.

84. Abrams JR, Lebwohl MG, Guzzo CA, et al. CTLA41g-mediated blockade of T-cell costimulation in patients with psoriasis vulgaris. J Clin Invest 1999; 103:1243-1252.

85. Krueger JG, Walters IB, Miyazawa M, et al. Successful in vivo blockade of CD25 (high-affinity interleukin 2 receptor) on T cells by administration of humanized anti-Tac antibody to patients with psoriasis. J Am Acad Dermatol 2000; 43:448-458.

86. Asadullah K, Sterry W, Trefzer U. Cytokine therapy in dermatology. Exp Dermatol 2002; 11:97-106.

12

Etanercept for Treatment of Psoriasis and Psoriatic Arthritis

Alice B. Gottlieb
University of Medicine and Dentistry of New Jersey–Robert Wood Johnson Medical School, New Brunswick, New Jersey, U.S.A.

I. INTRODUCTION

Etanercept (Enbrel, Amgen) is a recombinant human protein that has demonstrated efficacy as monotherapy for moderate to severe psoriasis (1) and is the first Food and Drug Administration-(FDA) approved treatment for psoriatic arthritis (2, 3). Etanercept acts as a competitive inhibitor of tumor necrosis factor (TNF), a proinflammatory cytokine implicated in the pathogenesis of psoriasis and psoriatic arthritis, and in several rheumatic diseases such as rheumatoid- and polyarticular-course juvenile rheumatoid arthritis, and ankylosing spondylitis (RA, JRA, and AS, respectively).

The designation of TNF as a key mediator of inflammatory processes in psoriasis and psoriatic arthritis derives not only from direct correlative data on its biological localization in these disease states, but also from a vast literature on its broad effects relevant to inflammation and immunity (4). TNF plays a critical role in the activation of the innate and acquired immune responses, but the persistence of the immune response and inappropriate production of TNF seen in patients with psoriasis leads to chronic inflammation, tissue damage, and excessive keratinocyte proliferation (5).

The downstream effects of excessive TNF production on various cell types and the clinical manifestations relevant to psoriasis and psoriatic arthritis are summarized in Table 1 (6, 7).

Table 1   Effects of Excessive TNF Production on Various Cell Types

Cell Type	Action of TNF	Effect
Macrophage	Increased proinflammatory cytokine production	Increased inflammation
	Increased chemokine production	Swelling of joints
Keratinocyte	Increased proliferation	Scale and thickness
Endothelial	Increased expression of adhesion molecules	Increased leukocyte infiltration into skin and joints
	Increased production of vascular endothelial growth factor	Increased angiogenesis and erythema
		Auspitz's sign
Hepatocyte	Increased acute-phase response	Increased C-reactive protein
Synoviocyte (fibroblastlike)	Increased metalloproteinase synthesis	Articular cartilage degradation
T lymphocyte	Increased proinflammatory cytokine production	Increased inflammation
	Increased nuclear transcription factor activation	
	T-cell activation	
Dendritic cell	Increased proinflammatory cytokine production	Increased inflammation
	Dendritic cell maturation	
	Increased dendritic cell migration from skin to lymph nodes	
	T-cell activation and differentiation	

II. STRUCTURE AND FUNCTION OF ETANERCEPT

A. Structure

The initiation of TNF-mediated events requires binding of TNF homotrimers to cell-surface receptors, multimerization of these receptors, and subsequent

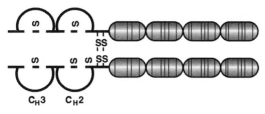

Fc region of   **Extracellular domain of**
human IgG1   **human p75 TNF receptor**

Figure 1   Structure of Etanercept.

signal transduction through the receptor's intracellular domains (8, 9). Soluble forms of the TNF receptors have been shown to exist naturally and are capable of acting as competitive inhibitors for binding of TNF to cell surface receptors (10). The presence of these natural antagonists, however, is not sufficient to block the activity of elevated TNF protein levels observed in most inflammatory diseases (5).

Etanercept is a fully human dimeric fusion protein consisting of the extracellular ligand-binding domain of the human 75 kilodalton (kD) TNF receptor linked to the Fc portion of human immunoglobulin 1 (IgG1). Etanercept does not promote complement-mediated cell lysis in vitro, and has been shown to have a very low (<2%) incidence of immunogenicity in patients with psoriasis, psoriatic arthritis, rheumatoid arthritis, and congestive heart failure (11).

The protein is produced using recombinant DNA technology in a Chinese hamster ovary (CHO) expression system and consists of 934 amino acids, with an apparent molecular weight of 150 kD. A schematic diagram of etanercept is provided in Figure 1.

B. Mechanism of Action

Etanercept inhibits the activity of TNF by competitively binding to this proinflammatory cytokine and preventing interactions with its cell-surface receptors. The dimeric nature of etanercept permits binding of the protein to two free, or receptor-bound molecules of TNF at an affinity 50–1000 times that of soluble monomeric forms of the TNF receptor (12). The increased binding affinity of etanercept is likely to play a key role in the increased TNF-inhibitory activity observed with dimeric forms of the recombinant receptor compared to naturally occurring monovalent forms (13).

Etanercept has been shown to affect animal models of inflammation, including murine collagen-induced arthritis (14, 15), and has demonstrated significant clinical efficacy in the treatment of psoriasis, psoriatic arthritis, RA, JRA, and ankylosing spondylitis (see section on Clinical Use) (1–3, 16–22). Clinical trials with etanercept are also underway in patients with other inflammatory diseases.

Elevated levels of TNF have been found in psoriatic skin lesions, and in synovial explants and fluid from patients with psoriatic arthritis (23–25). The levels of TNF in the serum of patients with plaque psoriasis (26) and in blister fluids of involved psoriatic skin (27) have also been shown to be higher than in those of controls. These values were significantly correlated with the psoriasis area and severity index (PASI) scores (see Table 2 for definition of PASI scores) (26, 27) and related to erythema scores (27).

The predominant source of TNF during inflammation in the rheumatoid arthritic joint is the monocyte/macrophage (28). However, in stimulated skin, keratinocytes, dermal dendritic cells, mast cells, and activated T cells are all capable of TNF production (5). The synthesis and release of TNF is an early event in inflammatory skin processes such as psoriasis (29). Following activation, levels of TNF increase cytokines such as IL-1, IL-2, granulocyte–macrophage colony-stimulating factor GM-CSF, and interferon (IFN)-gamma (30). TNF subsequently increases the expression of other inflammatory mediators and substances such as superoxide anions, prostaglandin E_2, metalloproteinases, and adhesion molecules

Table 2 Definition of the Psoriasis Area and Severity Index (PASI)

	0	1	2	3	4	5	6
Extent (%)	none	up to 10	10–30	3–50	50–70	70–90	> 90
Severity (E,I,S)	none	low	medium	high	very high		

The PASI score derives from a publication by Fredriksson and Pettersson in 1978 (60) and takes into account the localization, extent, and severity of the findings. The head (H), trunk (T), arms (A), and legs (L) are differentiated in terms of localization. Erythema (E), infiltration (I), and scaling (S) are differentiated for severity; and areas on the head (oH), on the trunk (oT), on the arms (oA), and on the legs (oL) are recorded separately for the extent (o) of foci.

Pairs of these terms are formed for each body section and added together, and then multiplied by the percentage body surface area for each body part, and by the extent, so that the calculation is as follows:

$$0.1 \times (E_H + I_H + T_H) \times oH = (1)$$
$$0.3 \times (E_T + I_T + T_T) \times oS = (2)$$
$$0.2 \times (E_A + I_A + T_A) \times oA = (3)$$
$$0.4 \times (E_L + I_L + T_L) \times oL = (4)$$
$$PASI = (1) + (2) + (3) + (4)$$

(5, 6, 31). These processes, as well as TNF-mediated stimulation of bone resorption, inhibition of bone formation, and inhibition of proteoglycan synthesis may all contribute to tissue and joint damage (32–34).

As with psoriasis and psoriatic arthritis, a primary role for TNF in the pathogenesis of RA has been established in vitro and in animal studies (35–39). Further evidence to support this role comes from observations of significant levels of TNF and TNF receptors in RA synovial tissue and fluid that appear to parallel the extent of inflammation and bone erosion (40–44). TNF contributes to the pathology of RA by activating synovial fibroblasts and osteoclasts within the joint, leading to increased collagenase and prostaglandin release, and increased bone resorption, respectively (31–33, 45).

Etanercept modulates biological responses that are induced or regulated by TNF, and are relevant to the improvements observed in patients with psoriasis, psoriatic arthritis, RA, and JRA, such as adhesion molecule expression, serum levels of cytokines, and serum levels of matrix metalloproteinases (15, 46).

C. Indications

Etanercept is indicated for use in reducing the signs and symptoms of active arthritis in psoriatic arthritis. Additional indications for etanercept for the treatment of rheumatoid and polyarticular-course juvenile rheumatoid arthritis (RA and JRA, respectively) are discussed later in this chapter, in the section on Clinical Use.

D. Diagnosis/Classification of Psoriatic Arthritis

Psoriatic arthritis is a progressive, chronic, inflammatory arthritis accompanied by the skin lesions of psoriasis that is usually seronegative for rheumatoid factor (47). The incidence of psoriatic arthritis among patients with psoriasis has been estimated to be between 7% and 42% (48). Although psoriatic arthritis may occur in almost 1% of the general population, the diagnostic criteria for this disease have not been strictly agreed upon (49). Moll and Wright have identified several patterns of joint involvement occurring in psoriatic arthritis that, while not true diagnostic schema, are most often used in classification/diagnosis of the disease (50). The five patterns most typically observed are symmetrical polyarthritis (rheumatoid-like), asymmetrical oligoarthritis, distal interphalangeal arthritis, spondylitis, and arthritis mutilans. The sensitivity of both these criteria and those proposed by the European Spondyloarthropathy Study Group (51) has been estimated to fall between 61% and 65% (52), pointing to the need for the development of more specific classification criteria for psoriatic arthritis.

Table 3 Radiological Features of Psoriatic Arthritis

Lack of juxta-articular osteopenia
Presence of pencil-in-cup change
Ankylosis
Periosteal reaction
Spur formation
Paramarginal erosions
Spondyloarthropathy
   Tendency for asymmetrical distribution of both
     sacroiliitis and syndesmophytes
   Syndesmophytes tend to be coarse, paramarginal,
     and not in consecutive vertebrae

The appearance of psoriatic skin lesions precedes arthritic symptoms in approximately 75% of patients with psoriatic arthritis. Between 10% and 15% of patients will experience psoriasis and psoriatic arthritis simultaneously, and 10–15% appear to show symptoms of arthritis prior to the appearance of psoriasis (47). Patients typically present with pain, stiffness, and swelling of affected joints. Approximately 80% of patients with psoriatic arthritis have nail involvement characterized by onycholysis, transverse ridging, and uniform nail pitting that may be accompanied by distal joint inflammation. Enthesitis, especially at the insertion of the Achilles tendon or plantar fascia, may be present clinically, or be detected radiologically. Additional radiological features of psoriatic arthritis are listed in Table 3 (49).

There are no diagnostic tests available specific for psoriatic arthritis. A summary of laboratory results often observed with psoriatic arthritis is provided in Table 4.

Table 4 Laboratory Results in Patients with Psoriatic Arthritis

Rheumatoid factor negative (most cases)
Erythrocyte sedimentation rate (ESR) increased
Complete blood count: Mild normocytic normochromic anemia
   and leukocytosis
Uric acid elevations (with increasing psoriasis severity)
Synovial fluid exam
   White blood cells (WBC) 2,000–15,000/mm^3
   High WBC seen with large effusions
Serum hemolytic complement elevated
Serum electrophoresis: Hypergammaglobulinemia

III. CLINICAL USE

A. Psoriatic Arthritis

The recommended dosage of etanercept for adults with psoriatic arthritis is 25 mg administered subcutaneously (SC) twice weekly at intervals of 72–96 h. For psoriatic arthritis, etanercept may be used as monotherapy or concomitantly with methotrexate (MTX), salicylates, nonsteroidal anti-inflammatory drugs (NSAIDs), or analgesics.

A phase II, randomized, double-blind, placebo-controlled 12 week study assessed the efficacy and safety of 25 mg twice-weekly subcutaneous injections of etanercept or placebo in 60 adult patients with psoriatic arthritis, defined as ≥3 swollen joints and ≥3 tender joints, and psoriasis (2). Patients must have had an inadequate response to NSAIDs, and were allowed to continue on stable dosages of MTX (≤25 mg/week) or corticosteroids (≤10 mg/day). Topical therapies, oral retinoids, and phototherapy for psoriasis were discontinued prior to treatment.

The study endpoints for psoriatic arthritis were the proportion of patients who met the psoriatic arthritis response criteria (PsARC) and American College of Rheumatology 20% criteria (ACR20) for improvement in the number of tender and swollen joints, and in patient and physician assessments. These guidelines are outlined in Table 5 (53, 54). The endpoints for psoriasis were a 75% improvement in the PASI score, and improvements in prospectively identified individual target lesions (≥2 cm diameter).

The etanercept-treated group had statistically better outcomes for all clinical psoriatic arthritis endpoints. At 12 weeks, 87% of the etanercept-

Table 5 Psoriatic Arthritis Study Endpoint Criteria

PsARC	Improvement in two (at least one must be a joint score), and worsening of none of the following (scale: 0–5 units): Patient global assessment Physician global assessment Tender joint scores Swollen joint scores
ACR20	Requires at least 20% reductions in tender and swollen joint counts and in at least three of the following: Patient assessment of pain Patient global assessment Physician global assessment Patient assessment of disability Acute phase reactant (C-reactive protein)

treated patients achieved the PsARC compared with 23% of patients receiving placebo (p < 0.0001). The ACR20 was achieved by 73% of etanercept- and 13% of placebo-treated patients (p < 0.0001).

Etanercept also improved the psoriasis skin lesions in this trial. Nineteen patients were evaluable for psoriasis ($\geq$3% of body surface involvement) in each treatment group. At 12 weeks, 26% of the etanercept- and 0% of the placebo-treated patients had achieved a 75% improvement in PASI (p = 0.0154). The median response of a prospectively defined target lesions was 50% in the etanercept group compared to 0% in the placebo group (p = 0.0004).

An open-label extension of this study demonstrated that treatment with etanercept allowed the reduction or discontinuation of concomitant MTX and/or steroids in some patients.

The results of a larger, multicenter, randomized, double-blind, placebo-controlled phase III trial of the efficacy and safety of etanercept in psoriatic arthritis and psoriasis were similar to those in the phase II trial (3).

The phase III trial included 205 adult (aged between 18 and 70 years) patients with active psoriatic arthritis ($\geq$3 swollen joints and $\geq$3 tender joints) in one or more of the following forms: distal interphalangeal (DIP) involvement (n = 104); polyarticular arthritis (absence of rheumatoid nodules and presence of psoriasis; n = 173); arthritis mutilans (n = 3); (4) asymmetrical psoriatic arthritis (n = 81); or ankylosing spondylitis-like (n = 7). Patients also had plaque psoriasis with a qualifying target lesion $\geq$2 cm in diameter. Patients treated with MTX could continue at a stable dosage of $\leq$25 mg/week. Patients received 25 mg twice-weekly subcutaneous injections of etanercept or placebo for 6 months.

Arthritis severity was measured by ACR20 and PsARC criteria. Psoriasis activity was measured by improvement in target lesion score, and, in a subset of patients who had plaque psoriasis involvement of at least 3% of their body surface area (n = 62 for placebo; n = 66 for etanercept), by the PASI score.

Etanercept-treated patients with psoriatic arthritis experienced significant improvements in symptoms at 6 months, and significantly greater improvements in ACR20, 50, and 70 responses compared to those treated with placebo. The skin lesions in the subset of evaluable patients with psoriasis also improved as measured by the percentage of patients achieving improvements in the PASI. The ACR and PsARC responses are summarized in Figure 2. The subset of patients with psoriasis who were evaluated using the PASI score showed a median improvement of 47% in patients receiving etanercept, while no improvement was seen in those receiving placebo.

ACR Response at 24 Weeks

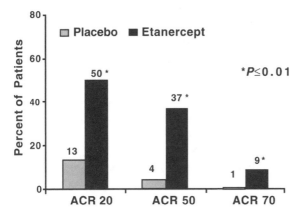

PsARC at 24 Weeks

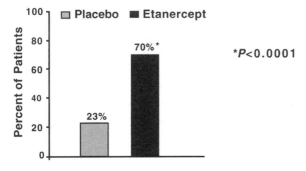

Figure 2 Phase III psoriatic arthritis trial: percentage improvement in psoriatic arthritis disease activity at 6 months.

B. Psoriasis

Phase II and III clinical trials of etanercept for the treatment of psoriatic arthritis and psoriasis have demonstrated consistent efficacy for this drug in clearing of chronic plaque psoriasis (2, 3). Data from a phase II psoriasis trial were presented at the 2002 annual meetings of the American Academy of Dermatology (55) and Society for Investigative Dermatology (1), and are briefly summarized below.

The phase II etanercept monotherapy trial was a 24 week, multicenter, double-blind, randomized, placebo-controlled study. The trial enrolled 112 patients with chronic, stable plaque psoriasis over ≥10% of their body surface area, and who had received at least one systemic psoriasis therapy previously. Patients who had skin conditions that might interfere with the evaluation of the effect of etanercept on psoriasis (e.g., eczema) were excluded from the study. Systemic psoriasis therapies and systemic corticosteroids were discontinued within 4 weeks of entering the study. Topical psoriasis therapies were discontinued within 2 weeks of the first dose of study drug, with the exception of stable, moderate-strength topical corticosteroids for the scalp, axillae, and groin.

Patients received 25 mg etanercept (n = 57) or placebo (n = 55) SC twice weekly. Thirty percent and 56% of patients receiving etanercept achieved at least a 75% improvement in the PASI score (PASI 75) at 12 and 24 weeks, respectively. Only 2% and 5% of placebo-treated patients achieved a PASI 75 at 12 and 24 weeks, respectively.

C. Rheumatoid Arthritis

Etanercept has been studied for use in RA for many years and has been available for clinical use in the United States since late 1998. It is indicated for reducing the signs and symptoms and inhibiting the progression of structural damage in patients with moderately to severely active RA. Etanercept can be used as monotherapy, or in combination with MTX in patients with inadequate responses to MTX alone. Clinical responses to etanercept generally begin to occur within 1–2 weeks after initiation of therapy, and a dose of 25 mg administered SC twice weekly has been shown to be more effective than 10 mg etanercept, and significantly better than placebo in all components of the ACR criteria as described below. These response rates were maintained for up to 5 years in clinical trials (16). In addition, long-term treatment with etanercept has been shown to allow the dosage reduction of discontinuation of concomitant MTX or corticosteroids in some RA patients (16).

The safety and efficacy of etanercept have been assessed in three randomized, double-blind controlled studies. The ACR response rates from these trials are summarized in Table 6 (15).

Study I (17) evaluated 234 patients (≥18 years) with active RA who had failed to respond to therapy with at least one but no more than four disease-modifying antirheumatic drugs, who had ≥12 tender joints, ≥10 swollen joints, and erythrocyte sedimentation rate (ESR) ≥28 mm/hour, CRP > 2.0 mg/dl, or morning stiffness ≥45 min. Etanercept (10 or 25 mg) was administered SC twice weekly for 6 consecutive months. Results from patients receiving 25 mg etanercept are summarized in Table 6.

Study II (18) evaluated 89 patients with similar inclusion criteria to Study I, but patients in this study had also received MTX for at least 6 months with a stable dosage for at least 4 weeks, and had six tender or swollen joints. Patients in Study II received either 25 mg etanercept or placebo SC twice weekly for 6 months in addition to MTX.

Study III (19) compared the efficacy of 10 or 25 mg etanercept SC twice weekly for 12 months with MTX in 632 adult ($\geq$18 years) patients with early active RA (disease duration $\leq$3 years duration). MTX tablets (increased from 7.5 mg/week to a maximum of 20 mg/week over the first 8 weeks of the trial) or placebo tablets were given once a week on the day of etanercept injection. The patients in the study had never received treatment with MTX, had $\geq$12 tender joints, $\geq$10 swollen joints, and ESR $\geq$28 mm/hour, CRP $>$ 2.0 mg/dl, or morning stiffness for $\geq$45 min. The study was unblinded after all patients had completed at least 12 months (median 17.3 months) of therapy. Most patients remained in the study through 2 years. Results from patients receiving 25 mg etanercept are summarized in Table 6.

Table 6 ACR Responses in Adult RA Trials (%)

	Study I		Study II		Study III	
	Placebo (n = 80)	Etanercept (n = 78)	MTX/Placebo (n = 30)	MTX/Etanercept (n = 59)	MTX (n = 217)	Etanercept (n = 207)
ACR20						
Month 3	23	62[a]	33	66[a]	56	62
Month 6	11	59[a]	27	71[a]	58	65
Month 12	NA	NA	NA	NA	65	72
ACR50						
Month 3	8	41[a]	0	42[a]	24	29
Month 6	5	40[a]	3	39[a]	32	40
Month 12	NA	NA	NA	NA	42	49
ACR70						
Month 3	4	15[a]	0	15[a]	7	13[b]
Month 6	1	15[a]	0	15[a]	14	21[b]
Month 12	NA	NA	NA	NA	22	25

[a] p < 0.01, etanercept vs. placebo.
[b] p < 0.05, etanercept vs. MTX.

D. Polyarticular-Course Juvenile Rheumatoid Arthritis

Etanercept has been shown to be well tolerated by pediatric patients, and treatment with 0.4 mg/kg etanercept SC twice has been shown to lead to significant improvements in patients with active JRA who have had inadequate response to one or more disease-modifying antirheumatic drugs (20).

The safety and efficacy of etanercept were assessed in a multicenter trial of children with a variety of JRA onset types, who were unable to tolerate or who had had an inadequate response to MTX (20). Patients aged 4–17 years received 0.4 mg/kg etanercept SC twice weekly for up to 3 months in the initial, open-label part of the trial. Patients who responded to treatment at study day 90 entered a double-blind study and were randomly assigned to receive either placebo or etanercept for 4 months or until a flare of the disease occurred. A response was defined as an improvement of 30% or more in at least three of six indicators of disease activity, with no more than one indicator worsening by more than 30%. Indicators included active joint count, limitation of motion, physician and patient/parent global assessments, functional assessment, and ESR (56). Disease flare was defined as a $\geq 30\%$ worsening in three of the six JRA indicators and $\geq 30\%$ improvement in not more than one of the six indicators and a minimum of two active joints.

At the end of the open-label study, 74% of the etanercept-treated patients had responded. In the double-blind portion of the study 77% of the patients receiving placebo and 24% of the patient receiving etanercept experienced a disease flare ($p = 0.007$). Eighty-one percent of the patients receiving placebo withdrew due to disease flare compared to 28% of those receiving etanercept ($p = 0.003$). The median time to disease flare was 28 days for placebo- and 116 days for etanercept-treated patients ($p < 0.001$). There were no significant differences in the adverse events between the two groups (20).

IV. SAFETY

The safety of etanercept has been demonstrated in nearly 120,000 patients in both controlled clinical trials and in postmarketing surveillance. In controlled trials, the only adverse event that occurred more frequently in patients treated with etanercept compared to placebo was mild to moderate injection site reactions, erythema, and/or itching, pain, or swelling. Approximately 37% of patients receiving etanercept experienced injection site reactions in these trials. These reactions tended to occur in the first month, subsequently decreased in frequency, and did not generally result in discontinuation of the drug. The mean duration for reactions was 3–5 days. Seven percent of patients experienced redness at a previous injection site (15). Application of cool compresses and 1% hydrocortisone ointment are helpful to alleviate discomfort associated with injection-site reactions.

A study presented at the 2001 meeting of the American College of Rheumatology demonstrated the global long-term safety of etanercept in 2054 patients from North America and the European Union who have received treatment for up to 5 years (57). The rates of infection requiring hospitalization or intravenous antibiotics were 0.04 per patient-year in the total population, which is comparable to the control group (0.04 per patient-year) in controlled trials. Postmarketing reports have, however, included reports of serious infections and sepsis, including fatalities with the use of etanercept. Patients who are taking concomitant immunosuppressive therapies, or patients who may be predisposed to infections, may be at an increased risk of infection when administered etanercept. Caution should be used when considering etanercept for patients with a history of recurring infections, and etanercept should not be administered to patients with sepsis or active infections, including chronic or localized infections.

The long-term data (up to 5 years) in patients with RA also suggested that the incidence of malignancies was not increased in the etanercept group compared to the expected number from the National Cancer Institute's (NCI) Surveillance, Epidemiology, and End Results (SEER) database (41 observed vs. 42 predicted) (57). There was no predominance in subtype of malignancy. The NCI SEER database does not include information on nonmelanoma skin cancers. However, the incidence of squamous cell carcinomas (SCC) in the etanercept clinical safety database (n = 2) is well below conservative benchmark estimates of the incidence of SCC in the general population (n = 5.1–11.5) based on studies done in Olmstead County, Minnesota (58), and southern Arizona (59).

In postmarketing surveillance there have been rare reports of new onset or exacerbation of central nervous system demyelinating disorders and pancytopenia in patients treated with etanercept. However, the causal relationship to etanercept remains unclear. Caution should be exercised when considering the use of etanercept in patients with pre-existing or recent-onset central demyelinating disorders. Discontinuation of etanercept therapy should be considered in patients with confirmed significant hematological abnormalities.

The impact of long-term treatment with etanercept on the development of autoimmune diseases is unknown. A subset of patients with active RA were evaluated for antinuclear antibodies (ANA) in three clinical trials (17–19). In two of these trials, the percentage of patients developing new positive ANA (titer $\geq 1:40$) was higher in patients treated with etanercept (11%) than in placebo-treated patients (5%). The percentage of patients developing antinuclear and anticardiolipin antibodies was also increased in the etanercept-treated group compared to patients receiving placebo in these trials (17, 18). There was no pattern of increased autoantibody development observed in patients treated with etanercept compared to those treated with MTX in the third trial (19). Rare adverse events have been described in patients with rheumatoid factor-positive and/or erosive RA who have developed additional autoantibodies in conjunction with rash suggestive of a lupuslike syndrome. This syndrome has been seen to resolve with discontinuation of therapy.

Most patients receiving etanercept have been shown to be capable of mounting B-cell immune responses to pneumococcal polysaccharide vaccine, but titers in aggregate were moderately lower and fewer patients had twofold rises in titers compared to patients not receiving etanercept (15). Patients receiving etanercept may receive concurrent vaccinations, except for live vaccines.

Etanercept has been listed as category B for pregnancy. Although there has been no evidence of harm to the fetus in developmental toxicity studies of etanercept performed in rats and rabbits, there have been no studies in pregnant women and, therefore, etanercept should be used during pregnancy only if clearly needed. Likewise, it is unknown if etanercept is excreted in human milk or absorbed systemically after ingestion. A decision to discontinue nursing or to discontinue etanercept treatment should be made by nursing mothers. Etanercept has not demonstrated mutagenic activity when tested in vitro and in vivo (15).

V. HOW TO USE ETANERCEPT

Etanercept is supplied as a sterile, white, lyophilized powder that requires reconstitution with 1 ml supplied sterile bacteriostatic water for injection (BWFI), USP (containing 0.9% benzyl alcohol).

Self-administration of etanercept by patients is appropriate with medical follow-up and only after counseling by qualified healthcare professionals on proper injection technique.

Etanercept is supplied in a carton containing four dose trays. Each tray contains one 25 mg multiple-use vial of etanercept, one syringe with diluent (1 ml sterile BWFI), one plunger, and two alcohol swabs. Etanercept dose trays should be stored at 36–42° F (2–8° C) both before and after mixing. Solutions of etanercept should be refrigerated within 4 h of diluting and must be used within 14 days. The stability and sterility of etanercept solutions

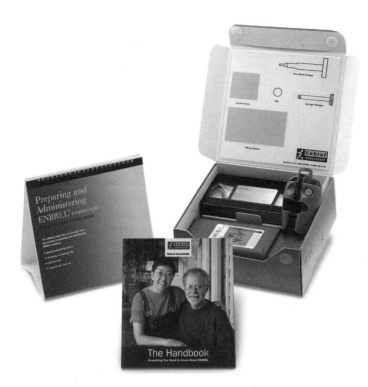

Figure 3 Etanercept *dosing system* starter kit.

cannot be guaranteed after 14 days, and any unused portions should be discarded after that time. Etanercept must not be frozen.

Mixing of etanercept may be accomplished by one of three methods recommended by the manufacturer and described in detail below: the free-hand method, the mixing station method, or the dose preparation guide method. The dosing system starter kit (see Fig. 3) contains tools to help the patient prepare and administer etanercept. Each kit contains a so-called mixing station device that helps keep the needle of the syringe in line with the center of the vial stopper to ensure that the needle is inserted correctly. This kit is available at no charge. Alternatively, after emptying the contents of the tray, and turning it over, the underside of the tray can become the dose preparation guide (see Fig. 4), and is specially designed to hold the vial and syringe in place while the etanercept solution is prepared. The mixing station and dose preparation guide methods are suggested as alternatives for those patients who may be unable to use the free-hand method due to arthritis of the hands.

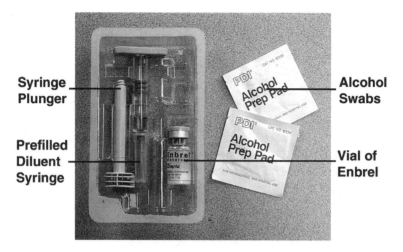

Syringe Plunger — ———

Prefilled Diluent Syringe — ———

Alcohol Swabs

Vial of Enbrel

Figure 4   Etanercept dose tray.

The first step in setting up for an injection is the selection of a clean, well-lit, flat working surface, followed by removal of the etanercept dose tray from the refrigerator and placement on the flat surface. After thoroughly washing hands with soap and water, and inspecting the dose tray for the required components (etanercept vial, syringe with diluent, plunger, and two alcohol swabs), the paper seal should be peeled from the tray, and expiration dates on both the vial and syringe label carefully inspected. If these dates are not the current month and year (or later), or if any of the components of the dose tray are missing, this dose should not be used and a pharmacist should be consulted.

Injection sites should be chosen on the thighs, abdomen, or upper arms, and should be rotated with each injection. Each new injection should be made at least one inch from the previous site, and should never be given in areas where the skin shows any sign of bruising or infection. An injection site should be prepared by wiping the alcohol swab over the skin in a circular motion. Care should be taken to not touch this site again prior to injection.

Use of the free-hand method for diluting etanercept involves first removing the plastic cap (not the gray stopper or metal ring) from the etanercept vial and cleaning the gray stopper with a new alcohol swab. The vial of etanercept should then be placed upright on the flat surface. After sliding the plunger into the syringe, it should be turned clockwise until a slight resistance is felt. The cover of the needle should then be removed.

With the vial of etanercept sitting upright on the flat surface, the needle is then inserted straight down through the center ring of the gray stopper. If the needle has been inserted correctly, there should be a slight resistance followed by a "pop" as the needle goes through. The entire volume of diluent in the syringe should then be slowly added to the vial by pushing down on the plunger. Adding the liquid too quickly will result in foaming.

With the syringe in place, a gentle swirling motion should be used to dissolve the powder. Do not shake the solution to facilitate the process. Complete dissolution may take up to 10 min, and should produce a clear, colorless preparation. Solutions containing visible particulate matter after 10 min should not be injected.

The vial should be turned upside down with the needle still in place. While holding the vial at eye level, the plunger should be slowly drawn back to the appropriate ml dose mark on the side of the syringe. The needle may need to be partially withdrawn as the level of the solution in the vial drops. Some white foam may remain in the vial and is not abnormal.

The syringe should be checked for the presence of air bubbles while still in the vial. These may be removed by gently tapping the syringe, and then slowly pressing the plunger to force them out into the vial. If solution is accidentally pushed back into the vial at this point, it must be slowly drawn back into the syringe. The needle should then be completely removed from the vial, and not allowed to touch any surface.

The mixing station is provided in the dosing system starter kit and is available to patients at no charge through their physicians by calling 1-888-4ENBREL. A videotape and Step-by-Step Visual Guide are also provided in the dosing system. Patients choosing to use the mixing station method for diluting etanercept should follow the instructions on the videotape and in the visual guide.

The dose preparation guide method for diluting etanercept involves using the preparation guide located on the underside of the dose tray. After the cap is removed from the etanercept vial, and the gray stopper is wiped with alcohol, the vial should be pressed into the space marked with ↓V in the dose preparation guide. The gray stopper must face the center of the tray, and the open stopper window should face upwards.

After the needle-cover is removed, the needle should be pointed at the gray stopper, and the 0.5 mL mark on the syringe should be lined up with the edge of the dose preparation guide. The needle should not touch the tray. The syringe should be slid into the dose preparation guide until the needle touches the center ring of the gray stopper. Again, if the needle is correctly aligned, there should be a slight resistance and then a "pop" as the needle enters the vial. The needle tip can be visualized within the vial by looking through the stopper window.

The plunger should then be slid into the syringe and turned clockwise until a slight resistance is felt. The entire volume of diluent should then be slowly added to the vial of etanercept by pushing down on the plunger. While holding the syringe in place, the entire dose tray should be lifted so that the vial is in an upright position, and the tray should be swirled gently in a circular motion. The appropriate dose can then be withdrawn while the dose tray is held at eye level, with the vial upside down. Bubbles can be removed as previously described. The syringe should then be slid out of the tray without allowing the needle to touch any surface.

To inject etanercept, patients should gently pinch and firmly hold the preciously cleaned site. The syringe should be held at a 45 degree angle to the skin with the other hand. A quick short motion should be used to push the needle into the skin, while the other hand releases the skin. The free hand should then push down the plunger to inject the etanercept, and the needle should be removed at the same angle as insertion. Cotton balls may be pressed over the injection site for 10 s if needed. Patients should not rub the injection site, and bandages are optional.

Patients should be advised on how to obtain sharps disposal containers. State and local laws for disposing of needles vary, and patients should be advised to contact a local hospital or health/sanitation department to determine appropriate disposal methods. As an alternative, patients may wish to use a service that provides containers (for a fee) that can be shipped to an approved disposal facility.

As with all injectable medications, patients who are traveling by air must carry a letter of authorization stating that they are receiving a physician-prescribed, self-administered, injectable therapy. Coolers for transporting etanercept while traveling can be obtained from the manufacturer by contacting Enliven services (1-888-4ENBREL; 1-888-436-2735). No specific laboratory monitoring is required for patients receiving etanercept.

VI. REIMBURSEMENT

Etanercept is reimbursed by most private insurance payers and Medicaid, but reimbursement levels may vary. If your patient is not sure of the coverage he or she has, or for specific information, the private or government-sponsored insurer may be contacted directly. Patients and healthcare providers can also call Enliven services (1-888-4ENBREL). Information on medical coding for reimbursement is available from the manufacturer insurance specialists at the ENLIVEN hot line. Sample preauthorization letters and reimbursement codes can be found in Appendix 12.A.

VII. CONCLUSION

Etanercept has demonstrated consistent efficiency in the treatment of inflammatory diseases such as psoriasis, psoriatic arthritis, RA, and JRA. Research on the potential future use of etanercept in other inflammatory diseases is now underway. The rapid and significant clinical responses to this agent underscore both the central role of TNF in contributing to the pathology of these diseases and the potent inhibitory effects of etanercept on its ability to do so. Etanercept is well tolerated by both adult and pediatric patient populations, and long-term data on the use of etanercept have demonstrated an excellent safety profile.

REFERENCES

1. Gottlieb AB, Matheson RT, Lowe NJ, Zitnik RJ. Efficacy of Enbrel in patients with psoriasis. J Invest Dermatol 2002; 119:234.
2. Mease PJ, Goffe BS, Metz J, VanderStoep A, Finck B, Burge DJ. Etanercept in the treatment of psoriatic arthritis and psoriasis: a randomised trial. Lancet 2000; 356(9227):385–390.
3. Mease P, Kivitz A, Burch F, Siegel E, Cohen S, Burge D. Improvement in disease activity in patients with psoriatic arthritis receiving etanercept (ENBREL): results of a phase 3 multicenter clinical trial [abstract]. Arthritis Rheum 2001; 44(suppl):S90–A 226.
4. Robert C, Kupper TS. Inflammatory skin diseases, T cells, and immune surveillance. N Engl J Med 1999; 341(24):1817–1828.
5. Baugh JA, Bucala R. Mechanisms for modulating TNFα in immune inflammatory disease. Curr Opin Drug Disc Dev 2001; 4:635–650.
6. Bonifati C, Ameglio F. Cytokines in psoriasis. Int J Dermatol 1999; 38: 241–251.
7. Krueger JG. The immunologic basis for the treatment of psoriasis with new biologic agents. J Am Acad Dermatol 2002; 46(1):1–23.
8. Smith RA, Baglioni C. The active form of tumor necrosis factor is a trimer. J Biol Chem 1987; 262(15):6951–6954.
9. Pennica D, Kohr WJ, Fendly BM, Shire SJ, Raab HE, Borchardt PE, Lewis M, Goeddel DV. Characterization of a recombinant extracellular domain of the type 1 tumor necrosis factor receptor: evidence for tumor necrosis factor-alpha induced receptor aggregation. Biochemistry 1992; 31(4): 1134–1141.
10. Aderka D, Engelmann H, Maor Y, Brakebusch C, Wallach D. Stabilization of the bioactivity of tumor necrosis factor by its soluble receptors. J Exp Med 1992; 175(2):323–329.
11. Foerder CA, Rogge MC. Immunogenicity of Enbrel (Etanercept): clinical trial observations. EULAR 2002; abstract THU0032.

12. Mohler KM, Torrance DS, Smith CA, Goodwin RG, Stremler KE, Fung VP, Madani H, Widmer MB. Soluble tumor necrosis factor (TNF) receptors are effective therapeutic agents in lethal endotoxemia and function simultaneously as both TNF carriers and TNF antagonists. J Immunol 1993; 151(3): 1548–1561.

13. Peppel K, Crawford D, Beutler B. A tumor necrosis factor (TNF) receptor-IgG heavy chain chimeric protein as a bivalent antagonist of TNF activity. J Exp Med 1991; 174(6):1483–1489.

14. Wooley PH, Dutcher J, Widmer MB, Gillis S. Influence of a recombinant human soluble tumor necrosis factor receptor FC fusion protein on type II collagen-induced arthritis in mice. J Immunol 1993; 151(11):6602–6607.

15. Enbrel (etanercept) [package insert]. 05/2002. 2002. Seattle, Washington, Immunex Corporation and Wyeth-Ayerst Pharmaceuticals.

16. Moreland LW, Cohen S, Fleischmann RM, Baumgartner SW, Schiff MH, Burge DJ. Safety and efficacy of up to 5 Years of Etanercept (Enbrel) therapy in rheumatoid arthritis. EULAR 2002; abstract FRI0078.

17. Moreland LW, Schiff MH, Baumgartner SW, Tindall EA, Fleischmann RM, Bulpitt KJ, Weaver AL, Keystone EC, Furst DE, Mease PJ, Ruderman EM, Horwitz DA, Arkfeld DG, Garrison L, Burge DJ, Blosch CM, Lange ML, McDonnell ND, Weinblatt ME. Etanercept therapy in rheumatoid arthritis. A randomized, controlled trial. Ann Intern Med 1999; 130(6):478–486.

18. Weinblatt ME, Kremer JM, Bankhurst AD, Bulpitt KJ, Fleischmann RM, Fox RI, Jackson CG, Lange M, Burge DJ. A trial of etanercept, a recombinant tumor necrosis factor receptor:Fc fusion protein, in patients with rheumatoid arthritis receiving methotrexate [see comments]. N Engl J Med 1999; 340(4):253–259.

19. Bathon JM, Martin RW, Fleischmann RM, Tesser JR, Schiff MH, Keystone EC, Genovese MC, Wasko MC, Moreland LW, Weaver AL, Markenson J, Finck BK. A comparison of etanercept and methotrexate in patients with early rheumatoid arthritis. N Engl J Med 2000; 343(22):1586–1593.

20. Lovell DJ, Giannini EH, Reiff A, Cawkwell GD, Silverman ED, Nocton JJ, Stein LD, Gedalia A, Ilowite NT, Wallace CA, Whitmore J, Finck BK. Etanercept in children with polyarticular juvenile rheumatoid arthritis. Pediatric Rheumatology Collaborative Study Group [see comments]. N Engl J Med 2000; 342(11):763–769.

21. Gorman JD, Sack KE, Davis JC, Jr. Treatment of ankylosing spondylitis by inhibition of tumor necrosis factor alpha. N Engl J Med 2002; 346(18): 1349–1356.

22. Marzo-Ortega H, McGonagle D, O'Connor P, Emery P. Efficacy of etanercept in the treatment of the entheseal pathology in resistant spondylarthropathy: a clinical and magnetic resonance imaging study. Arthritis Rheum 2001; 44(9):2112–2117.

23. Ritchlin C, Haas-Smith SA, Hicks D, Cappuccio J, Osterland CK, Looney RJ. Patterns of cytokine production in psoriatic synovium. J Rheumatol 1998; 25:1544–1552.

24. Partsch F, Steiner G, Leeb BF, Dunky A, Broll H, Smolen JS. Highly increased levels of tumor necrosis factor-alpha and other proinflammatory cytokines in psoriatic arthritis synovial fluid. J Rheumatol 1997; 24:518–523.

25. Ettehadi P, Greaves MW, Wallach D, Aderka D, Camp RD. Elevated tumour necrosis factor-alpha (TNF-alpha) biological activity in psoriatic skin lesions. Clin Exp Immunol 1994; 96(1):146–151.

26. Mussi A, Bonifati C, Carducci M, D'Agosto G, Pimpinelli F, D'Urso D, D'Auria L, Fazio M, Ameglio F. Serum TNF-alpha levels correlate with disease severity and are reduced by effective therapy in plaque-type psoriasis. J Biol Regul Homeost Agents 1997; 11(3):115–118.

27. Bonifati C, Carduci M, Cordiali Fei P, Trento E, Sacerdoti G, Fazio M, Ameglio F. Correlated increases of tumour necrosis factor-alpha, interleukin-6 and granulocyte monocyte-colony stimulating factor levels in suction blister fluids and sera of psoriatic patients—relationships with disease severity. Clin Exp Dermatol 1994; 19(5):383–387.

28. Wakefield PE, James WD, Samlaska CP, Meltzer MS. Tumor necrosis factor. J Am Acad Dermatol 1991; 24(5 Pt 1):675–685.

29. Nickoloff BJ. The cytokine network in psoriasis. Arch Dermatol 1991; 127(6):871–884.

30. Aggarwal BB, Natarajan K. Tumor necrosis factors: developments during the last decade. Eur Cytokine Network 1996; 7(2):93–124.

31. Dayer JM, Beutler B, Cerami A. Cachectin/tumor necrosis factor stimulates collagenase and prostaglandin E2 production by human synovial cells and dermal fibroblasts. J Exp Med 1985; 162(6):2163–2168.

32. Bertolini DR, Nedwin GE, Bringman TS, Smith DD, Mundy GR. Stimulation of bone resorption and inhibition of bone formation in vitro by human tumour necrosis factors. Nature 1986; 319(6053):516–518.

33. Saklatvala J. Tumour necrosis factor alpha stimulates resorption and inhibits synthesis of proteoglycan in cartilage. Nature 1986; 322(6079):547–549.

34. Shinmei M, Masuda K, Kikuchi T, Shimomura Y. The role of cytokines in chondrocyte mediated cartilage degradation. J Rheumatol Suppl 1989; 18:32–34.

35. Buchan G, Barrett K, Turner M, Chantry D, Maini RN, Feldmann M. Interleukin-1 and tumour necrosis factor mRNA expression in rheumatoid arthritis: prolonged production of IL-1 alpha. Clin Exp Immunol 1988; 73(3):449–455.

36. Brennan FM, Chantry D, Jackson AM, Maini RN, Feldmann M. Cytokine production in culture by cells isolated from the synovial membrane. J Autoimmun 1989; 2 Suppl:177–186.

37. Feldmann M, Brennan FM, Maini RN. Role of cytokines in rheumatoid arthritis. Annu Rev Immunol 1996; 14:397–440.

38. Thorbecke GJ, Shah R, Leu CH, Kuruvilla AP, Hardison AM, Palladino MA. Involvement of endogenous tumor necrosis factor alpha and transforming growth factor beta during induction of collagen type II arthritis in mice. Proc Natl Acad Sci USA 1992; 89(16):7375–7379.

39. Williams RO, Feldmann M, Maini RN. Anti-tumor necrosis factor ameliorates joint disease in murine collagen-induced arthritis. Proc Natl Acad Sci USA 1992; 89(20):9784–9788.

40. Saxne T, Palladino MA, Jr., Heinegard D, Talal N, Wollheim FA. Detection of tumor necrosis factor alpha but not tumor necrosis factor beta in rheumatoid arthritis synovial fluid and serum. Arthritis Rheum 1988; 31(8):1041–1045.

41. Husby G, Williams RC, Jr. Synovial localization of tumor necrosis factor in patients with rheumatoid arthritis. J Autoimmun 1988; 1(4):363–371.

42. Brennan FM, Maini RN, Feldmann M. TNF alpha—a pivotal role in rheumatoid arthritis? Br J Rheumatol 1992; 31(5):293–298.

43. Neidel J, Schulze M, Lindschau J. Association between degree of bone-erosion and synovial fluid-levels of tumor necrosis factor alpha in the knee-joints of patients with rheumatoid arthritis. Inflamm Res 1995; 44(5):217–221.

44. Deleuran BW. Cytokines in rheumatoid arthritis. Localization in arthritic joint tissue and regulation in vitro. Scand J Rheumatol Suppl 1996; 104:1–34.

45. Maini RN, Taylor PC. Anti-cytokine therapy for rheumatoid arthritis. Annu Rev Med 2000; 51:207–229.

46. Catrina AI, Lampa J, Ernestam S, Af Klint E, Bratt J, Klareskog L, Ulfgren AK. Anti-tumour necrosis factor (TNF)-alpha therapy (etanercept) down-regulates serum matrix metalloproteinase (MMP)-3 and MMP-1 in rheumatoid arthritis. Rheumatology (Oxford) 2002; 41(5):484–489.

47. Mease PJ. Tumour necrosis factor (TNF) in psoriatic arthritis: pathophysiology and treatment with TNF inhibitors. Ann Rheum Dis 2002; 61(4): 298–304.

48. Gladman DD. Psoriatic arthritis. In: Maddison PJ, Isenberg DA, Glass DN, eds. Oxford Textbook of Rheumatology. Oxford: Oxford University Press, 1998: 1071.

49. Gladman DD. Psoriatic arthritis. Rheum Dis Clin North Am 1998; 24(4): 829–844.

50. Moll JM, Wright V. Psoriatic arthritis. Semin Arthritis Rheum 1973; 3(1): 55–78.

51. Dougados M, van Der LS, Juhlin R, Huitfeldt B, Amor B, Calin A, Cats A, Dijkmans B, Olivieri I, Pasero G, et al. The European Spondylarthropathy Study Group preliminary criteria for the classification of spondylarthropathy. Arthritis Rheum 1991; 34(10):1218–1227.

52. Salvarani C, Lo Scocco G, Macchioni P, Cremonesi T, Rossi F, Mantovani W, Battistel B, Bisighini G, Portioli I. Prevalence of psoriatic arthritis in Italian psoriatic patients. J Rheumatol 1995; 22(8):1499–1503.

53. Felson DT, Anderson JJ, Boers M, Bombardier C, Chernoff M, Fried B, Furst D, Goldsmith C, Kieszak S, Lightfoot R et al. The American College of Rheumatology preliminary core set of disease activity measures for rheumatoid arthritis clinical trials. The Committee on Outcome Measures in Rheumatoid Arthritis Clinical Trials. Arthritis Rheum 1993; 36(6):729–740.

54. Clegg DO, Reda DJ, Mejias E, Cannon GW, Weisman MH, Taylor T, Budiman-Mak E, Blackburn WD, Vasey FB, Mahowald ML, Cush JJ,

Schumacher HR Jr, Silverman SL, Alepa FP, Luggen ME, Cohen MR, Makkena R, Haakenson CM, Ward RH, Manaster BJ, Anderson RJ, Ward JR, Henderson WG. Comparison of sulfasalazine and placebo in the treatment of psoriatic arthritis. A Department of Veterans Affairs Cooperative Study. Arthritis Rheum 1996; 39(12):2013–2020.

55. Gottlieb AB, Lowe NJ, Matheson RT, Lebsack ME. Efficacy of etanercept in patients with psoriasis. Presented at the American Academy of Dermatology, New Orleans, LA, Feb 22–27, 2002.

56. Giannini EH, Ruperto N, Ravelli A, Lovell DJ, Felson DT, Martini A. Preliminary definition of improvement in juvenile arthritis. Arthritis Rheum 1997; 40(7):1202–1209.

57. Klareskog L, Moreland LM, Cohen SB, Sanda M, Burge DJ. Global safety and efficacy of up to five years of etanercept (Enbrel®) therapy [abstract]. Arthritis Rheum 2001; 44(suppl):S77–Abstract 150.

58. Gray DT, Suman VJ, Su WP, Clay RP, Harmsen WS, Roenigk RK. Trends in the population-based incidence of squamous cell carcinoma of the skin first diagnosed between 1984 and 1992. Arch Dermatol 1997; 133(6):735–740.

59. Harris RB, Griffith K, Moon TE. Trends in the incidence of nonmelanoma skin cancers in southeastern Arizona, 1985–1996. J Am Acad Dermatol 2001; 45(4): 528–536.

60. Fredriksson T, Pettersson U. Severe psoriasis—oral therapy with a new retinoid. Dermatologica 1978; 157(4):238–244.

APPENDIX 12.A

SAMPLE LETTER OF MEDICAL NECESSITY
Psoriatic Arthritis

Date
[Insurer Name]
[Attn:]
[Address]

Re: *[Patient Name]*
        [Policy Number]

Dear *[Insurer]*:

I am writing on behalf of *[Patient Name]* to document the medical necessity of administering ENBREL® (etanercept) to treat psoriatic arthritis. This letter provides information about the patient's medical history and diagnosis, a statement summarizing my treatment rationale, and a copy of the product's labeling.

ENBREL® is an injectable used to treat active psoriatic arthritis. It is generally administered via subcutaneous injection twice weekly and may be used in alone or in combination with other therapies.

Tumor necrosis factor (TNF) is found at increased levels in psoriatic arthritis patients and exerts its effects in part through triggering the release of tissue-destroying substances. The symptoms of psoriatic arthritis include pain, swelling, fatigue, stiffness, joint destruction, and functional decline. ENBREL®, the first biologic response modifier (BRM) to be approved by the U.S. Food and Drug Administration (FDA) for the treatment of psoriatic arthritis, is thought to act in part through inhibiting TNF's actions rendering TNF biologically inactive. The U.S. Food and Drug Administration cleared ENBREL® for marketing on November 2, 1998 for rheumatoid arthritis and expanded the label to include psoriatic arthritis on January 16, 2002.

[Discuss patient's diagnosis, treatment history, degree of illness, and need for ENBREL® therapy.]

[You may want to include clinical information, relevant compendia listings, or other pertinent materials specific to patient's condition.]

In light of this clinical information, and this patient's condition, the use of ENBREL® is medically necessary and warrants coverage. Please contact me if you require additional information.

Sincerely,

[Physician's Name]

Figure 12.A.1   Sample preauthorization letter.

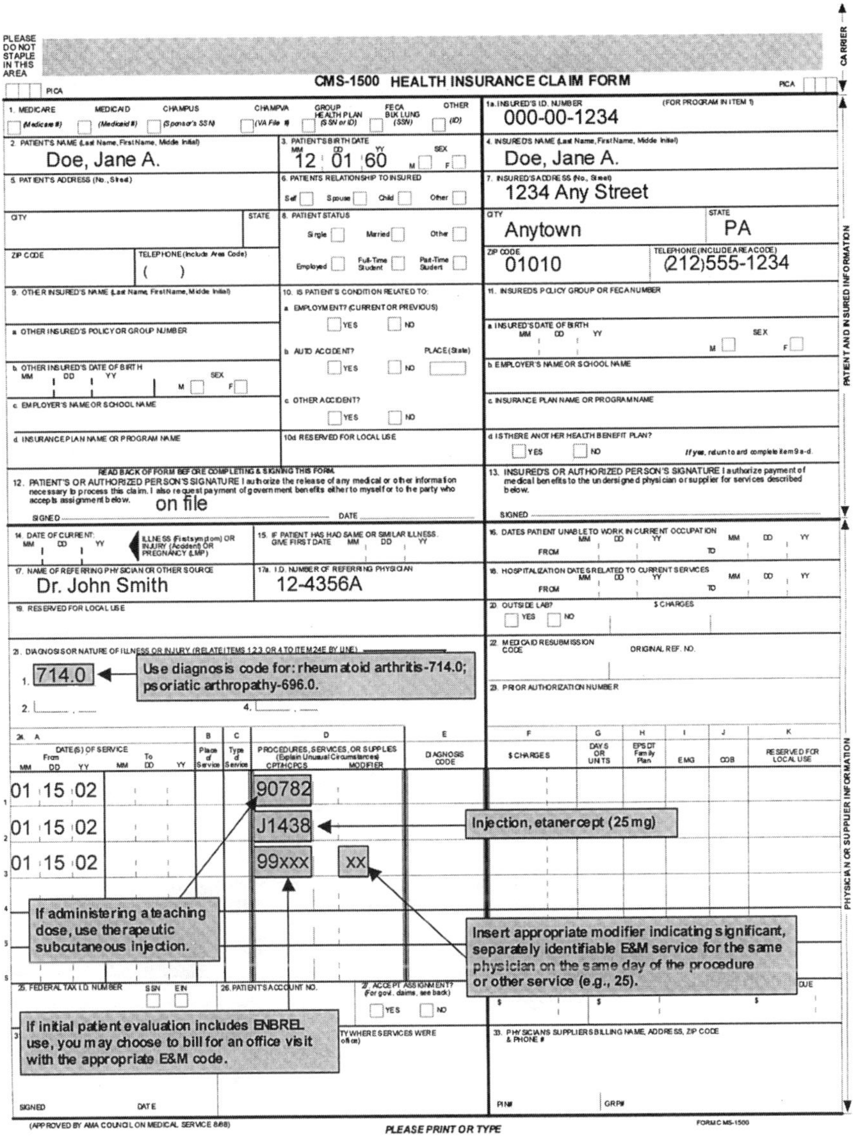
PLEASE DO NOT STAPLE IN THIS AREA

CMS-1500 HEALTH INSURANCE CLAIM FORM

1. MEDICARE MEDICAID CHAMPUS CHAMPVA GROUP HEALTH PLAN FECA BLK LUNG OTHER

1a. INSURED'S I.D. NUMBER: 000-00-1234

2. PATIENT'S NAME (Last Name, First Name, Middle Initial): Doe, Jane A.

3. PATIENT'S BIRTH DATE: 12 01 60

4. INSURED'S NAME (Last Name, First Name, Middle Initial): Doe, Jane A.

5. PATIENT'S ADDRESS (No., Street)

6. PATIENT'S RELATIONSHIP TO INSURED: Self Spouse Child Other

7. INSURED'S ADDRESS (No., Street): 1234 Any Street

CITY: Anytown STATE: PA

ZIP CODE: 01010 TELEPHONE (INCLUDE AREA CODE): (212)555-1234

8. PATIENT STATUS

9. OTHER INSURED'S NAME

10. IS PATIENT'S CONDITION RELATED TO:

11. INSURED'S POLICY GROUP OR FECA NUMBER

12. PATIENT'S OR AUTHORIZED PERSON'S SIGNATURE: on file

13. INSURED'S OR AUTHORIZED PERSON'S SIGNATURE

14. DATE OF CURRENT: ILLNESS (First symptom) OR INJURY (Accident) OR PREGNANCY (LMP)

15. IF PATIENT HAS HAD SAME OR SIMILAR ILLNESS, GIVE FIRST DATE

16. DATES PATIENT UNABLE TO WORK IN CURRENT OCCUPATION

17. NAME OF REFERRING PHYSICIAN OR OTHER SOURCE: Dr. John Smith

17a. I.D. NUMBER OF REFERRING PHYSICIAN: 12-4356A

18. HOSPITALIZATION DATES RELATED TO CURRENT SERVICES

19. RESERVED FOR LOCAL USE

20. OUTSIDE LAB? $ CHARGES

21. DIAGNOSIS OR NATURE OF ILLNESS OR INJURY (RELATE ITEMS 1,2,3 OR 4 TO ITEM 24E BY LINE)

1. 714.0

Use diagnosis code for: rheumatoid arthritis-714.0; psoriatic arthropathy-696.0.

22. MEDICAID RESUBMISSION CODE ORIGINAL REF. NO.

23. PRIOR AUTHORIZATION NUMBER

24. A DATE(S) OF SERVICE	B Place of Service	C Type of Service	D PROCEDURES, SERVICES, OR SUPPLIES CPT/HCPCS MODIFIER	E DIAGNOSIS CODE	F $ CHARGES	G DAYS OR UNITS	H EPSDT Family Plan	I EMG	J COB	K RESERVED FOR LOCAL USE
01 15 02			90782							
01 15 02			J1438							
01 15 02			99xxx xx							

Injection, etanercept (25 mg)

If administering a teaching dose, use therapeutic subcutaneous injection.

Insert appropriate modifier indicating significant, separately identifiable E&M service for the same physician on the same day of the procedure or other service (e.g., 25).

If initial patient evaluation includes ENBREL use, you may choose to bill for an office visit with the appropriate E&M code.

25. FEDERAL TAX I.D. NUMBER SSN EIN

26. PATIENT'S ACCOUNT NO.

27. ACCEPT ASSIGNMENT?

33. PHYSICIAN'S SUPPLIER'S BILLING NAME, ADDRESS, ZIP CODE & PHONE #

(APPROVED BY AMA COUNCIL ON MEDICAL SERVICE 8/88) PLEASE PRINT OR TYPE FORM CMS-1500

Figure 12.A.2 Sample claim form for Etanercept.

13

Alefacept to Treat Psoriasis

Gerald G. Krueger and Kristina P. Callis
University of Utah Health Sciences Center, Salt Lake City, Utah, U.S.A.

I. THE NEED FOR NEW SYSTEMIC APPROACHES TO TREAT PSORIASIS

As has been discussed in other chapters, we have systemic therapies for psoriasis that are quite effective. However all existing systemic therapies have safety and tolerability concerns. Cyclosporine causes hypertension and renal toxicity, which generally limits its use to < 1 year (1). Psoralen/ultraviolet A (PUVA) increases the risk of skin cancer with long-term use and is generally not the treatment of choice in patients with type I or II skin who have had more than 200 treatments (1). The most widely used agent, methotrexate, commonly causes asthenia and evidence of hepatotoxicity and, less commonly, bone marrow toxicity and pneumonitis. Chronically it can cause cirrhosis and portal fibrosis in significant numbers of patients (1). Curiously we can find no published reports in which psoriasis area severity index (PASI) endpoints were used to assess the efficacy of psoriasis treated with methotrexate. In a recent study to assess further its mechanism of action we assessed the efficacy, via PASI, of methotrexate in 25 consecutive patients requiring systemic therapy for psoriasis (K. Callis, 2002 Society of Investigative Dermatology, poster #220). In this study, 23 of 25 patients completed the aggressive treatment program starting at 15 mg/week and moving to as much as 30 mg/week over 6 months. A surprise was that although 65% had a ≥50% reduction in PASI, only 26% had a ≥75% reduction and only 3 (13%) achieved ≥95% reduction. We conclude from this study that methotrexate is less effective than is commonly believed (> 70% who tolerate the drug achieving > 75% improvement (2)) when assessed in a prospective fashion using PASI, the current standard of assessment of improvement. Thus, despite having several effective systemic agents for psoriasis there is an unmet need for psoriasis therapies that have long-lasting efficacy and few side effects.

II. T-CELL-MEDIATED IMMUNE RESPONSES IN PSORIASIS

Psoriasis is recognized as a T-cell-mediated immune disorder in which $CD4^+$ and $CD8^+$ memory T cells ($CD4^+CD45RO^+$ and $CD8^+CD45RO^+$) stimulate the hyperproliferation of keratinocytes (3, 4). Molecular definition of T-cell-mediated responses has given rise to pharmaceutical targets in the cascade of events triggered by such responses. The pathogenic events leading to psoriasis, the well-defined endpoints, and the size of the market have caused psoriasis to emerge as the prototypic T-cell-mediated disease in which to study rationally based intervention with biological agents targeted to specific components of T-cell-mediated pathways. Several strategies aimed at reducing or eliminating the pathogenic effects of T cells, described in this volume, are currently under investigation (5). One of these is alefacept (Biogen Inc., Cambridge, MA) approved by the FDA in January 2003 (at press time) for moderate-to-severe psoriasis. It is a fully human fusion protein consisting of the extracellular domain of lymphocyte function-associated antigen-3 (LFA-3) fused to the hinge, CH_2, and CH_3 sequences of immunoglobulin a_1. The Fc portion of IgG_1 binds to $Fc\gamma RIII$ on accessory cells (e.g., natural killer cells). The LFA-3 segment binds CD2 on the surface of T cells, which is upregulated on the surface of memory T cells (6–8).

III. MECHANISM OF ACTION OF ALEFACEPT

At least two signals are necessary for T cells to become activated to proliferate and secrete cytokines (5). The primary signal is provided by engagement of the T-cell receptor with antigen in association with major histocompatibility complexes on antigen-presenting cells (APCs). Costimulatory receptor–ligand pairs on the APC and the T cell provide the second signal. Interference with these molecular interactions disrupts costimulatory pathways and down-regulates T-cell responses and blocks the immune-mediated disease process. The mechanism of action of alefacept is illustrated in Figure 1 (9). Alefacept inhibits T-cell activation and proliferation by binding to CD2 on T cells and blocking the LFA-3/CD2 interaction (10). Alefacept also engages $Fc\gamma RI$ (on

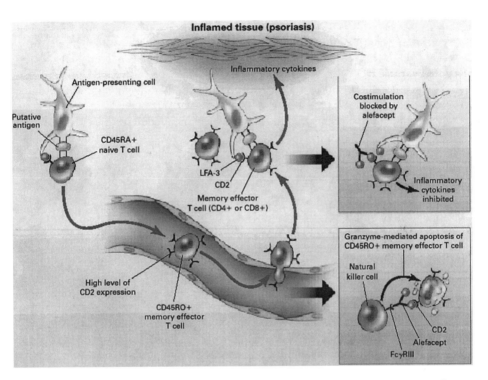

Figure 1 Proposed mechanism of action of alefacept. When T cells are present in the skin, hyperproliferation of keratinocytes and inflammation in lesional psoriasis may occur. Memory-effector T cells are generated when antigen-presenting cells (e.g., Langerhans or dermal dendritic cells) process antigen, migrate to regional lymph nodes, and interact with naïve T cells. The major MHC on antigen-presenting cells usually present antigen to T-cell receptors (TCR) on naïve T-cells. The antigen in psoriasis is not known, and the TCR–MHC interaction in psoriasis may be nonspecific. For naïve T cells (having CD45RA surface molecules) to become activated $CD4^+$ or $CD8^+$ memory-effector cells (having CD45RO surface molecules), costimulatory molecules on the T cell and the antigen-presenting cells (including CD2 and LFA-3, respectively) must interact. Memory-effector T cells proliferate and circulate, and those that reach the skin express CLA. When such memory-effector T cells interact with antigen-presenting cells, they release TH1-type cytokines IFN-γ and TNF-α, prolonging and intensifying the inflammatory response. Psoriasis-mediating T cells are subject to the action of alefacept (insets). Alefacept inhibits T-cell activation by blocking the costimulatory CD2 - LFA-3 interaction. Also, when alefacept binds CD2 on memory-effector T cells and interacts with FCγRIII receptors on natural killer cells, granzyme-mediated apoptosis (programmed cell death) of T cells is facilitated. (Reprinted with permission of the N Engl J Med.)

macrophages) and FcγRIII (on natural killer cells and neutrophils) IgG receptors, resulting in apoptosis of those T cells expressing high levels of CD2 (11). Because CD2 expression is higher on activated memory-effector ($CD4^+CD45RO^+$ and $CD8^+CD45RO^+$) than on naïve ($CD45RA^+$) T-cells, alefacept produces a selective apoptotic reduction in memory-effector T cells (13).

Figure 2 depicts the alefacept dose–response reduction in circulating CD4 T cells as well as those expressing the memory effector (CD4 + CD45RO +) and the naïve (CD4 + CD45RA +) phenotype. As reported, this reduction correlates (p < 0.001) with efficacy (9). James G. Krueger reported at the 2002 Society of Investigative Dermatology Meeting that reduction in memory effector T cells in skin is eight fold greater than in the circulation in the > 65% who responded to a 12 week course of intravenous (IV) alefacept. Thus, the reduction in the circulation noted in Figure 2 only partially reflects the pharmacological effects at the level of the lesion of psoriasis.

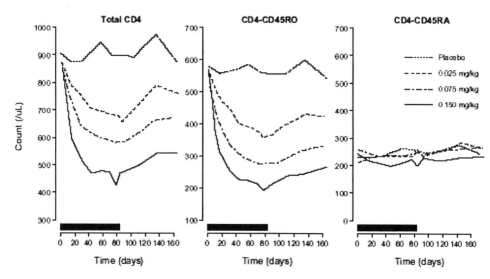

Figure 2 Peripheral lymphocyte subset counts. Mean counts of $CD4^+$ T lymphocytes, $CD4^+CD45RO^+$ memory-effector T lymphocytes, and $CD4^+$ $CD45RA^+$ naïve T lymphocytes vs. time by dose group. The bar represents the treatment period. All evaluable patients in the intent-to-treat analysis, including patients who received concomitant medications in the follow-up period, are included. The profiles for $CD8^+$ memory-effector and naïve T lymphocytes were nearly identical to those of $CD4^+$ cells (data not shown). (Reprinted with permission of the N Engl J Med.)

IV. CLINICAL TRIALS

A. Efficacy of IV Alefacept

Early studies showed that 0.075 mg/kg given weekly as a 30 s IV bolus for 12 weeks was most the most effective dose (9). Additional pharmacokinetic and pharmacodynamic studies predicted that a non-weight-adjusted dose (7.5 mg), as an IV bolus would be as effective as a weight-adjusted dose. For the pivotal phase III trial one dose was used for all patients ≥50 kg; if the patient weighed < 50 kg, the dose was decreased by 33%. The IV pivotal trial was a randomized, double-blind, placebo-controlled, parallel-group study of two treatment courses, each with a 12 week treatment period (once weekly alefacept 7.5 mg or once weekly saline placebo administered as a 30-second IV bolus) and a 12 week treatment-free follow-up phase. Patients were randomized to three cohorts: cohort 1 received two courses of alefacept, cohort 2 received an alefacept course followed by a placebo course, and cohort 3 received a placebo course followed by an alefacept course.

A total of 490 (89%) of 553 patients completed course 1 treatment and follow-up. A total of 401 (89%) of 449 patients completed course 2 treatment and follow-up. Most patients who dropped from study did so due to voluntary withdrawal, disease worsening, and being lost to follow-up. Very few patients discontinued because of adverse events.

In both courses, mean PASI scores progressively decreased in those receiving alefacept during the 12 week treatment period and continued to decrease further after the last dose (Fig. 3). In course 1, the maximum mean reduction from baseline PASI was 47% in the combined alefacept group (cohorts 1 and 2) and 20% in the placebo group (cohort 3).

Improvement continued after alefacept administration was stopped with the mean maximal reduction in PASI occurring 8 weeks after the last dose of alefacept. A second course of alefacept therapy provided additional benefit. Patients who received two courses of alefacept (cohort 1) had a maximum mean reduction from baseline PASI of 54% at 6 weeks posttreatment of course 2 (Fig. 3).

Alefacept significantly improved clinical outcomes and severity of psoriasis in both courses, regardless of the definition of response. For the primary endpoint, a significantly greater percentage of patients in the combined alefacept group (cohorts 1 and 2) than in the placebo group (cohort 3) achieved a ≥75% reduction in PASI from baseline at 2 weeks after the last dose of course 1 (14% vs 4%, p < 0.001). Because many patients do not achieve maximal benefit until after the last dose, the overall response rate is a more meaningful endpoint. The overall response rate reflects improvement at any time after the first dose (i.e., during the dosing period as well as the 12 week follow-up period). A comparison of this assessment of improvement

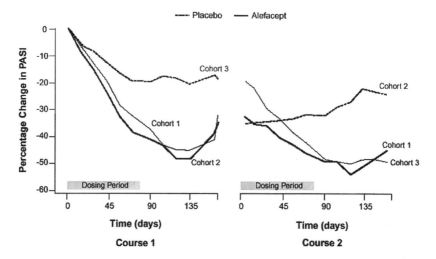

Figure 3 Mean percentage reduction in PASI over both courses. (Reprinted with permission of the J Am Acad Dermatol.)

is presented in Table 1. The analysis of overall response rates also demonstrates significance for patients receiving alefacept versus placebo (p < 0.001). A second course offered additional benefit (12).

In the other phase III trial study, 507 patients were randomized to receive a fixed dose of either 10 mg or 15 mg alefacept (or placebo) administered intramuscularly (IM) once weekly over 12 weeks with a 12 week follow-up. For the primary endpoint—the percentage of patients achieving a

Table 1 Comparison of Overall Response Rates

Route of delivery	% with ≥50% reduction in PASI	% with ≥75% reduction in PASI	% with Clear/Almost clear
IV 1 course 7.5 mg	56	28	23
IV 2 courses 7.5 mg	71	40	32
IV placebo	24	8	6
IM 1 course 15 mg	57	33	24
IM 2 courses 15 mg	69	43	31
IM placebo	35	13	8

Results in patients receiving one or two courses of alefacept 7.5 mg/week IV or 15 mg/week IM with no other systemic therapy used between the two alefacept courses.

≥75% reduction in PASI 2 weeks after the last dose—the 15 mg dose was significantly more effective than placebo (21% vs 5%, p < 0.001). The response rates for the 15 mg dose are listed in Table 1; significance levels were those of the IV dose (12a).

Most patients in the IM trial were crossed over to a second course of alefacept after the 12 weeks of follow-up. Similar to the IV study, a second course of alefacept provided incremental benefit over the first course (Table 1) (12a).

B. Duration of Response with IV and IM Alefacept

Response to alefacept was durable. Duration has been determined in several ways. It is the authors' opinion that the most meaningful interpretation

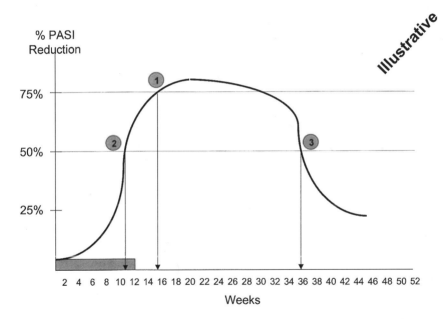

Figure 4 An illustration of the method used to calculate duration of response, defined as the time that patients maintained a ≥50% reduction from baseline PASI for those who achieved a ≥75% reduction from baseline PASI at any time during the study without the use of phototherapy or systemic therapies. 1, Time point at which a ≥75% reduction in PASI was noted; 2, time at which this patient achieved ≥50% reduction in PASI; 3, time point at which the patient's level dropped below this reduction. The total time spent at ≥50% improvement is duration of response. (Reprinted with permission of the J Am Acad Dermatol.)

of durable is the time patients maintained clinically significant improvement, defined as a ≥50% reduction in PASI relative to baseline during or after treatment. Durability was best delineated in cohort 2; these patients received a single 12 week course of alefacept (see Fig. 3) and were then evaluated in study for an additional 36 weeks: 12 weeks of follow-up, 12 weeks of placebo, and 12 more weeks of follow-up. The method for determining duration of response is illustrated in Figure 4. The median duration of a ≥50% reduction in PASI for patients who achieve ≥75% reduction in PASI is 216 days and for patients who achieve "clear" or "almost clear" status during or after treatment it is 241 days. The duration of response was longer following a second course of alefacept therapy (Fig. 5). Among patients who received two courses of alefacept (cohort 1) and achieved a ≥75% reduction in PASI (or a Physician's global assessment [PGA] of "clear" or "almost clear") during either treatment or follow-up period, the median duration of response could not be determined because > 50% of these patients had maintained their ≥50% improvement status at the final endpoint, which was nearly 1 year after the first dose of study drug. These differences are significant (p < 0.01) and indicate that two courses provided a greater duration of response than a single course. The protocols for the IM studies do not allow for a direct comparable

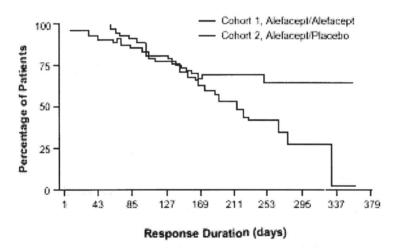

Figure 5 Duration of a ≥50% reduction in PASI from baseline in patients who achieved a ≥75% reduction in PASI during or after treatment plotted as a survival curve. Log-rank test p = 0.019, for cohort 1 (two courses of IV alefacept) vs. cohort 2 (one course of IV alefacept followed by placebo). (Reprinted with permission of the J Am Acad Dermatol.)

analysis; however, durability after one course is equivalent to that of the IV route of administration.

C. Safety and Tolerability

At least one course of alefacept has been given to 1357 patients during controlled trials, leading to the Biologics License Application (BLA) for and subsequent FDA approval of alefacept for the treatment of psoriasis (12a).

Alefacept was well tolerated in all of the trials. Adverse events were similar between the two routes of administration. In the largest of the pivotal phase III trial (the IV trial) the incidence of each adverse event was comparable or lower during the second course. The only adverse event in course 1 that had a ≥5% higher incidence in the combined alefacept group (cohorts 1 and 2) vs. the placebo group (cohort 3) was chills (10% vs. 1%). Chills tended to occur soon after dosing (> 90% within 24 h of treatment) and were limited to one or two occasions early during treatment and rarely occurred in the second course. In course 2, the only adverse events that occurred with a ≥5% higher incidence in the alefacept group than the placebo group were accidental injury (20% vs. 15%) and pharyngitis (16% vs. 11%). The majority of accidental injuries were minor events, such as sprains. Infections were generally mild and responsive to conventional therapy. The vast majority of episodes coded to the term "infection" were common colds (12).

In these pivotal trials, patients who were scheduled to receive alefacept received placebo if their CD4 counts dropped below a predefined and arbitrarily set limit of 250 cells/μl. Alefacept was permanently substituted with placebo if the $CD4^+$ lymphocyte count remained below 250 cells/μl for four or more consecutive visits. With one course of alefacept, 10% of patients had at least one placebo substitution and < 2% (7) had permanent placebo substitutions. In course 2, placebo was substituted at least once in ≈ 7% of patients. There was only one permanent placebo substitution in course 2 (12).

Throughout the study, no opportunistic infections and no association of infections with $CD4^+$ T-cell counts < 250 cells/μl were observed. Laboratory parameters were measured at baseline and at the end of the treatment and follow-up periods. No consistent statistically significant abnormalities were recorded during either the first or second course of the pivotal trail or in the phase II safety and dose-ranging trials (12a).

No clinically important changes in vital signs or physical examinations were observed. Antialefacept antibodies were detected in ≤1% of patients in each cohort throughout the study; titers were low (<1:40) and did not correlate with dosage, length of therapy, or any adverse events (13). No immune hypersensitivity reactions were observed. Analysis also revealed no evidence for rebound of disease after alefacept therapy was stopped (12a). No patient experienced signs or symptoms referable to cytokine release syndrome or capillary leak syndrome (13).

Malignancies were diagnosed in five patients: adenocarcinoma of the colon in a patient with a family history of colon cancer and a recent medical history of guaiac-positive stools; adenocarcinoma of the lung in a patient with a history of heavy smoking; and squamous cell carcinoma of the skin in three patients who had previously received PUVA and methotrexate for long-standing psoriasis (13). None were considered to be related to the study drug.

Alefacept selectively reduces levels of specific T-cell subsets. Thus the ability of host defenses to mount an adequate response to pathogens was of concern. The integrity of T-cell-dependent immune responses to challenge with neoantigen and recall antigen was tested in a multicenter, randomized, open-label, parallel-group study (12a). In this study, psoriasis patients treated with alefacept 7.5 mg IV bolus once weekly for 12 weeks received immunizations with a harmless foreign neoantigen, ϕX174 as a surrogate pathogen, as well as a recall antigen: tetanus toxoid. Controls were untreated patients with psoriasis. To create the most rigorous test possible, the first and second immunizations of ϕX174 were performed at time points that coincided with the period of maximal reductions in CD4 and CD8 memory effector T cells. Mean anti-ϕX174 antibody titers were comparable in both groups. Consistent with an acquired immune response, antibody titers rose rapidly after immunization with tetanus toxoid. The percentage of patients with twofold or greater increase in antitetanus titer 3 weeks after immunization was comparable between the alefacept (89%) and control (91%) groups. Although alefacept has demonstrated positive effects in an immune-mediated disease, it does not blunt immune responses to novel and recall antigens and, based on currently available data, does not increase susceptibility to infectious disease or malignancy.

V. COMMON QUESTIONS ON THE CLINICAL USE OF ALEFACEPT

A. How Should Clinicians and Patients Interpret Response Data from Clinical Trials on Patients with Moderate to Severe Disease?

Most dermatologists have not used PASI (14) or PGA enough to be able to translate these findings to the clinic. On the other hand, they are very facile in interpreting the patient's assessment. It is the authors' opinion that physicians respond to patients' needs. If patients are satisfied with their treatment, it is likely that the physician will not alter treatment unless, as commonly occurs currently, cumulative side effects dictate a different response. Because the patient's attitude is central, it seems reasonable in this day of evidence-based medicine that one turn to quality of life (QOL) assessments generated as part of determining drug efficacy. In the alefacept trials, the Dermatology Life Quality Index (DLQI) was used. We compared DLQI results from patients who achieved the status of clear or almost clear by PGA with patients who achieved a ≥75% reduction in PASI and a reduction in PASI of ≥50% relative to baseline in the phase III alefacept trials. It is noteworthy that the DLQI in the clear, almost clear, and the ≥75% reduction in PASI groups are nearly equivalent with slightly greater than 70% improvement in DLQI scores. Not expected is the fact that those with a lesser clinical response (the ≥50% reduction in PASI) also had a significant improvement (60%) in their DLQI. These improvements in QOL persisted at the end of the 12 week treatment-free follow-up period. This supports the notion that a ≥50% reduction in PASI must be considered to be a positive therapeutic event when coupled with maintenance at this level of response. The median duration of ≥50 reduction in PASI by those who achieved ≥50% reduction in PASI was more than 4 months (140 days), which was achieved in ≈ 70% of subjects treated with alefacept.

B. Who Should Be Treated with Alefacept?

A 1998 survey of over 17,000 members of the National Psoriasis Foundation reveals that approximately 20% of these patients have severe psoriasis (15). Unless comfort measures are the goal of therapeutic intervention, systemic therapy or light-based therapies are the most reasonable options for these patients. These have acute and/or cumulative side effects. We estimate that there are at least 5 million people in the United States with psoriasis. At least 10% of patients with moderate to severe psoriasis are either not responding to current therapy and/or have concerns about its cumulative side effects (15). All of these patients (~500,000 in the United States) are reasonable candidates for intervention with agents such as alefacept that currently have lower toxicity profiles and are designed to attack specific targets of the pathogenic processes that lead to psoriasis. Others to be considered for these new agents are patients who have run out of reasonable therapeutic options.

This section would not be complete without a review of what defines mild, moderate, and severe disease. For reasons that are not clear, the Food and Drug Administration has maintained that this is best defined as percentage of body surface area (BSA) covered with disease. Currently BSA has to be 10% for patients with psoriasis to be entered on a trial for moderate to severe disease. While BSA is a consideration, neither patients nor physicians classify severity of chronic skin disease on the basis of how much of the body is covered with disease.

For patients and their physicians severity is inexorably linked to the impact psoriasis has on the quality of life. Treatment decisions need to focus on the complex interplay between the severity of skin lesions and their impact on the patient, and on the costs and risks to the patient relative to the expected benefits. Recently the Medical Advisory Board of the National Psoriasis Foundation (NPF) wrote a position paper on what defines mild, moderate, and severe disease (16). They take the defensible position that severity of psoriasis is linked to how the disease alters the QOL. The key elements describing severity are as follows:

Mild: Disease does not alter QOL.
Moderate: Disease does alter QOL, therapies are expected to improve QOL, and have minimal risk.
Severe: Disease does alter QOL, response to treatments with minimal risks is ineffective, and patients will accept life-altering side effects to achieve better QOL.

A desire of all patients would be for an effective therapy without acute or cumulative toxicities. If such an agent were available, all psoriasis would be considered mild to moderate. The new biological response modifiers, such as alefacept, appear to offer many patients this option.

C. Is There a Preference for the IV or IM Alefacept Formulation?

The FDA has approved both the IM and the IV formulation of alefacept for the treatment of moderate to severe psoriasis. Experience may dictate otherwise, but it is predicted that both will gain advocates. The cost of generating and purifying the current biological agents coming to the market for psoriasis is considerable. For alefacept the IM route requires twice (15 mg/week) the amount that the IV route (7.5 mg/week) takes to have the same impact on disease. The IM route will require no more expertise than is required for an IM injection of triamcinolone. The IV route will require some additional training for the staff in many dermatologists' offices. Alefacept, when given IV, can be given as a bolus over a 30 s time period. The following steps are suggested:

1. Reconstitute alefacept using instructions in package insert and draw into appropriate-size syringe.
2. Select a vein for intravenous access.
3. Clean the area with antiseptic.

4. Apply tourniquet.
5. Gain intravenous access with a 19 gauge butterfly needle. Attach syringe with alefacept. Withdraw small amount of blood to establish that venous access has been obtained. Infuse drug and blood into the patient over 30 s, after completion, withdraw 1 cc blood and reinfuse to clear the line of residual alefacept.
6. Remove infusion line, apply pressure to control bleeding, and manage as routine venipuncture.

Note: it is possible to draw blood for laboratory testing through this same line. If this is to be done, it is necessary that it be drawn *before* infusion of drug. This is most easily accomplished by attaching a disposable two-way stopcock to the 19 gauge butterfly and use one port to withdraw blood and the other to infuse the drug.

D. What is the Most Effective Way to Assess Improvement?

Important decisions will hinge on assessment of improvement. Two approaches are suggested. The authors' preferred way is to take advantage of the patient's memory. We have learned that patients can consistently recall the worst their disease has ever been and most know what it is like to have no disease. On the other hand, patients and doctors are notoriously inaccurate in recalling the severity of disease 12 or more weeks after they have started a course of therapy. We suggest the following approach. At the baseline visit, ask the patient to rate their psoriasis on a scale of 1–10, with 10 defined as the worst their psoriasis has ever been and 1 as no disease. With encouragement and use in the routine decision making by staff and physician at every visit, the patient's evaluation of their psoriasis will become an invaluable tool to assess progress. The second approach is to use PASI (14) or the newly developed NPF Psoriasis Score (July–August 2002 issue of the National Psoriasis Foundation Physicians Forum). The latter has the advantage of having incorporated into it both a dynamic patient's global assessment (relative to the worst they have ever been) and a static physician's global assessment.

E. Who Should Receive a Second Course and Is a 12 Week Rest Period Necessary after Each Course?

The answer to these questions likely will change with clinical experience. Because of the prolonged remissions produced by alefacept, it is unlikely that patients who achieve clear or near-clear status will want or would benefit from a second course until their disease returns. It is possible, but currently not known, that alefacept at infrequent intervals (e.g. every 4–12 weeks) might prevent recurrence. Improvement in the first course makes additional benefit with a second course likely (see Table 1). Data from phase III trials show that those patients have an 80% likelihood of achieving at least the same response seen in course 1. Even patients with less than 50% improvement in course 1 have about a 40% likelihood of achieving clinically relevant improvement ($\geq 50\%$ reduction in PASI) with a second course.

Even those patients who have had no benefit, defined as less than a 25% improvement from baseline, from one course, have been noted to experience improvement with a second course.

The FDA-approved prescribing information (package insert) states that alefacept is to be given weekly, IV or IM, for 12 weeks, and is to be followed by a 12 week observation period. There are two reasons for the rest period. First, it can be generally predicted that there will be continued improvement after this treatment is stopped, (~ 8 weeks after last dose for median peak improvement). Second, we do not have data on what would happen to the lymphocyte counts without this rest period. It is possible that they could decline to levels that could have untoward consequences. There will be questions stemming from these guidelines: What if the patient is getting worse at 4 weeks into the rest period? What if lymphocyte counts are still going down at the end of the 12 week rest period? These and other questions will cause physicians to alter the recommended guidelines. To do this they will rely on training, assessment of the patient's history, the physical findings, as well as the laboratory parameters. A combination of phase 4 studies and clinicians' experience treating patients with alefacept will address many of the outstanding questions that remain in terms of future modifications to the FDA-approved package insert.

F. When Should the Second and Repeat Courses Be Given?

The second course of alefacept can be given any time after 12 weeks of treatment-free follow-up of a 12-week course of therapy. It is possible that time to retreatment can be extended with vigorous topical management; a vigorous hydration program with heavy emollients, systemic anti-itch agents, topical treatment with agents that have proven efficacy (see Chapter 2 on topical agents); as well as light-based therapy. It is our experience that most patients will want a repeat course when they have lost $> 50\%$ of their maximal improvement.

At this time ~ 50 patients have had five or more courses of alefacept. There has been no evidence of cumulative toxicity, increased infections, increased antibodies to drug, and no further suppression of memory effector cells in the circulation (12a).

G. What Is the Safest Way to Increase the Dosage?

There are no data to guide in the use of higher dosages of alefacept. With time these data will become available. If indicated, a rational approach would be to give alefacept for longer courses rather than to raise the dosage. In phase II trials the cohort with the highest dosage (0.15 mg/kg/week) had doses substituted with placebo more often because lymphocyte subset counts dropped below the predefined limits. Thus we consider that the most rational way to increase the dosage will be to give it for longer periods of time (i.e., for 14, 16, 18, or more weeks). If this is necessary, lymphocyte and lymphocyte subset (total T-cell counts, and CD4 counts) testing will need to be done. If these fall more than two standard deviations below the lower limits of normal for that laboratory, it is our recommendation that dosing be interrupted. When alefacept is given to baboons the T-cell counts respond in a fashion similar to humans. When baboons are given alefacept at dosages 45 times the dosage currently recommended for treating psoriasis, their T-cell counts do not drop below 20% of pretreatment levels (data on file at Biogen). How this relates to using higher dosages in humans is unknown, but it does suggest that there is a lower limit that cannot be bridged with this drug.

H. What Other Agents Are Predicted to Be Compatible, and How and When Should They Be Used?

As this and other chapters in this text note, alefacept and light therapy (PUVA, broad- and narrow-band UVB) work by selectively inducing apoptosis of activated T cells in psoriatic lesions. It follows that light therapy would be addictive, possibly synergistic, and therefore compatible. Because nonaugmented light therapy (e.g. narrow-band UVB) is the safest of the systemic therapies for psoriasis, it is predicted that this will be the first concomitant therapy to be used. We do not have any knowledge that would suggest how or if the dosage or frequency of light or the monitoring T cells needs to be altered in the patient receiving alefacept and light therapy. Caution and careful observation are appropriate as experience is gained; there is the possibility that this combination could increase the risk of cutaneous malignancy. However, the patients who had previously received light therapy for psoriasis and been treated in alefacept trials, and then followed for up to 1 year, had no increased incidence of skin cancer.

Cyclosporine inhibits the generation of cytokines by activated T cells; thus, it would also be predicted to be compatible (1). It has been suggested that an effective approach to speed response and cause more patients to move to a high level of response (> 75% reduction in disease activity) is to give a 4–8 week course of cyclosporine at an aggressive dosage: 4–5 mg/kg/ day. Once significant improvement, which will be variable (25–75% reduction in 8 weeks) (1), has occurred the cyclosporine would be discontinued or tapered over 4 weeks. Whether this approach would move the number of people achieving ≥75% improvement or alter long-term remission is unknown. Again there are no data to assist in decisions for monitoring interactive toxicity. Caution and careful observation are appropriate as experience is gained.

Methotrexate is thought to exert its antipsoriatic effects via action on activated T cells (1). Although methotrexate can induce a rapid response, maximal effect is generally seen after 3 months of therapy. As noted earlier, our methotrexate study indicates only 13% achieved clear or almost clear status, 26% achieved > 75% reduction in PASI, and 65% achieved a > 50% reduction in PASI after 6 months of use. The number who achieved > 75% improvement was less than expected; our recent review of the literature notes that over 70% of subjects will have substantial clearing (2). We believe that the reason for not seeing this level of improvement in our study is secondary to the fact that methotrexate has never been evaluated in a prospective fashion using PASI. The foregoing emphasize the fact that a 50–75% reduction in PASI constitutes clinically meaningful improvement. In our methotrexate trial there were no significant decreases in circulating total or subsets of lymphocyte counts, (T cells, memory T cells: CD4 and C8, natural killer cells) and there was no correlation with T-cell counts and response to treatment. Although this suggests that alefacept and methotrexate might be safely used in combination, there are no data to assist in decisions for monitoring for interactive toxicity. Caution and careful observation are appropriate as experience is gained.

Drugs with a beneficial effect for psoriasis that are known to be myelosuppressive (1, 17), (e.g., fumaric acid, 6 thioguanine, hydroxyurea, etc.), if used in combination with alefacept, need to be administered with additional caution. Other agents with antipsoriatic effects, such as Soriatane and CellCept, are not expected to have added toxicity and might have added beneficial effects.

I. What Laboratory Testing Is Required?

This chapter went to press only days after the FDA approved the use of alefacept for psoriasis. The FDA-approved package label recommends weekly monitoring of CD4+ T lymphocyte counts during the 12-week dosing period to guide dosing. The FDA recommends that patients whose CD4+ T cell counts fall below 250 cells/μl should have their next dose withheld, and that alefacept should be discontinued if the counts remain below that level for one month. During the phase III trials, lymphocyte counts were determined at weekly intervals. The need for assessing counts while off drug or in the follow-up period between courses does not seem to be indicated unless the lymphocyte counts are depressed significantly, (e.g., >33% below the lower limits of normal) (see Table 2). Data show that the maximum reduction in T-cell counts generally occurs within 6 weeks of initiating alefacept. By 3 months following alefacept administration, CD4 memory-effector cells (one of the T-cell subsets affected by alefacept) are above the lower limits of normal in near 90% of subjects (12a). If reduced lymphocyte counts persist, monitoring may be indicated at less frequent intervals (e.g., every 8 weeks) until counts return to normal range (see Fig. 2). An advantage to early monitoring is that an indication of response can be gained. Patients with the greatest drop in memory effector cells in the circulation are most likely to achieve a >75% improvement. Of patients with the greatest reduction (top 25th percentile) in circulating memory effector T cells in the first 4 weeks of therapy, more than 60% went on to achieve >75% improvement (data on file at Biogen, 2002). Required monitoring can therefore be presented to the patient in a positive manner.

Table 3 lists the changes seen in total lymphocyte and subsets as a consequence of one or two courses of IV alefacept. In general it can be stated that a reduction in total lymphocyte count mirrors that of the specific subsets. Because the CD4 and CD8 memory-effector T cells had the biggest changes, assessment of one of these subsets at 1 or 2 week intervals while on treatment seems most informative and appropriate until we have more experience. If these selected subsets cannot be measured, a T-cell count or possibly a total lymphocyte count can be substituted to guide dosing. If current safety is maintained, we predict that the monitoring requirements will be less burdensome (e.g., at baseline, 4, 8, and 12 weeks).

Some patients will have CD4 or CD8 memory-effector T-cell, total T-cell, or total lymphocyte counts below the lower limit of normal when they

Table 2 Normal Range of Lymphocyte Counts (cells/μl) at the Associated and Regional University Pathology Laboratories (Salt Lake City, UT, USA)

	Total lymphocytes/μl	Total T cells/μl	CD4 T-cells/μl
Normal range	910-4280	723-2737	404-1612

Table 3 Comparison of Percentage Decrease in Total and Selected Subsets
of Lymphocytes

	Total lymphocytes	CD4 T cells	CD8 T cells	CD4 memory effector T cells	CD8 memory effector T cells
1	23	36	40	48	59
2	21	33	41	51	66

Results in patients receiving two courses of alefacept 7.5 mg/week IV × 12, with a 12 week rest
period between courses.

are first considered for therapy with alefacept. To gain further perspective
we determined how many patients were screening failures (199 of 1294, 15%)
for the 2 phase III trials. An interesting finding was that 18 of 199 (9%) were
treatment failures because their CD4 counts were below the lower limits of
normal (< 400/µl). The frequency of such patients in the general population
is not known. Since becoming aware of this we have found that there are
number of otherwise healthy people who have varying degrees of leukopenia. We estimate that at least 2% of patients with psoriasis have suppressed
lymphocyte counts. The analysis of the foregoing screening failures suggests
that it could be significantly more. It is our assessment that these subjects do
not have increased infections, are not necessarily infected with human
immunodeficiency virus (HIV), and regard themselves as otherwise healthy.
The safety and efficacy of alefacept in patients with psoriasis with suppressed
lymphocyte counts and who are otherwise healthy are unknown. Recommendations are difficult. We think that if a thorough evaluation for underlying causes of the lymphocytopenia reveals no apparent cause, alefacept
could be used cautiously. If this treatment is chosen, the indicated monitoring of lymphocytes and lymphocyte subsets would offer an additional
measure of safety.

J. How Should Alefacept Be Used in Subsets of Patients for Whom There Is No Clinical Trial Experience?

Clinical trials with alefacept excluded the following groups of patients: those
whose lymphocytes were below the lower limits of normal, those who were
HIV$^+$, those with hepatitis B and/or C infection, and those with erythrodermic or pustular psoriasis. Arguments can be generated for not giving a drug
that lowers CD4 counts in a disease in which CD4 counts are suppressed, (e.g.,
HIV$^+$ patients with clinical manifestations of acquired immunodeficiency
syndrome). There is no rational reason for not using alefacept in patients with

erythrodermic or pustular psoriasis. Determining hepatitis B and C status seems an unnecessary burden, given that patients receiving alefacept generate normal primary and secondary immune responses (12a). However, if a patient has abnormal liver functions on entry that are without apparent cause, hepatitis status should be determined. If hepatitis is present with a clinically relevant viral load, it is our opinion that alefacept not be given until safety in this population has been determined.

During the phase 3 trials, patients who developed a clinically significant infection (in the investigator's judgment) while receiving alefacept had drug withheld until the infection had cleared. Until countermanding data are available, it is recommended that patients with clinically significant infection have alefacept held until the infection has resolved or brought under control with appropriate antimicrobial agents.

VI. SUMMARY

One or more courses of alefacept significantly improve psoriasis and produce durable clinical remissions, without rebound following treatment cessation. The incremental effectiveness of a second course of alefacept provides strong support for its use as an intermittent therapy for this chronic disease. Because psoriasis is a chronic disease with a fluctuating course of remissions and flares that is frequently managed with agents that display significant toxicity, it is predicted that alefacept will help meet the unmet need for a safe and effective remittive therapy.

REFERENCES

1. Lebwohl M, Ali S. Treatment of psoriasis. Part 2. Systemic therapies. J Am Acad Dermatol 2001; 45(5): 649–661.
2. Tristani-Firouzi P, Krueger GG. Efficacy and safety of treatment modalities for psoriasis. Cutis 1998; 61(2 Suppl): 11–21.
3. Friedrich M, et al. Flow cytometric characterization of lesional T-cells in psoriasis: intracellular cytokine and surface antigen expression indicates an activated, memory/effector type 1 immunophenotype. Arch Dermatol Res 2000; 292(10): 519–521.
4. Bos JD, De Rie MA. The pathogenesis of psoriasis: immunological facts and speculations. Immunol Today 1999; 20(1): 40–46.
5. Gordon KB, West DP. Biologic therapy in dermatology. In: Wolverton SE, ed. Comprehensive Dermatologic Drug Therapy. Philadelphia: WB Saunders, 2001: 928–942.

6. Chisholm PL, et al. The effects of an immunomodulatory LFA3-IgG1 fusion protein on nonhuman primates. Ther Immunol 1994; 1(4): 205–216.
7. Miller GT, et al. Specific interaction of lymphocyte function-associated antigen 3 with CD2 can inhibit T-cell responses. J Exp Med 1993; 178(1): 211–222.
8. Meier W, et al. Immunomodulation by LFA3TIP, an LFA-3/IgG1 fusion protein: cell line dependent glycosylation effects on pharmacokinetics and pharmacodynamic markers. Ther Immunol 1995; 2(3): 159–171.
9. Ellis CN, Krueger GG. Treatment of chronic plaque psoriasis by selective targeting of memory effector T lymphocytes. N Engl J Med, 2001; 345(4): 248–255.
10. Majeau GR, et al. Mechanism of lymphocyte function-associated molecule 3-Ig fusion proteins inhibition of T-cell responses. Structure/function analysis in vitro and in human CD2 transgenic mice. J Immunol 1994; 152(6): 2753–2767.
11. Sanders ME, et al. Human memory T lymphocytes express increased levels of three cell adhesion molecules (LFA-3, CD2, and LFA-1) and three other molecules (UCHL1, CDw29, and Pgp-1) and have enhanced IFN-gamma production. J Immunol 1988; 140(5): 1401–1407.
12. Krueger GG, et al., A randomized, double-blind, placebo-controlled phase III study evaluating efficacy and safety of two courses of alefacept in patients with chronic plaque psoriasis. J Am Acad Dermatol 2002; 47: 821–833.
12a. Biogen briefing document FDA Dermatology Advisory Meeting, Bethesda, MD, May 2002.
13. Krueger GG. Selective targeting of T-cell subsets: focus on alefacept—a remittive therapy for psoriasis. Expert Opin Biol Ther 2002; 2(4): 431–441.
14. Fredriksson T, Pettersson U. Severe psoriasis—oral therapy with a new retinoid. Dermatologica 1978; 157(4): 238–244.
15. Krueger G, et al., The impact of psoriasis on quality of life: results of a 1998 National Psoriasis Foundation patient-membership survey. Arch Dermatol 2001; 137(3): 280–284.
16. Krueger GG, et al., Two considerations for patients with psoriasis and their clinicians: what defines mild, moderate, and severe psoriasis? What constitutes a clinically significant improvement when treating psoriasis? J Am Acad Dermatol 2000; 43(2 Pt 1): 281–285.
17. Mason C, Krueger GG. Thioguanine for refractory psoriasis: a 4-year experience. J Am Acad Dermatol 2001; 44(1): 67–72.

14

Infliximab in the Treatment of Psoriasis

Alice B. Gottlieb

University of Medicine and Dentistry of New Jersey–Robert Wood Johnson Medical School, New Brunswick, New Jersey, U.S.A.

I. INTRODUCTION

Advances in psoriasis therapy have been made over the last two decades based on a greater understanding of the pathogenesis of psoriasis. In particular, we now know that psoriasis shares a common pathophysiology with many disorders involving a hyperactive inflammatory response, and, like other immune-mediated inflammatory disorders (IMIDs), psoriasis has a genetic component that predisposes certain people or families to the disease. Based on this IMID principle, a triggering event causes the immune system to respond inappropriately, inducing hyperproliferation of epidermal cells. A novel approach to treating psoriasis blocks crucial steps in the underlying immune system process that result in the dermatological symptoms associated with this immune-mediated disorder.

As opposed to drugs such as methotrexate and cyclosporine that can cause broad immunomodulation, a new class of drugs, termed biotherapeutics, targets specific steps in the immune cascade. Infliximab, the subject of this chapter, targets the activity of tumor necrosis factor α (TNFα) and, by interrupting the inflammatory cascade, has the potential to relieve the signs and symptoms of psoriasis. Other biotherapeutics are discussed in other chapters of this book.

II. PATHOPHYSIOLOGY OF PSORIASIS

Psoriasis is an inflammatory, T-cell-mediated disease; however, the cause of T cell activation is still unknown. Although the precise causes and pathogenesis of psoriasis are unclear, immunological, genetic, and environmental factors are known to have important roles (1). The development of psoriasis can be classified into three phases: trafficking, migration, and inflammation (Fig. 1).

A. Trafficking

When antigenic material is captured by Langerhans cells (the antigen-presenting cells of the skin), they travel to the lymph nodes where they present

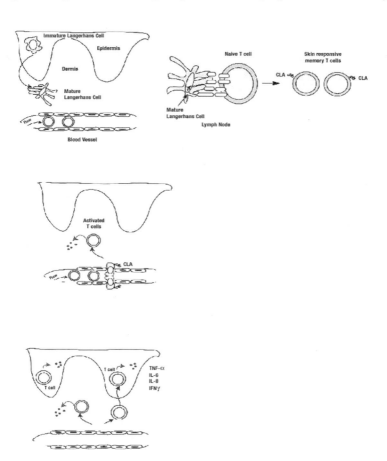

Figure 1 Three phases in the development of psoriasis.

antigen to naive T cells and convert them to memory T cells. Subsequently, skin-homing memory T cells are released to travel back to the epidermis (2).

B. Migration

To be effective, the activated T cells must leave the blood vessel and migrate to the affected area of the skin. T cells must adhere to the lining of the blood vessels prior to passing through the vessel wall into the dermis. During the activation process, the T cells acquire the cell surface expression of cutaneous lymphocyte-associated antigen (CLA), which promotes access into the relevant portion of the skin. Chemokines produced in the skin facilitate adhesion to the vessel wall, as does the presence of adhesion molecules in the affected skin regions: intracellular adhesion molecules (ICAM) and vascular cell adhesion molecules (VCAM). Once the activated T cells have left the blood vessel, they are attracted by chemokines, migrating through the dermis to the epidermis, where they activate local inflammatory processes.

C. Inflammation

In the epidermal layers, activated T cells and possibly other cell types, such as Langerhans cells, cause the epidermal hyperproliferation with abnormal differentiation and inflammation that is characteristic of psoriasis (3–6). These cells release chemokines and cytokines including TNFα, interleukin (IL)-6, IL-8, IL-12, granulocyte–macrophage colony-stimulating factor (GM-CSF), and interferon-gamma (IFNγ), which ultimately cause the clinical manifestations of psoriasis. Levels of TNFα, γ-interferon, IL-12, IL-6, IL-8, and other inflammatory cytokines are elevated in psoriatic lesions but not in the normal skin of patients with psoriasis (7–12).

III. ROLE OF TNFα IN PSORIASIS

TNFα appears to be central to, or able to modify, each of the three components of the disease process: trafficking, migration, and inflammation.

TNFα can promote *trafficking* by stimulating Langerhans cells to migrate from the skin to the lymph nodes. One possible mechanism involves E-cadherin. This adhesion molecule, residing in the epidermis, promotes Langerhans cell binding to keratinocytes, thereby retaining keratinocyte-bound Langerhans cells in the epidermis. TNFα decreases E-cadherin expression (13), which then allows Langerhans cells to travel from the skin to lymph nodes and subsequently activate T cells.

TNFα promotes *migration* of the T cells from the bloodstream into the skin by inducing expression of the adhesion molecules ICAM-1 and VCAM-1 on endothelial cells and keratinocytes, which directly results in the migration of inflammatory cells into the dermis and epidermis (14, 15). Leukocyte migration into skin could also be promoted by the induction of vascular endothelial growth factor by TNFα (16).

Lastly, TNFα increases *inflammation* associated epidermal hyperplasia by increasing keratinocyte proliferation and production of Type I vasoactive intestinal peptide (VIP) receptor mRNA in keratinocytes. Subsequent binding of VIP to its receptor also promotes keratinocyte proliferation in addition to stimulating the synthesis of inflammatory cytokines such as IL-6 and IL-8, and regulated upon activation normal T cells expressed and secreted (RANTES) (17, 18). In addition, TNFα increases plasminogen activator inhibitor type 2 (PAI-2), a serine proteinase inhibitor that is thought to protect cells from apoptosis (19). The prevention of apoptosis could lead to increased longevity of keratinocytes. Thus, TNFα results in excessive production of keratinocytes that survive longer and consequently thicken the epidermis. The accumulated data suggest that TNFα contributes to many of the clinical and histological phenotypes characteristic of psoriasis and related diseases.

IV. THE ROLE OF TNFα IN PSORIATIC ARTHRITIS

Arthritis occurs in 5–7% of people with psoriasis, but it may affect up to 40% of hospitalized patients with extensive skin involvement (20). The skin condition generally precedes the onset of arthritis symptoms, but in approximately 10% of patients arthritic symptoms occur first. TNFα figures prominently in the development of psoriatic arthritis, and preliminary findings strongly suggest that the same immune-mediated mechanism is involved in the pathogenesis of psoriasis.

As in psoriasis, elevated concentrations of cytokines secreted by activated monocytes/macrophages (TNFα, IL-1, IL-6, and IL-8) are seen in psoriatic arthritis. Additionally, cytokines associated with Th1 cells (IL-2, IFNγ, and lymphotoxin α) are also found in the synovial fluids and membranes of patients with psoriatic arthritis (21–23). These findings suggest that the pathology of psoriatic arthritis may involve interactions between monocytes/macrophages and Th1 cells (23). Along with being involved in the overall inflammatory process, TNFα also is directly associated with bone and cartilage destruction, which is a feature of psoriatic arthritis.

V. ROLE OF TNFα IN OTHER IMMUNE-MEDIATED INFLAMMATORY DISORDERS

The accumulated data point to a key role for TNFα in the pathogenesis of not only psoriasis and psoriatic arthritis but also rheumatoid arthritis (RA), Crohn's disease (CD), and other IMIDs.

Patients with RA have increased levels of TNFα and IL-1 in the synovial fluid, which are known to contribute substantially to the clinical spectrum of RA. Within the immunological microenvironment of the synovium, these cytokines exert a proinflammatory effect by recruiting leukocytes and causing inflammation (24). In turn, recruited leukocytes release other proinflammatory mediators, including IL-6, IL-11, IL-15, IL-17, and a host of proteolytic enzymes (25). These molecules activate osteoclasts, which cause bone and cartilage destruction that is characteristic of RA. TNFα and IL-1 also mediate cartilage destruction by stimulating the secretion of collagenases by articular chondrocytes, and activating synovial fibroblasts, which subsequently secrete additional enzymes including matrix metalloproteinases (25).

In CD, TNFα is known to play a central role in the pathological inflammatory process. In these patients, macrophages and Th-1 cells secrete excessive quantities of TNFα, IL-1, IL-6, IL-8, IL-12, and IFNα in the affected intestinal mucosae (26). Mucosal tissue biopsies from patients with CD are characterized by an increased expression of TNFα, both at transcriptional and translational levels (25). The excessive expression of proinflammatory cytokines is reflected in the secretion of further proinflammatory mediators, destructive enzymes, and free radicals, which produce the tissue injury, increased mucosal permeability, diarrhea, and fibrosis characteristic of CD (27). Patients with CD have a higher incidence of psoriasis than the general population, and patients with psoriasis are approximately seven times more likely to develop CD than the general population (28). In a genome scan for psoriasis susceptibility loci, Nair et al. identified a region on chromosome 16 conferring susceptibility to psoriasis that appeared to overlap with a region previously identified as associated with susceptibility to CD (28).

TNFα-targeting therapies have been shown to be effective in treating ankylosing spondylitis, suggesting that this disorder is at least partially mediated by TNFα (29–31). Case reports and case series describing patients with other IMIDs, including uveitis, Sjögren's syndrome, giant cell arteritis, graft vs. host disease, sarcoidosis, hidradenitis suppuritiva, and pyoderma gangrenosum who have been successfully treated with anti-TNFα therapy further support the IMID approach to therapy. Thus, rather than considering these disorders as separate entities in nonoverlapping therapeutic areas, the common pathogenesis suggests that they should be grouped together as IMIDs (32–49).

VI. ANTI-TNFα THERAPY

Given the central role that TNFα is believed to play in the pathophysiology of psoriatic disease, it is reasonable to expect that inhibition of this cytokine would alter the course of the disease, and that the TNFα pathway presents a key target for pharmacological intervention in psoriasis.

TNFα has a unique chemical structure and activity profile. TNFα exists as either an inactive monomer or as an active complex of three monomers, called a trimer. In blood plasma, soluble TNFα exists in both monomeric and trimeric form. In contrast, transmembranous TNFα only exists in the trimeric form (50).

The availability recombinant DNA technology led to the development of highly specific biopharmaceuticals that were less likely to elicit undesirable responses than nonspecific immunosuppressants such as methotrexate or cyclosporine. To date, two anti-TNFα biopharmaceuticals have been developed using such recombinant DNA technology: etanercept (Enbrel) and infliximab (Remicade). Although both are anti-TNFα agents, their structures (Fig. 2), binding specificities, and mechanisms of action are distinctly different. An important difference is that infliximab inactivates all types of TNFα, whether monomeric or trimeric and whether soluble in plasma or in transmembranous form, while etanercept binds only soluble TNF (50–56).

Infliximab is a chimeric monoclonal antibody specific for TNFα, comprising the human antibody constant regions and murine antibody variable regions (57). It has a molecular weight of 149,100 daltons and a binding specificity for human TNFα. Currently, infliximab is approved for the treatment of RA, CD, and fistulizing CD. The remainder of this chapter

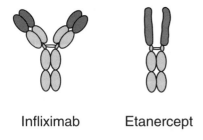

Infliximab   Etanercept

Figure 2   Structures of etanercept and infliximab.

summarizes current clinical data on the use of infliximab in these approved indications, as well as in patients with psoriatic diseases.

VII. INFLIXIMAB

A. Mechanism of Action

Infliximab interferes with the actions of TNFα by directly binding to soluble and transmembrane TNFα molecules both in plasma and diseased tissue. Because of its unique structure, each infliximab molecule can bind to two TNFα molecules, with one on each arm, as shown in Figure 3A. As shown in Figure 3B, as many as three infliximab molecules can bind to a single trimer of TNFα, thereby blocking all of its receptor-binding sites. Furthermore, these bonds appear to be stable, with no dissociation observed under experimental conditions (58). Once fully blocked by infliximab, TNFα will not be available to bind to its receptor (50, 57–59) and propagate postreceptor signal transduction and the subsequent dysregulation of the immune response collectively underlying IMIDs.

In addition to neutralizing TNFα directly, it has been suggested that infliximab may prevent or reduce formation of the biologically active trimer by binding to monomeric TNFα (50). Infliximab has a human IgG1 isotype and, therefore, once bound it would be expected to neutralize the effects of soluble TNFα and cause antibody-dependent killing or complement-mediated killing of cells expressing transmembrane TNFα.

Infliximab has been shown to bind to transmembrane TNFα and trigger apoptosis through a noncomplement pathway in CD3/CD28-acti-

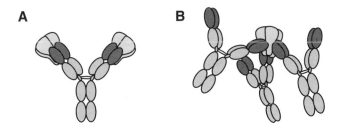

Infliximab/TNF complex

Figure 3   Interaction of infliximab with TNFα. A. A single infliximab molecule can bind to two TNFα molecules. B. Three infliximab molecules can bind to trimeric TNFα, blocking all active sites.

vated peripheral blood lymphocytes (60). By binding to transmembrane TNFα, infliximab reduces adhesion and neutralizes signaling to the proinflammatory cytokines that lead to cell proliferation and increased production of inflammatory mediators. In addition, infliximab may lyse TNF-producing cells and may lead to the apoptosis of T lymphocytes (50, 58, 61). It has also been suggested that when infliximab binds to transmembranous TNFα, it could switch off activated T cells (33). Thus, infliximab not only inhibits TNFα but also blocks activated T cells.

B. Clinical Indications

The potential benefits associated with using infliximab to block TNFα pathways have led to its evaluation in the treatment of a variety of disorders. The results of clinical trials with infliximab in RA and CD demonstrated considerable suppression of disease activity and led to Food and Drug Administration (FDA) approval of infliximab for the treatment of these chronic conditions (62–64).

1. Rheumatoid Arthritis

Infliximab is administered in combination with methotrexate for both acute (induction) and maintenance therapy for moderately to highly active RA to reduce the signs and symptoms of disease, inhibit the progression of structural damage, and improve physical function in patients who have had an inadequate response to methotrexate alone.

In the RA clinical trial entitled the Anti-TNF Trial in Rheumatoid Arthritis with Concomitant Therapy and known by its acronym as the ATTRACT Study, 428 patients with active RA, who had an inadequate response to treatment with methotrexate dosages of 12.5 mg/week or higher, were randomly assigned to receive their entry dosage of methotrexate in combination with placebo or 3 or 10 mg/kg infliximab. There were five treatment groups in this study: a placebo group and four infliximab groups. Two infliximab groups (3 and 10 mg/kg) received an induction regimen consisting of infusions at weeks 0, 2, and 6 with subsequent infusions administered every 4 weeks. The placebo group likewise received infusions of placebo at weeks 0, 2, and 6 with subsequent infusions every 4 weeks. The other two infliximab groups (3 and 10 mg/kg) received the induction regimen at weeks 0, 2, and 6 with subsequent infusions administered every 8 weeks; however, placebo infusions were administered during interim 4 week visits to maintain the blind. After both 30 and 54 weeks of therapy, infliximab therapy significantly improved disease outcomes compared with methotrexate alone, as indicated by clinical markers, radiographic progression, physician assessments, and quality of life assessments (62, 63).

2. Crohn's Disease

Infliximab is the only anti-TNFα therapy approved for the treatment of patients with CD to reduce the signs and symptoms (i.e., induce remission). It is indicated as monotherapy for patients who have moderately to highly active disease, and who have had an inadequate response to conventional treatment (64). Infliximab also has been shown to maintain remission when administered every 8 weeks (65). In cases of fistulizing CD, infliximab reduced the number of enterocutaneous fistulas in patients who were unresponsive to conventional therapy (66).

The CD clinical trial was entitled A Crohn's Disease Clinical Trial Evaluating Infliximab in a New Long-Term Treatment Regimen and is known by its acronym as the ACCENT I Study. In this trial, 545 patients with moderate to severe CD (defined by a baseline Crohn's disease activity index [CDAI] score ≥220) received a 5 mg/kg intravenous infusion of infliximab at week zero. Individuals responding to treatment by week 2 were randomly assigned to receive repeat infusions of placebo or induction therapy with 5 mg/kg of infliximab at weeks 2 and 6, followed by maintenance therapy every 8 weeks (at weeks 14, 22, 30, 38, and 46) or induction therapy with 5 mg/kg of infliximab at weeks 2 and 6 followed by maintenance therapy with 10 mg/kg of infliximab every 8 weeks through week 46. Study results showed that 311 of 545 of patients (57%) responded to a single infliximab infusion after 2 weeks of treatment. Among responders, significantly more patients receiving a maintenance regimen of 5 mg/kg infliximab every 8 weeks achieved and maintained clinical remission (39% vs. 25% for placebo) (65).

Noncomparative studies with infliximab in pediatric patients with refractory CD have indeed shown significant clinical efficacy (67, 68). Anecdotal evidence suggests that clinical response in children may be greater than that of adults because of their higher metabolism (69). A formal clinical trial in pediatric patients with CD is underway.

3. Future Indications

In addition to the currently approved indications of RA and CD, infliximab is in clinical development for the treatment of psoriasis (33), and has been investigated for efficacy in the treatment of psoriatic arthritis (32), juvenile arthritis (70), ankylosing spondylitis, (29–31), and ulcerative colitis (71–73).

C. Clinical Trial of Infliximab in Psoriatic Disease

During a CD clinical trial, when a patient with both CD and psoriasis was treated with 5 mg/kg of infliximab, the investigators noted that both disorders remitted and relapsed at the same time (74). In addition, infliximab was been shown to be effective in the treatment of psoriasis in an open-label trial (36). These findings led to the design of a study to evaluate the safety and efficacy of infliximab in the treatment of psoriasis.

Results of a 10-week, placebo-controlled, double-blinded clinical evaluation of infliximab 33 patients with plaque-type psoriasis (33) demonstrated that significant relief of signs and symptoms could be achieved with infliximab treatment. Long-term, open-label follow-up data obtained from the 10-week study indicate that infliximab, particularly the higher dosage of 10 mg/kg, may provide sustained, high-level relief with intermittent administration of infliximab (75).

1. Placebo-Controlled, Double-Blind Phase

In the placebo-controlled, double-blind phase of the study (33), patients were evaluated who had at least a 6 month history of plaque-type psoriasis that had been insensitive to treatment with topical corticosteroids, and whose psoriasis covered at least 5% of the body. Patients were randomly assigned to receive intravenous placebo (n = 11), 5 mg/kg infliximab (n = 11), or 10 mg/kg infliximab (n = 11), infused over 2 h and repeated after 2 and 6 weeks. Efficacy and other clinical and laboratory measures were recorded at screening, baseline, and every 2 weeks thereafter until 10 weeks after initiating treatment. Patients were not permitted to take other prescription medications during the study.

2. Efficacy Evaluations

The Psoriasis Area Severity Index (PASI) score (76) was determined at baseline and at week 10, for which time point a favorable response to treatment was defined as an improvement of at least 75%. At the end of a 10 week treatment period, 82% of patients in the 5 mg/kg infliximab group and 73% of patients in the 10 mg/kg infliximab group demonstrated a 75% or greater improvement in PASI scores, compared with 18% of patients in the placebo group. PASI scores determined over the course of the study showed a rapid response to infliximab therapy, with a significant benefit evident by week 2 and a median time to response of 4 weeks (Fig. 4).

The physician's global assessment (PGA) also was performed at baseline and week 10 to determine the response to treatment or extent of improvement in psoriatic plaques relative to baseline. A response to treatment

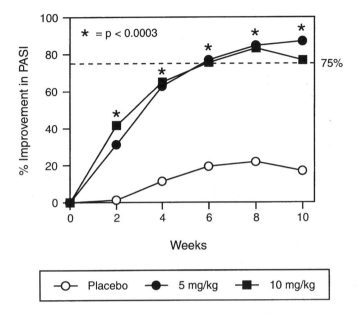

Figure 4 75% PASI score improvements from baseline.

was defined as a PGA rating of good (50–74% clearing with moderate improvement), excellent (75–99% clearing with striking improvement), or clear (100% clearing). A nonresponse to treatment was a PGA rating of fair (25–49% clearing with slight improvement), poor (0–24% clearing with little or no change), or worse.

At week 10, 82% of patients who received 5 mg/kg infliximab and 91% of those who received 10 mg/kg infliximab had responded to treatment, compared with 18% of patients who received placebo (Fig. 5). Many patients experienced an excellent response to treatment, with some showing resolution and clearing of their cutaneous manifestations (Fig. 6).

Biopsy results supported clinical findings (77). Patients who received 5 or 10 mg/kg infliximab or placebo at weeks 0, 2, and 6 showed rapid and dramatic decreases in epidermal inflammation and normalization of keratinocyte differentiation in psoriatic plaques, as shown by immunohistochemical analysis of lesional biopsies at weeks 0, 2, 10, and nonlesional biopsies at week 0. A notable finding was that these cellular changes preceded maximal clinical response. Indeed, the magnitude and rapid onset of response to infliximab therapy in these initial studies have been substantial, similar to those achieved with cyclosporine; however in contrast with cyclosporine, improvements in PASI have been maintained. Unlike cyclosporine therapy,

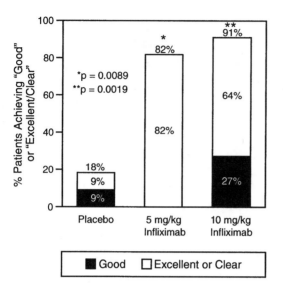

Figure 5 PGA score improvements from baseline after 10 weeks of infliximab treatment (p values for comparison of each treatment arm vs. placebo).

there is no targeted organ toxicity observed with infliximab therapy. Infliximab monotherapy has been shown to normalize keratinocyte proliferation and differentiation and markedly decrease epidermal inflammation, whereas cyclosporine does not consistently alter these cellular processes despite apparent clinical remission. These results further demonstrate the role of TNF-α in the pathogenesis of psoriasis and argue for the clinical development of infliximab for the treatment of psoriasis.

3. Open-Label Follow-Up Phase

At the end of the double-blind phase of the study, nonresponder patients in the placebo group were randomly assigned to receive 5 mg/kg infliximab (n = 5), or 10 mg/kg of infliximab (n = 4) at weeks 10, 12, and 16. After 26 weeks from the date of the first infusion, PASI assessments were performed again for all patients in the original infliximab treatment arms, as well as those who received infliximab from week 10 to 16. Through week 26, a total of 16 patients received 5 mg/kg infliximab, and 15 patients received 10 mg/kg infliximab. At week 26, among the 16 patients who received 5 mg/kg infliximab, 40% maintained at least 50% improvement, and 33% maintained at least 75% improvement in PASI scores relative to baseline. Among the 15 patients who received 10 mg/kg infliximab, 73% maintained at least 50%

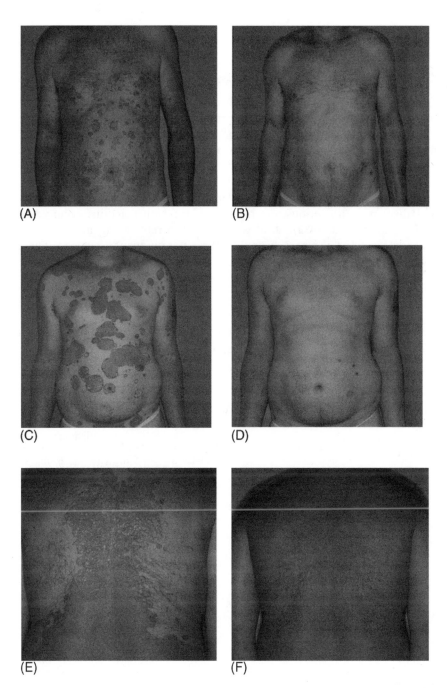

Figure 6 Photographic record of infliximab therapy.

improvement and 67% maintained at least 75% improvement in PASI scores at week 26 relative to baseline.

4. Infliximab Safety Profile in Psoriasis

In the double-blind portion of the study (i.e., through week 10), patients in the infliximab group exhibited a safety profile similar to that observed in the placebo group. Accordingly, headache was the only adverse event recorded more frequently in the 10 mg/kg infliximab group than in the placebo group (Table 1).

In the open-label follow-up phase of the trial (unpublished data), the majority of adverse events were considered mild in nature by the investigator, and there were no serious adverse events. Infusion reactions occurred in 3 of the 33 patients (9%), all of whom received retreatment infusions. No infusion reactions occurred during the three-dose induction regimen. These reactions were generally mild and transient in nature and were preventable with the prophylactic measures.

5. Conclusions

In the double-blind, placebo-controlled portion of this study, patients with psoriasis experienced a high degree of clinical benefit from infliximab therapy,

Table 1 Adverse Events Reported by Two or More Patients

| | | Infliximab | |
Adverse event	Placebo (n = 11)	5 mg/kg (n = 11)	10 mg/kg (n = 11)
Headache	2	1	7
Upper respiratory tract infection	4	2	3
Abdominal bloating/pain (nonspecific)	1	2	1
Infection	2	1	1
Increased AST	1	0	2
Sore throat	0	1	2
Dysesthesia	1	1	0
Fever	0	0	2
Myalgia	0	1	1
Positive antinuclear antibody titer	0	2	0
Pruritus	2	0	0
Rhinitis	1	1	0

Source: Ref. 33.

with 82% and 73% of patients in the 5 and 10 mg/kg infliximab dosage groups, respectively, achieving at least a 75% reduction in PASI scores at week 10. Furthermore, the response time was rapid, as demonstrated by a clinically meaningful benefit by week 2 (33). Results of the open-label extension of this study demonstrate that the clinical response achieved with three dosages of infliximab at weeks 0, 2 and 6 was sustained through 26 weeks. Overall, 57% of infliximab-treated patients maintained at least 50% improvement in their PASI scores from baseline and 48% maintained at least 75% improvement in their PASI scores through week 26. Those who received 10 mg/kg infliximab were more likely to maintain their response following the induction period.

Selection of the appropriate dosage regimen of infliximab involves consideration of efficacy in achieving and maintaining clearance as well as safety, particularly with chronic or repeated administration. An appropriate regimen to consider may be an induction regimen followed by infrequent maintenance infusions, which offer the advantage of continual suppression of psoriasis and may be preferable to episodic treatment based of recurrence. Multicenter trials are underway to evaluate further various dosage regimens, and dosage selection must be based on efficacy, patient safety, total drug exposure, and quality-of-life issues.

D. Clinical Evaluation of Infliximab in Psoriatic Arthritis

As mentioned earlier, a subset of patients with psoriasis will develop psoriatic arthritis, possibly as a result of common pathology. A preliminary, open-label study of infliximab in the treatment of six patients with severe psoriatic arthritis who had an inadequate response to methotrexate therapy (administered at a dosage of 15–25 mg/week) showed substantial clinical and radiological benefit from 5 mg/kg infliximab administered at weeks 0, 2, and 6. All six patients showed rapid and sustained response as determined by a 50% improvement in the American College of Rheumatology (ACR) Criteria (78)* at week 10, with five of the six patients achieving a 70% ACR

---

*A specified percentage of ACR response (e.g., 20%, 50%, or 70%) is defined as the corresponding percentage improvement in the number of tender and swollen joints among 28 or more joints evaluated in addition to the same specified percent improvement in 3 or more of the following: patient's assessment of pain; physician's global assessment of disease status and patient's global assessment of disease status (assessed by visual analog scale); patient's assessment of disability (assessed by a validated instrument such as the Health Assessment Questionnaire); and acute-phase reactants such as erythrocyte sedimentation rate and C-reactive protein levels.

response. In addition, improvements in specific measures of clinical response were as follows: 88% in swollen joint count, 85% in tender joint count, 85% in PGA; 71% in PASI scores; 78% in Health Assessment Questionnaire scores; 91% in c-reactive protein (CRP) levels; and 77% in erythrocyte sedimentation rate (ESR) (32).

Similar results were attained in a retrospective analysis or 29 patients with both active psoriasis and psoriatic arthritis. Stevens et al. reported that all patients treated with infliximab for psoriasis experienced significant improvement in their psoriatic arthritis, with the mean numbers of swollen and tender joints decreasing from 14.6 to 3.1 and from 15.5 to 2.5, respectively (79). Based on these and other open-label studies with similar findings (39, 80, 81), a clinical trial program is underway to evaluate formally the use of infliximab in the treatment of psoriatic arthritis. The results of a multicenter, double-blind, placebo-controlled trial in approximately 100 patients with psoriatic arthritis support open-label efficacy and safety of infliximab in this indication. The results of this study will be published shortly.

E. Infliximab Safety Profile

The safety of infliximab has been established both in the clinical trial setting and through an extensive postmarketing safety database (more than 280,000 patients). It is noteworthy that many patients receiving infliximab have long histories of receiving one or more immunosuppressive therapies.

1. Adverse Events

During the long-term, prospective, safety follow-up evaluation of patients treated with infliximab in clinical trials (82), fewer than 2% of 771 infliximab-treated patients had infusion reactions that required discontinuation of therapy. While the incidence of mild infections, primarily upper respiratory infections, was increased in this patient population relative to placebo controls, there was no increase in the incidence of serious infections among infliximab-treated patients. Although low titers of autoantibodies can occur with infliximab treatment (in less than 10% of patients in this population), drug-induced lupus occurred infrequently and was reversible with discontinuation of therapy. Table 2 shows the most common adverse events observed among patients in these RA and CD clinical trials.

Infliximab has continued to demonstrate a favorable safety profile in more recent clinical trials. In the ACCENT I trial (65), maintenance therapy with infliximab was well tolerated in 573 patients with CD, among whom 188 received a single infusion and 385 received maintenance therapy with

Table 2 Incidence of Adverse Events (%) Observed in Clinical Trials of Infliximab in Rheumatoid Arthritis and Crohn's Disease

	Rheumatoid Arthritis		Crohn's Disease	
	Placebo (n = 133)	Infliximab (n = 555)	Placebo (n = 56)	Infliximab (n = 199)
Average weeks of follow-up	52	68	15	27
Respiratory				
Upper respiratory tract infections	23	33	9	16
Coughing	7	16	0	5
Sinusitis	6	16	2	5
Pharyngitis	9	14	5	9
Rhinitis	8	11	4	6
Bronchitis	9	11	2	7
Dyspnea	3	6	0	3
Gastrointestinal				
Nausea	20	21	4	17
Diarrhea	14	16	2	3
Abdominal pain	9	15	4	12
Vomiting	11	11	0	9
Dyspepsia	6	9	0	5
Ulcerative stomatitis	2	7	4	2
Other				
Headache	16	26	21	23
Rash	6	15	5	6
Urinary tract infection	8	13	4	3
Dizziness	11	12	9	8
Pain	12	12	5	9
Arthralgia	5	11	2	5
Fever	8	11	7	10
Back pain	4	10	4	5
Fatigue	5	10	5	11
Hypertension	5	8	2	1
Pruritus	2	8	2	5
Worsening of RA	7	8	N/A	N/A
Peripheral edema	6	7	2	1
Chest pain	5	6	5	6
Depression	3	6	0	2
Moniliasis	2	6	0	5
Urticaria	1	6	0	3

5 mg/kg or 10 mg/kg infliximab through week 46. Although more patients who received maintenance therapy discontinued treatment because of adverse events than those who received the single-dose regimen of infliximab, the incidences of serious adverse events and infections were similar between patients who received only a single infliximab infusion and those who received multiple infliximab infusions. Two patients died of sepsis; however, both cases of sepsis were ruled probably not related to infliximab. The risk–benefit ratio for patients at high risk for infection should be considered prior to initiating infliximab therapy. In particular, the development of a case of tuberculosis in this trial is a cause for concern. Despite the absence of controlled data, it appears there may be an association between infliximab treatment and reactivation of latent or dormant tuberculosis (83). This potential is consistent with the putative biological activity of TNF in controlling intracellular pathogens.

As in patients with CD, the combination of infliximab and methotrexate was well tolerated by the 342 patients with RA who received 3 mg/kg or 10 mg/kg infliximab every 4 or 8 weeks in the ATTRACT trial. In this trial, 86 patients receiving methotrexate alone served as the control group (62). There was no increase in the incidence of serious infections, and the overall frequency of cancers was similar to that predicted from the Surveillance, Epidemiology, and End Results database (84).

2. Contraindications and General Precautions for Infliximab

Because infliximab is administered by infusion, patients should be monitored closely for infusion-related reactions for 2 h after treatment. Emergency treatments should be available in the event of acute infusion reactions. Patients who have received previous infusions of infliximab should be monitored for delayed hypersensitivity reactions. These events have been observed infrequently in clinical studies and postmarketing surveillance with retreatment intervals up to 1 year.

Treatment should be discontinued if lupuslike symptoms occur. In clinical studies, three patients with RA and three with CD had diagnoses of a possible lupuslike syndrome. All six patients improved following discontinuation of therapy and appropriate medical treatment. No cases of lupuslike reactions have been observed in up to 3 years of follow-up.

Because anti-TNFα therapy or any immunomodulatory therapy alters the immune response, it may affect susceptibility to infection or allow reemergence of infection. Consequently, such therapies are associated with an increased risk of infection that can be serious or even fatal.

Tuberculosis, invasive fungal infections, and other opportunistic infections have been observed in patients receiving infliximab. Patients should be evaluated for the presence of a latent tuberculosis infection with a tuberculin skin test and should be treated for latent tuberculosis infection prior to therapy with infliximab.

During postmarketing surveillance, rare instances of tuberculosis have been reported, as has the occurrence of demyelinating disorders (such as multiple sclerosis). However, because these events are reported voluntarily from a population of uncertain size, and many of them are receiving concomitant immunosuppressive therapy, it is not always possible to estimate reliably their frequency or to establish a causal relationship to infliximab therapy. Of note, the majority of tuberculosis cases have been reported in Europe where the tuberculosis vaccine is not routinely administered.

The manufacturer of infliximab implemented a tuberculosis awareness education program in 2001, which highlighted the need for tuberculin testing and appropriate treatment of latent tuberculosis. As a result of the program, the number of reported cases of tuberculosis declined, despite an increase in the use of infliximab (85).

Patients should be monitored for infections during and after treatment, and treatment should be discontinued if serious infection occurs. Patients with mild congestive heart failure (CHF, New York Heart Association [NYHA] Class I/II) should be carefully monitored, and infliximab therapy should be withdrawn in patients whose CHF worsens or who experience new symptoms. Patients with pre-existing or recent-onset central nervous system demyelinating or seizure disorders should be carefully monitored. Caution should be taken when treating the elderly and patients with renal or hepatic insufficiency.

Because of the paucity of data in pregnant women, use in pregnancy should be reserved for patients in whom there is a strong clinical need for treatment with infliximab. Breastfeeding while women are being treated with infliximab is not recommended.

3. Safety Conclusions

Safety is a major consideration when considering a treatment for psoriasis. Evaluation of infliximab in a limited number of patients with psoriasis in a placebo-controlled trial indicated that infusion reactions were generally mild and transient and that there were no serious infections or obvious increase in infections in infliximab-treated patients compared to placebo patients. It will be important to characterize the adverse event profile of infliximab in a large number of patients with psoriasis. It is advantageous that infliximab has been administered to over 280,000 patients worldwide, which is substantially more than most biologicals currently being evaluated for psoriasis.

VIII. SUMMARY

Psoriasis and psoriatic arthritis are chronic disorders of the skin and joints that share a common pathogenesis with other IMIDs such as RA and CD. Significant progress has already been made in the development of safe and effective biological therapy for long-term use in patients with RA and CD. Now these biologicals are proving to be safe and effective in psoriatic diseases. Perhaps one of the most promising approaches is anti-TNFα therapy.

One anti-TNF agent, infliximab, provides rapid, significant, and lasting relief of the signs and symptoms of psoriasis and psoriatic arthritis. Given the unique structure and mechanism of action of infliximab, it appears to have a high degree of efficacy and specificity and may be able rapidly to control both psoriasis and psoriatic arthritis.

REFERENCES

1. Mease PJ. Tumour necrosis factor (TNF) in psoriatic arthritis: pathophysiology and treatment with TNF inhibitors. Ann Rheum Dis 2002;61:298–304.
2. Gottlieb AB. Psoriasis: immunopathology and immunomodulation. Dermatol Clin 2002;19:649–657.
3. Baker BS, Fry L. The immunology of psoriasis. Br J Dermatol 1992;126:1–9.
4. Bos JD, DeRie MA. The pathogenesis of psoriasis: immunological facts and speculations. Immunol Today 1999;1:40–45.
5. Gottlieb AB. Immunopathogenesis of psoriasis. Arch Dermatol 1997;133:781–782.
6. Ortonne JP. Aetiology and pathogenesis of psoriasis. Br J Dermatol 1996; 135(Suppl 49):1–5.
7. Trepicchio W, Ozawa M, Walters IB. IL-11 is an immune-modulatory cytokine which downregulates IL-12, Type 1 cytokines, and multiple inflammation-associated genes in patients with psoriasis. J Invest Dermatol 1999;112:598.
8. Austin L, Ozawa M, Kikuchi T, Krueger G. Intracellular TNF-alpha, IFN-gamma, and IL-2 identify TC1 and TH1 effector populations in psoriasis vulgaris plaque lymphocytes: single-cell analysis by flow cytometry. J Invest Dermatol 1998;110:649.
9. Grossman RM, Krueger J, Yourish D. Interleukin-6 (IL-6) is expressed in high levels in psoriatic skin and stimulates proliferation of cultured human keratinocytes. Proc Natl Acad Sci USA 1989;86:6367–6371.
10. Sticherling M, Bornscheuer E, Schroder JM, Christophers E. Localization of neutrophil-activating peptide-1/interleukin-8-immunoreactivity in normal and psoriatic skin. J Invest Dermatol 1991;96:26–30.
11. Livden JK, Nilsen R, Bjerke JR, Matre R. In situ localization of interferons in psoriatic lesions. Arch Dermatol Res 1989;281:392–397.

12. Ettehadi P, Greaves MW, Wallach D, Aderka D, Camp RD. Elevated tumour necrosis factor-alpha (TNF-alpha)biological activity in psoriatic skin lesions. Clin Exp Immunol 1994; 96:146–151.

13. Schwarzenberger K, Udey MC. Contact allergens and epidermal proinflammatory cytokines modulate Langerhans cell E-cadherin expression in situ. J Invest Dermatol 1996;106:533–558.

14. Norris DA. Cytokine modulation of adhesion molecules in the regulation of immunologic cytotoxicity of epidermal targets. J Invest Dermatol 1990;95: 111S–120S.

15. Griffiths CEM, Voorhees JJ, Nickoloff BJ. Characterization of intercellular adhesion molecule-1 and HLA-DR expression in normal and inflamed skin: modulation by recombinant gamma interferon and tumor necrosis factor. J Am Acad Dermatol 1989;20:617–629.

16. Sato N, Nariuchi H, Tsuruoka N. Actions of TNF and IFN-gamma on angiogenesis in vitro. J Invest Dermatol 1990;95:85S–89S.

17. Nickoloff BJ. The cytokine network in psoriasis. Arch Dermatol 1991;127:871–884.

18. Kakurai M, Fujita N, Murata S, Furukawa Y, Demitsu T, Nakagawa H. Vasoactive intestinal peptide regulated its receptor expression and functions of human keratinocytes via type I vasoactive intestinal peptide receptors. J Invest Dermatol 2001;116:743–749.

19. Wang Y, Jensen PJ. Regulation of the level and glycosylation state of plasminogen activator inhibitor type 2 during human keratinocyte differentiation. Differentiation 1998;63:93–99.

20. Cuellar ML, Silveria LH, Espinoza LR. Recent developments in psoriatic arthritis. Curr Opin Rheumatol 1994;6:378–384.

21. Danning CL, Illei GG, Hitchon C, Greer MR, Boumpus DT, McInnes IB. Macrophage-derived cytokine and nuclear factor *B* p56 expression in synovial membrane and skin of patients with psoriatic arthritis. Arthritis Rheum 2000; 43:1244–1256.

22. Partsch G, Wagner E, Leeb BF, Broll H, Dunky A, Smolen JS. T cell derived cytokines in psoriatic arthritis synovial fluids. Ann Rheum Dis 1998;57:691–693.

23. Ritchlin C, Haas-Smith SA, Hicks D, Cappuccio J, Osterland CK, Looney RJ. Patterns of cytokine production in psoriatic synovium. J Rheumatol 1998; 25:1544–1552.

24. Feldmann M, Maini RN. Anti-TNF alpha therapy of rheumatoid arthritis: what have we learned? Annu Rev Immunol 2001;19:163–196.

25. Song XR TTGD. Coming of age: anti-cytokine therapies. Mol Interv 2002; 2:36–46.

26. Papadakis KA, Targan SR. Role of cytokines in the pathogenesis of inflammatory bowel disease. Ann Rev Immunol 2000;51:289–298.

27. Fiocchi C. Inflammatory bowel disease: etiology and pathogenesis. Gastroenterology 1998;115:182–205.

28. Nair RP, Henseler T, Jenisch S, Stuart P, Bichakjian CK, Lenk W, Westphal E, Guo SW, Christophers E, Voorhees JJ, Elder JT. Evidence for two psoriasis

susceptibility loci (HLA and 17q) and two novel candidate regions (16q and 20p) by genome-wide scan. Hum Mol Genet 1997;6:1349–1356.

29. Gorman JD, Sack KE, Davis JC. Treatment of ankylosing spondylitis by inhibition of tumor necrosis factor alpha. N Engl J Med 2002;(346):1349–1356.

30. Braun W, Brandt J, Listing J, Zink A, Alten R, Golder W, et al. Treatment of active ankylosing spondylitis with infliximab: a randomised controlled multi-centre trial. Lancet 2002;359:1187–1193.

31. Brandt J, Haibel H, Cornely D, Golder W, Gonzalez J, Reddig J, Thriene W, Sieper J, Braun J. Successful treatment of active ankylosing spondylitis with the anti-tumor necrosis factor alpha monoclonal antibody infliximab. Arthritis Rheum 2000;43:1346–1352.

32. Antoni C, Deschant C, Lorenz HM, Wendler J, Olgilvie A. Successful treatment of psoriatic arthritis with infliximab in a MRI-controlled study. Ann Rheum Dis 2000;59(Suppl 1)200.

33. Chaudhari U, Romano P, Mulcahy LD, Dooley LT, Baker DG, Gottlieb AB. Efficacy and safety of infliximab monotherapy for plaque-type psoriasis: a randomized trial. Lancet 2001;357:1942–1947.

34. Elewski BE. Infliximab for the treatment of severe pustular psoriasis: a case report. American Academy of Dermatology, Annual Meeting, 2002.

35. Menter A JSCJ. Successful treatment of pediatric psoriasis with infliximab. American Academy of Dermatology, 60th Annual meeting, 2002:P545.

36. Schopf RE, Aust H, Knop J. Treatment of psoriasis with the chimeric mono-clonal antibody against tumor necrosis factor alpha, infliximab. J Am Acad Dermatol 2002;46:886–891.

37. Tan MH. Improvement of pyoderma gangrenosum and psoriasis associated with Crohn disease with anti-tumor necrosis factor alpha monoclonal antibody. Arch Dermatol 2001;137:930–933.

38. O'Quinn RP, Miller JL. The effectiveness of tumor necrosis factor alpha anti-body (infliximab) in treating recalcitrant psoriasis. Arch Dermatol 2002;138:644–648.

39. Mang R, Stege H, Ruzicka T, Krutmann J. Response of severe psoriasis to infliximab. Dermatology 2002;204:156–157.

40. Braughman RPI, Lower EE: Inflximab for refractory sarcoidosis. Sarcoidosis Vasc Diffuse Lung Dis 2001;18:70–74.

41. Botros N, Pickover L, Das KM. Image of the month. Pyoderma gangrenosum caused by ulcerative colitis. Gastroenterology 2000;118:654.

42. Campbell S, Ghosh S. Infliximab therapy for Crohn's disease in the presence of chronic hepatitis C infection. Eur J Gastroenterol Hepatol 2001;Feb 13:191–192.

43. Couriel DR, Hicks K, Giralt S, Champlin RE. Role of tumor necrosis factor-alpha inhibition with infliximab in cancer therapy and hematopoietic stem cell transplantation. Curr Opin Oncol 2000;12:582–587.

44. Declercq E. Perspectives for the chemotherapy of AIDS. Anticancer Res 1987;7:1023–1038.

45. Fabrizio C, Niccoli L, Salvarani C, Padula A, Olivieri. Treatment of long-standing active giant cell arteritis with infliximab: report of four cases. Arthritis Rheum 2001;44:2933–2935.

46. Martinez F, Nos P, Benlloch S, Ponce J. Hidradenitis suppurativa and Crohn's disease: response to treatment with infliximab. Inflamm Bowel Dis 2001;7:323–326.

47. Schothorst AA, Evers LM, Noz KC, Filon R, van Zeeland AA. Pyrimidine dimer induction and repair in cultured human skin keratinocytes or melanocytes after irradiation with monochromatic ultraviolet radiation. J Invest Dermatol 1991;96:916–920.

48. Smith JR, Levinson RD, Holland GN, Jabs DA, Robinson MR, Whitcup SM, Rosenbaum JT. Differential efficacy of tumor necrosis factor in the management of inflammatory eye disease and associated rheumatic disease. Arthritis Rheum 2001;45:252–257.

49. Steinfeld SD, Demols P, Salmon I, Kiss R, Appelboom T. Infliximab in patients with primary Sjogren's syndrome: a pilot study. Arthritis Rheum 2001; 44:2371–2375.

50. Scallon B, Cai A, Solowski N, Rosenberg A, Song XY, Shealy D, Wagner C. Binding and functional comparisons of two types of tumor necrosis factor antagonists. J Pharmacol Exp Ther 2002;301:418–426.

51. Sandborn WJ, Hanauer SB. Antitumor necrosis factor therapy for inflammatory bowel disease: a review of agents, pharmacology, clinical results, and safety. Inflamm Bowel Dis 1999;5(2):119–133.

52. Agnholt J, Kaltoft K. Infliximab downegulates interferon-γ production in activated gut T-lymphocytes from patients with Crohn's disease. Cytokine 2001;15:212–222.

53. Mohler KM, Torrance DS, Smith CA, Goodwin RG, Stremler KE, Fung VP, Madani H, Widmer MB. Soluble tumor necrosis factor (TNF) receptors are effective therapeutic agents in lethal endotoxemia and function simultaneously as both TNF carriers and TNF antagonists. J Immunol 1993;151:1548–1561.

54. Bathon JM, Martin RW, Fleischmann RM, Tesser JR, Schiff MH, Keystone EC, Genovese MC, Wasko MC, Moreland LW, Weaver AL, Markenson J, Finck BK. A comparison of etanercept and methotrexate in patients with early rheumatoid arthritis. N Engl J Med 2000;243:1586–1593.

55. Mease PJ, Goffe BS, Metz J, VanderStoep A, Finck B, Burge DJ. Etanercept in the treatment of psoriatic arthritis and psoriasis: a randomized trial. Lancet 2000;356:385–390.

56. Weinblatt ME, Kremer JM, Bankhurst AD, Bulpitt KJ, Fleischmann RM, Fox RI, Jackson CG, Lange M, Burge DJ. A trial of etanercept, a recombinant tumor necrosis factor receptor/Fc fusion protein, in patients with rheumatoid arthritis receiving methotrexate. N Engl J Med 1999;340:253–259.

57. Knight DM, Trinh H, Le J, Siegel S, Shealy D, McDonough M, Scallon B, Moore MA, Vilcek J, Daddona P, et al. Construction and initial characterization of a mouse-human chimeric anti-TNF antibody. Mol Immunol 1993; 20:1443–1453.

58. Scallon BJ, Moore MA, Trinh H, Knight DM, Ghrayeb J. Chimeric anti-TNF monoclonal antibody cA2 binds recombinant transmembrane TNFa and activates immune effector functions. Cytokine 1995;7:251–259.

59. Siegel SA, Shealy DJ, Nakada MT, Le J, Woulfe DS, Probert L, Kollias G, Ghrayeb J, Vilcek J, Daddona PE. The mouse/human chimeric monoclonal antibody cA2 neutralizes TNF in vitro and protects transgenic mice from cachexia and TNF lethality *in vivo*. Cytokine 1995;7:15–25.

60. Ten Hove T, Van Montfrans C, Peppelenbosch MP, Van Deventer SJ. Infliximab treatment induces apoptosis of lamina propria T lymphocytes in Crohn's disease. Gut 2001;50:206–211.

61. Choy EHS, Panayi GS. Cytokine pathways and joint inflammation in rheumatoid arthritis. N Engl J Med 2001;344:907–916.

62. Lipsky PE, van der Heijde DM, St Clair EW, Furst DE, Breedveld FC, Kalden JR, Smolen JS, Weisman M, Emery P, Feldmann M, Harriman GR, Maini RN; Anti-Tumor Necrosis Factor Trial in Rheumatoid Arthritis with Concomitant Therapy Study Group. Infliximab and methotrexate in the treatment of rheumatoid arthritis. Anti-tumor necrosis factor trial in rheumatoid arthritis with concomitant therapy study group. N Engl J Med 2000;343:1594–1602.

63. Maini R, St Clair EW, Breedveld F, Furst D, Kalden J, Weisman M, Smolen J, Emery P, Harriman G, Feldmann M, Lipsky P. Infliximab (chimeric anti-tumour necrosis factor alpha monoclonal antibody) versus placebo in rheumatoid arthritis patients receiving concomitant methotrexate: a randomized phase III trial. ATTRACT study group. Lancet 1999;354:1932–1939.

64. Targan SR, Hanauer SB, van Deventer SJ, Mayer L, Present DH, Braakman T, DeWoody KL, Schaible TF, Rutgeerts PA. A short-term study of chimeric monoclonal antibody cA2 to tumor necrosis factor alpha for Crohn's disease. Crohn's disease cA2 study group. N Engl J Med 1997;337:1029–1035.

65. Hanauer SB, Feagan BG, Lichtenstein GR, Mayer LF, Schreiber S, Colombel JF, Rachmilewitz D, Wolf DC, Olson A, Bao W, Rutgeerts P, ACCENT I Study Group. Maintenance infliximab for Crohn's disease: the ACCENT I randomized trial. Lancet 2002;359:1541–1549.

66. Present DH, Rutgeerts P, Targan S, Hanauer SB, Mayer L, van Hogezand RA, Podolsky DK, Sands BE, Braakman T, DeWoody KL, Schaible TF, van Deventer SJ. Infliximab for the treatment of fistulas in patients with Crohn's disease. N Engl J Med 1999;340:1398–1405.

67. Vasiliauskas EA, Schaffer S, Dezenberg CV, et al. Collaborative experience of open-label infliximab in refractory pediatric Crohn's disease. Gastroenterology 2000;118(Suppl 2):A178.

68. Kugathusan S, Werlin SL, Martinez A, et al. Prolonged duration of response to infliximab in early but not late pediatric Crohn's disease. Am J Gastroenterology 2000;95:3189–3194.

69. Baldassano RN. Surpassing conventional therapies: the role of biologic therapy. J Pediatr Gastroenterol Nutr 2001;33:519–526.

70. Elliott MJ, Woo P, Charles P, Long-Fox A, Woody JN, Maini RN. Suppression of fever and the acute-phase response in a patient with juvenile

chronic arthritis treated with monoclonal antibody to tumour necrosis factor-alpha (cA2). Br J Rheumatol 1997;36:589–593.
71. Chey WY, Hussain A, Ryan C, Potter GD, Shah A. Infliximab for refractory ulcerative colitis. Am J Gastroenterol 2001;96:2373–2381.
72. Sands BE, Tremain WJ, Sandborn WJ, Rutgeerts PJ, Hanauer SB, Mayer L, Targan SR, Podolsky DK. Infliximab in the treatment of severe, steroid-refractory ulcerative colitis: a pilot study. Inflamm Bowel Dis 2001;7:83–88.
73. Mamula P, Markowitz JE, Brown KA, Hurd LB, Piccoli DA, Baldassano RN. Infliximab as a novel therapy for pediatric ulcerative colitis. J Pediatr Gastroenterol Nutr 2002;34:307–11.
74. Oh CS, Das KM, Gottlieb AB. Treatment with anti-tumor necrosis factor alpha monoclonal antibody dramatically decreases the clinical activity of psoriasis lesions. J Am Acad Dermatol 2000;42:829–830.
75. Gottlieb AB, Chaudhari U, Mulcahy LD, Li S, Dooley LT, Baker DG. Infliximab monotherapy provides rapid and sustained benefit for plaque-type psoriasis. J Amer Acad Dermatol, in press.
76. Fredrikksson T, Pettersson U. Severe psoriasis: oral therapy with a new retinoid. Dermatologica 1978;157:238–244.
77. Gottlieb AB, Masud S, Ramamurthi R, Abdulghani A, Romano P, Chaudhari U Dooley LT, Fasanmade AA, Wagner, CL. Pharmacodynamic and pharmacokinetic response to anti-tumor necrosis factor monoclonal antibody (Infliximab) treatment of moderate to severe psoriasis vulgaris. J Am Acad Dermatol 2003;48:68–75.
78. Felson D, Anderson J, Boers M, et al. Preliminary definition of improvement in rheumatoid arthritis. Arthritis Rheum 1995;38:727–735.
79. Stevens M. Infliximab in the treatment of psoriatic arthritis and psoriasis. Proc World Congress Dermatol July 2002;p2029.
80. Ogilvie AL, Antoni C, Dechant C. Treatment of psoriatic arthritis with anti-tumour necrosis factor-α antibody clears skin lesions or psoriasis resistant to treatment with methotrexate. Br J Dermatol 2001;144:587–589.
81. O'Quinn RP, Miller JL. The effectiveness of tumor necrosis factor antibody (infliximab) in treating recalcitrant psoriasis: a report of 2 cases. Arch Dermatol 2002;138:644–648.
82. Schaible TF. Long term safety of infliximab. Can J Gastroenterol 2000;14 (Suppl C):29C–32C.
83. Keane J, Gershon S, Wise R, Mirabile-Levens E, Kasznica J, Schwieterman WD, Siegel JN, Braun MM. Tuberculosis associated with infliximab, a TNF-alpha neutralizing agent. N Engl J Med 2001;345:1098–1104.
84. Parker SL, Tong T, Bolder S, Wingo P. Cancer statistics, 1997. CA Cancer J Clin 1997;47:5–27. (Erratum, CA Cancer J Clin 1997;47:68).
85. Schaible TF, Keenan GF, Hendricks DF, Tynan K, Curry S. The impact of a tuberculosis (TB) awareness education program on TB testing by physicians in a RA population. Proc Am Coll Rheumatol 2002 (abstract).

15
Treatment of Psoriasis Using Efalizumab

Craig L. Leonardi
St. Louis University School of Medicine, St. Louis, Missouri, U.S.A.

I. INTRODUCTION

Immunological studies have vastly improved our understanding of the pathogenesis of psoriasis. It is now clear that psoriasis results from an immunological response that involves multiple T-cell–mediated events (1, 2). A key element in the initiation and maintenance of this chronic disease involves T-cell activation. Full T-cell activation requires two events (3). The first involves presentation of antigen bound to the major histocompatibility complex (MHC) on the surface of the antigen-presenting cell (APC) to a T-cell receptor (TCR). The second is stabilization of the APC–T cell interaction through binding of secondary receptor–ligand pairs to form an immunological synapse (4).

Numerous receptor–ligand pathways have been implicated in the genesis of psoriasis, but one that has been well characterized is the interaction of lymphocyte function-associated antigen-1 (LFA-1) and intercellular adhesion molecule-1 (ICAM-1). LFA-1, a cell surface glycoprotein in the β_2 integrin receptor family, promotes intercellular adhesion in immunological and inflammatory reactions and also in T-cell activation (5, 6). LFA-1 is a heterodimeric protein with two subunits, a unique α subunit (CD11a) and a β subunit (CD18), and it is expressed on various cells types, including lymphocytes. ICAM-1, an adhesion molecule, is one of several ligands for LFA-1, and is thought to play an important role in psoriasis (5). A wide variety of in vitro findings have highlighted the importance of LFA-1 and ICAM-1 in the

333

pathogenesis of psoriasis and other inflammatory skin disorders. LFA-1 expression has been shown to be elevated on memory T cells, a factor that may influence T-cell response during restimulation (6). Also, although keratinocytes in patients with immunological skin disorders express ICAM-1, those found in healthy skin do not (7). In the early 1990s, research indicated that LFA-1/ICAM-1 interactions are a prerequisite for full T-cell activation by activating the T-cell costimulatory pathways (8). LFA-1/ICAM-1 interactions also promote the trafficking of inflammatory cells into the epidermis, a process that is common to various inflammatory skin diseases, including psoriasis (9). These findings have led to the hypothesis that the LFA-1/ICAM-1 pathway is an attractive target for immunosuppressive therapies in diseases of unknown antigenic origin, as in the case for psoriasis (10).

Efalizumab (Raptiva, anti-CD11a, or hu1124) is a humanized anti-CD11a monoclonal IgG_1 antibody. It is the humanized version of the murine antihuman CD11a monoclonal antibody MHM24 and has been shown to inhibit effectively various T-cell functions including target cell lysis, T-cell adhesion, T-cell activation, and T-cell proliferation (11, 12). Efalizumab was developed by grafting the murine complementarity-determining (CDR) hypervariable sequences into a human framework consisting of consensus human IgG_1 κ heavy and light chains (Fig. 1) (12). Efalizumab's binding affinity to CD11a and dissociation constants (Kd) are comparable to those of MHM24 (12). Humanized monoclonal antibodies are generally less immu-

Binding Site for CD11a

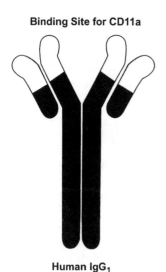

Human IgG₁

Figure 1   Structure of efalizumab.

nogenic, safer, and remain in the circulation longer than their murine counterparts (13).

By binding to CD11a and inhibiting LFA-1/ICAM-1 interactions, efalizumab is believed to modulate several of the key T-cell-mediated processes in the inflammatory cascade that ultimately results in psoriasis. As depicted in Figure 2, blockade of LFA-1/ICAM-1 pairing can inhibit binding of T cells to endothelial cells (12), decrease the trafficking of T cells from the circulation into the dermis (14, 15), and prevent activation of T cells (12). The net effect is to decrease the release of inflammatory mediators in the skin, causing restoration of normal phenotype.

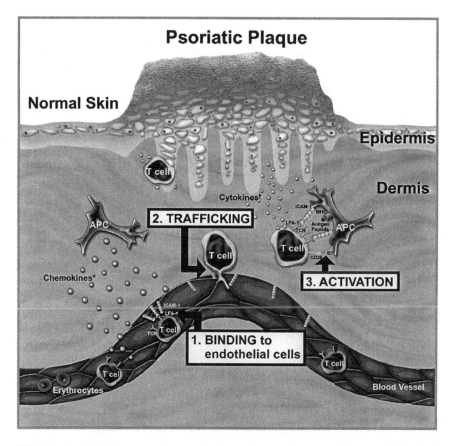

Figure 2 Critical steps in psoriasis pathogenesis targeted by efalizumab (simplified). APC, antigen-presenting cell; MHC, major histocompatibility complex; TCR, T-cell receptor.

II. SUMMARY OF PHASE I/II FINDINGS

Early clinical testing with efalizumab characterized the pharmacokinetic profile and provided immunobiological and histological evidence of activity in psoriasis patients. The pharmacokinetics and pharmacodynamics were determined in a dose-ranging study involving 31 psoriatic patients (16). The data showed that CD11a was saturated at an efalizumab concentration of 10 μg/ml, that CD11a expression on circulating lymphocytes rapidly decreased and remained decreased while efalizumab was detectable in the plasma, that CD11a expression returned to normal within 7–10 days of efalizumab clearance from plasma, and that antiefalizumab antibodies were not detected in any patients.

Next, the immunobiological and clinical effects of a single intravenous IV efalizumab infusion in psoriasis patients were explored (17). Dosages of efalizumab greater than 1.0 mg/kg resulted in complete blockade of CD11a staining in peripheral blood, and psoriatic plaques lasting at least 14 days. In addition, decreased epidermal thickness, decreased epidermal and dermal CD3+ T cells, and decreased ICAM-1 staining of keratinocytes and blood vessels in psoriatic plaques were observed. These data support the hypothesis that efalizumab inhibits T-cell trafficking *into* and decreases production of inflammatory cytokines *within* psoriatic lesions. Most important was that efalizumab resulted in clinical improvement as evidenced by a decreased psoriasis area and severity index (PASI) values compared to baseline. These, and other early findings provided proof of concept for the role of LFA-1/ICAM-1 interactions in the pathogenesis of psoriasis and demonstrated the correlation between CD11a downmodulation and clinical response (18).

A subcutaneous (SC) formulation of efalizumab was developed next to improve the convenience of administration. In an open-label phase I study, 57 patients received 8 weekly dosages of efalizumab ranging from 0.3 mg/kg/ wk to 2.0 mg/kg/week (19, 20). The mean half-life of SC efalizumab was 6.2 days and it was cleared from the plasma 3–5 weeks following the last dose. At the last dose, 55% and 64% of patients achieved ≥50% PASI improvement at the 1 and 2 mg/kg/week dosages respectively. In addition, 10% and 29% of patients achieved ≥75% PASI improvement at the 1 and 2 mg/kg/week dosages respectively. Roughly half of the patients demonstrated good or better improvement on the physician's global assessment (PGA). This clinical improvement was accompanied by decreased epidermal thickness, diminished dermal and epidermal T-cell infiltration, reduced keratinocyte K16 expression, and reduced CD11a expression on circulating T cells. The most frequent adverse events with this SC formulation were headache, pain, and rhinitis.

The safety and efficacy of 12 weeks of SC efalizumab were also evaluated in 61 patients with moderate to severe plaque psoriasis (21). At day 84, 90% of patients in the 1.0 mg/kg/wk and 70% in the 2.0 mg/kg/wk dosage groups experienced ≥50% PASI improvement. In addition, 30% of patients in the 1.0 mg/kg/wk group and 25% in the 2.0 mg/kg/wk group experienced ≥75% PASI improvement from baseline. Similar improvements in the good to better and excellent or better categories on PGA were observed for both dosage groups. Histological evidence confirmed the clinical activity and was consistent with observations in prior IV and SC studies. The adverse events were similar to those observed in prior SC studies and were primarily mild to moderate in severity. Given the evidence of clinical activity, safety and tolerability, and convenience associated with SC administration, the phase III trials evaluated the SC formulation.

III. PHASE III CLINICAL RESULTS

A. Study Design

Two phase III trials have recently been completed, and several more are underway to define further the optimal administration schedule for efalizumab. The results of these studies are being finalized and are expected to be published imminently. The safety and efficacy of efalizumab were evaluated in two phase III randomized, double-blind, parallel-group, placebo-controlled clinical trials involving more than 1000 patients. To qualify, patients must have had stable plaque psoriasis (PASI ≥12.0 and psoriatic body surface area [BSA] ≥10%) and were candidates for systemic therapy. Patients were randomized to receive SC efalizumab 1.0 mg/kg or 2.0 mg/kg or placebo weekly for 12 weeks (Fig. 3). Because these two studies had identical design

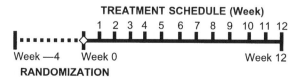

First Treatment (12 Weeks)
Randomized to either:
• Efalizumab
  • 1.0 mg/kg SC weekly (n = 394)
  • 2.0 mg/kg SC weekly (n = 409)
• Placebo (n = 292)

TREATMENT SCHEDULE (Week)
1 2 3 4 5 6 7 8 9 10 11 12
Week —4   Week 0   Week 12
RANDOMIZATION

Figure 3 Trial design.

for the first 12 weeks, the efficacy and safety data were pooled to provide a more precise estimation of outcome in a larger cohort of patients (22). A total of 1095 patients were randomized to efalizumab 1.0 mg/kg/wk (n = 394), efalizumab 2.0 mg/kg/week (n = 409), or placebo (n = 292) during the first 12 week treatment phase. At baseline, the treatment groups were well matched with respect to demographics and severity of disease.

B. Efficacy at 12 Weeks

Patients who received efalizumab experienced rapid clinical response as measured by PASI. The mean percentage PASI improvement in the efalizumab-treated patients began to diverge clearly from placebo by treatment day 14 (Fig. 4). A greater proportion of patients who received 1.0 mg/kg/wk or 2.0 mg/kg/wk efalizumab achieved ≥75% PASI improvement relative to baseline, compared to placebo (29.2% and 27.6%, respectively vs. 3.4) (Fig. 5). Although many studies utilize ≥75% PASI improvement as the primary efficacy measure, achieving ≥50% improvement in PASI scores is a clinically relevant and meaningful outcome that is worth careful evaluation. At 12 weeks, 55.6% and 54.5% of patients achieved ≥50% improvement in PASI at the 1.0 mg/kg/wk and 2.0 mg/kg/wk dosages, respectively (Fig. 5). In addition, the proportion of patients demonstrating improvement on secondary measures of efficacy, overall lesion severity (OLS) and PGA, was greater

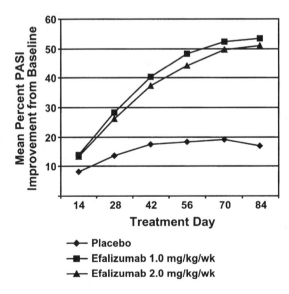

Figure 4 Percentage PASI improvement by visit (ACD2058g and ACD2059g).

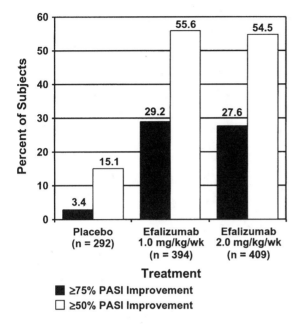

Figure 5 PASI improvement at 12 weeks (ACD2058g and ACD2059g).

in each efalizumab-treated group than in the placebo group (Fig. 6). Photos illustrating representative responses are shown in Figure 9.

C. Efficacy at 24 Weeks

Because psoriasis is a chronic disease requiring long-term treatment, a number of phase III trials have been designed to characterize the effects of continued efalizumab treatment and to determine the optimal dosing and administration schedule for long-term therapy. Trial ACD2059g evaluated the effects of an additional 12 weeks of efalizumab therapy and assessed the response to every other week dosing in patients achieving at least 50% PASI improvement at 12 weeks, to increasing the dosage for patients who had < 50% PASI improvement at 12 weeks, and to characterize the recurrence of psoriasis on abrupt discontinuation of efalizumab treatment.

Patients who were responders (≥75% PASI improvement) and partial responders (≥50% and < 75% PASI improvement) after 12 weeks of efalizumab treatment were rerandomized to an additional 12 weeks of treatment: efalizumab 2.0 mg/kg weekly, efalizumab 2.0 mg/kg every other week (qow), or placebo. For those patients who were nonresponders (< 50% PASI improvement) at 12 weeks, the efalizumab dosage was increased to 4.0 mg/kg

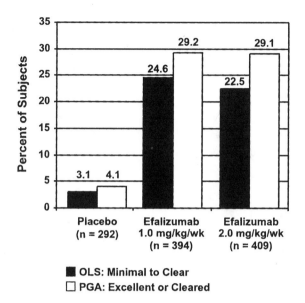

OLS: Minimal to Clear
PGA: Excellent or Cleared

Figure 6 Overall lesion severity (OLS) and PGA at 12 weeks (ACD2058g and ACD2059g).

weekly to determine whether continued treatment at a higher dosage could effect a response.

The results showed that extending treatment from 12 to 24 weeks both maintained the PASI responses achieved during the first 12-week treatment period and improved the response rate for those patients who had ≥50% and < 75% PASI improvement. In the responder group, an additional 12 weeks of efalizumab administered weekly or every other week maintained the ≥75% improvement in PASI scores achieved during the first 12 week treatment period. In addition, the majority of patients who received weekly and alternate-week efalizumab therapy achieved ≥50% PASI improvement at 24 weeks.

Of those patients who were partial responders (≥50% and < 75% PASI improvement) at week 12, extending the duration of efalizumab therapy increased the probability of their achieving ≥75% PASI improvement. While every other week dosing during extended treatment was sufficient to maintain the ≥75% PASI improvement the responders achieved at 12 weeks, for those subjects who achieved a partial response weekly efalizumab during extended treatment was more likely to result in ≥75% improvement in the PASI score. Finally, for those subjects who did not achieve a response (< 50% PASI improvement) after 12 weeks of treatment, increasing the dosage to 4.0 mg/kg weekly for an additional 12 weeks increased the likelihood of a response for some patients. Consistent with observations during the first 12 week treatment period, extended efalizumab treatment resulted in both maintenance and improvement of OLS and PGA responses for responders and partial responders, respectively.

The effects of efalizumab are reversible, and after cessation of therapy psoriasis returned with a median time to relapse (defined as loss of 50% of the PASI improvement) of 60–80 days (data on file, Genentech, Inc.). However, the trial design favored relapse because patients were abruptly discontinued from active therapy without taper or transition to alternative therapies as is typically seen in clinical settings. Throughout the efalizumab trials, some patients have shown exacerbation of psoriasis on quick withdrawal from active therapy. This rebound effect is similar to that seen when either cyclosporine or, to a lesser extent, methotrexate is abruptly discontinued. Several phase III studies are underway to determine the several strategies for withdrawal of efalizumab therapy. These approaches include slow tapering of efalizumab on a weekly basis, alternate week efalizumab dosing at standard dosages, and transition from efalizumab to other systemic agents in combination or rotation. Lastly, a trial now underway is evaluating the impact of more than 12 months of continuous therapy (see section below on prolonged efalizumab treatment).

D. Quality-of-Life Measures

Given the significant negative impact of psoriasis on quality of life, it is imperative that clinical trials assess quality of life in addition to the measures of clinical benefit. The impact of 12 weeks of efalizumab therapy on the patient-reported quality of life measures, dermatology life quality index (DLQI), and psoriasis symptom assessment (PSA) were pooled for the two phase III trials: ACD2058g and ACD2059g (23). The DLQI questionnaire measures the extent to which psoriasis affected quality of life during the previous week, with scores ranging from not at all to very much (24). The PSA scales, which were developed by Genentech, Inc., and based on the Skindex scale (25), assess the severity (ranging from never to always) and frequency (ranging from not at all to a great deal) of psoriasis symptoms. The pooled DLQI data revealed that at 12 weeks efalizumab-treated patients experienced significantly greater improvement in DLQI than those who received placebo. The mean improvement was greater in the 1.0 mg/kg/week and 2.0 mg/kg/week efalizumab groups (5.5 and 5.8, respectively vs. 1.9, $p < 0.001$) (Fig. 7). In addition, patients who received efalizumab reported greater improvement in the PSA frequency and severity scales than patients who received placebo (Fig. 8). The improvement in quality of life paralleled the improvements noted on the PASI, OLS, and PGA measures (Fig. 9).

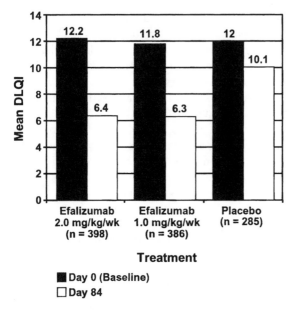

Figure 7 Dermatology life quality index (DLQI) improvement at 12 weeks (ACD2058g and ACD2059g).

E. Safety

Safety analyses demonstrated the safety and tolerability of SC efalizumab. Safety data from the first 12 weeks of the two phase III trials were pooled and evaluated. The adverse events most frequently reported included headache, nonspecific infection (e.g., common cold), nausea, chills, pain, and fever (Table 1) (22). Acute adverse events, defined as headache, chills, fever, nausea, vomiting, or myalgia that occurred on the day of injection or the following 2 days, occurred in 39% of all patients. Acute adverse events were most frequent following the first dose and were primarily mild to moderate in severity. The incidence of acute adverse events decreased with each subsequent dose. By the third dose, the overall incidence of acute adverse events was 5.1%, with no appreciable differences in incidence between the efalizumab and placebo groups (Fig. 10). Analysis of safety data from 24 weeks of efalizumab therapy from study ACD2059g indicates that, with the exception of the occurrence of acute adverse events, the 12 week and 24 week safety profiles were similar. During the second 12 week treatment period, the adverse event profile was similar to that of placebo (26, 27). The most common adverse events during the second 12 week treatment period were nonspecific infection (e.g., colds), psoriasis, headache, pain, rhinitis, pharyngitis, and

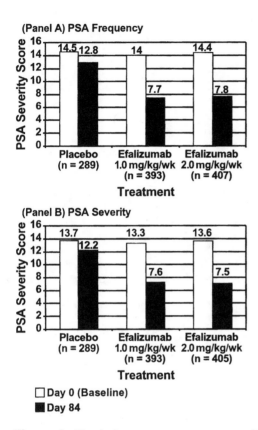

Figure 8 Psoriasis symptom assessment (PSA) improvement at 12 weeks (ACD2058g and ACD2059g). A. PSA frequency. B. PSA severity.

increased cough. Analysis of the psoriasis events indicated that more patients treated with placebo experienced psoriasis as an adverse event than did patients treated with efalizumab; fewer than 4% of efalizumab-treated patients reported psoriasis as an adverse event.

IV. PROLONGED EFALIZUMAB TREATMENT

It is likely that patients with psoriasis will derive the greatest clinical benefit from continuous efalizumab therapy. An open-label trial (ACD2243g) is assessing the safety, tolerability, and efficacy of 1–2 years of weekly SC efalizumab therapy in those patients who experience clinical benefit (defined as ≥50% PASI improvement) by day 84 (week 12). This trial is underway with

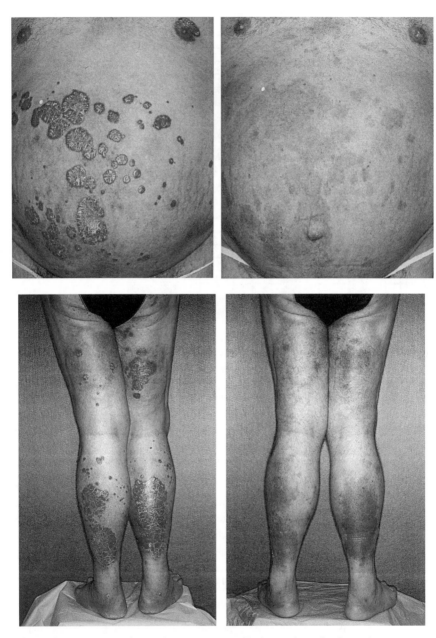

Figure 9   Representative patient responses. (Refer to the color insert.)

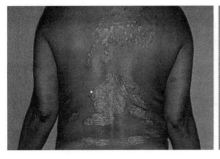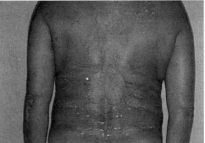

Figure 9 Continued

Table 1 Adverse events during first 12 weeks (ACD2058g and ACD2059g)

		Efalizumab	
Adverse Event	Placebo (%) (n = 292)	1.0 mg/kg/wk (%) (n = 396)	2.0 mg/kg/wk (%) (n = 407)
Headache	80 (27.4)	129 (32.6)	151 (37.1)
Infection, NOS	42 (14.4)	51 (12.9)	59 (14.5)
Nausea	27 (9.2)	48 (12.1)	56 (13.8)
Chills	13 (4.5)	58 (14.6)	53 (13.0)
Pain	20 (6.8)	56 (14.1)	45 (11.1)
Fever	15 (5.1)	39 (9.8)	46 (11.3)
Asthenia	24 (8.2)	34 (8.6)	38 (9.3)
Diarrhea	23 (7.9)	28 (7.1)	30 (7.4)
Myalgia	13 (4.5)	29 (7.3)	32 (7.9)
Pharyngitis	20 (6.8)	24 (6.1)	31 (7.6)
Accidental injury	15 (5.1)	28 (7.1)	27 (6.6)
Rhinitis	22 (7.5)	31 (7.8)	17 (4.2)
Back pain	6 (2.1)	20 (5.1)	25 (6.1)
Arthralgia	10 (3.4)	28 (7.1)	14 (3.4)
Dizziness	14 (4.8)	21 (5.3)	17 (4.2)
Peripheral edema	10 (3.4)	23 (5.8)	17 (4.2)
Pruritus	16 (5.5)	15 (3.8)	18 (4.4)
Sinusitis	7 (2.4)	22 (5.6)	14 (3.4)
Herpes simplex	15 (5.1)	18 (4.5)	25 (6.1)
Psoriasis	6 (2.1)	20 (5.1)	13 (3.2)

Includes all events occurring in ≥5% of any one group. Multiple occurrences of an event within a body system are counted once in the overall incidence.
NOS, not otherwise specified.

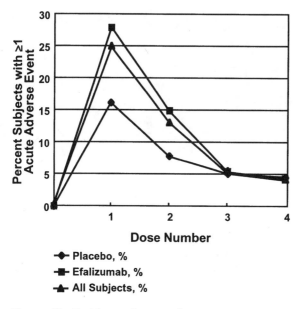

Figure 10   Incidence of acute adverse events.

more than 250 patients treated up to 1 year. Preliminary data from a cohort of patients who have completed 1 year of treatment was presented at the American Academy of Dermatology Annual Meeting 2002. These data indicate that approximately 80% of patients maintained ≥50% improvement in PASI scores for 1 year. These findings are preliminary in nature and they will be updated upon completion of the trial.

V. SUMMARY

Efalizumab represents a significant advance in the management of chronic plaque psoriasis. Several large phase III trials have demonstrated both safety and efficacy in both short- and long-term settings. With only slight increases in lymphocyte and white blood cells (WBC) counts during treatment, it is unlikely that any laboratory testing will be required to evaluate patients on efalizumab therapy. To date, there has been no evidence of drug interactions or organ toxicity (data on file, Genentech, Inc.).

With several biological agents in clinical development, it will be important to define how they should be used, to determine which patients are candidates for biological therapies, and to determine how these new therapies are to be administered. With efalizumab, the subcutaneous mode of delivery and the possibility of every other week dosing to maintain an established response offer patients a new level of dosing convenience.

Although efalizumab trials have enrolled only those patients with a PASI ≥ 12.0 and psoriatic BSA $\geq 10\%$, it is anticipated that patients with moderate to severe plaque psoriasis who have failed to respond to conventional therapies (systemic and/or phototherapy) and those patients who are not candidates for conventional therapies due to toxicity or tolerability limitations may derive clinical benefit from efalizumab therapy. In addition, patients with limited psoriasis whose disease has repeatedly failed to respond to conventional therapies also may achieve some measure of clinical benefit with efalizumab therapy.

The long-term efficacy of traditional psoriasis therapies is limited by a variety of factors including toxicity, inconvenient administration schedules or procedures, the need for specialized equipment, and noncompliance. These factors highlight the need for safer and effective therapies that can be administered long-term. Efalizumab represents an exciting potential addition to the management of psoriasis. Studies completed to date demonstrate that efalizumab has a rapid onset of action, results in significant benefit on measures of disease activity and quality-of-life measures, is convenient, and is safe and well tolerated. Clinical trials now underway will serve to define further the role of efalizumab in the management of psoriasis.

VI. PRACTICAL CONSIDERATIONS FOR USING EFALIZUMAB IN THE TREATMENT OF PSORIASIS

1. Patients should be educated in reconstitution of drug and self-administration by SC injection. Services will be provided when the product is marketed to assist with educational resources.
2. Stress compliance with the weekly dosing regimen. Efalizumab is a suppressive therapy that must be dosed continuously. Any changes in continuous therapy should be made under the careful direction of the prescribing doctor.
3. Efalizumab should be stored in the refrigerator. When released, the packaging will likely contain all items required for administration (syringe, needles, diluent, alcohol pads, instructions, phone numbers for assistance, etc).
4. A conditioning dose (0.7 mg/kg) is administered in the office on week 1 and the patient observed for 30 min. Should adverse events such as headache or myalgia occur in the first 24–48 h, expect them to be mild, transient, and easily managed with over-the-counter analgesics such as ibuprofen. These symptoms are usually not experienced after the second dose.

5. Continuous dosing at 1.0 mg/kg/week commences at the second dose. Patients should be instructed to rotate injection sites each week (e.g., arm → leg → abdomen).

6. Responders begin to experience clinical benefit as early as 2–4 weeks. Concomitant therapies (e.g., topicals) can be discontinued at the physician's discretion.

7. Patients achieving 50% improvement by week 12 may show continued response with additional 12 weeks of therapy. However, nonresponders at 24 weeks will require alternative treatments.

8. Once long-term control has been achieved, patients will occasionally experience breakthrough disease. Increasing the dosage of efalizumab to 2.0 mg/kg/week may be of benefit during these episodes. Once control has been re-established, it is usually possible to reduce the dosage back to 1.0 mg/kg/week.

9. A standard schedule for follow-up appointments has not been established. Since a need for continuous laboratory testing is not anticipated, patients may only have to be seen every 3–6 months to address specific concerns (e.g., resistant areas such as elbows, knees, scalp).

10. If efalizumab needs to be discontinued, alternative therapy should be instituted. Although rebound has been seen in a minority of patients, it always occurred in the setting of abrupt discontinuation, as was required in the trials. In practice, patients with moderate–severe psoriasis should be transitioned gradually onto an alternative therapy.

REFERENCES

1. Nickoloff BJ. The immunologic and genetic basis of psoriasis. Arch Dermatol 1999; 135:1104–1110.

2. Bos JD, De Rie MA. The pathogenesis of psoriasis: immunological facts and speculations. Immunol Today 1999; 20:40–46.

3. Reiser H, Stadecker MJ. Costimulatory B7 molecules in the pathogenesis of infectious and autoimmune disease. N Engl J Med 1996; 335:1369–1377.

4. Grakoui A, Bromley SK, Sumen C, Davis MM, Shaw AS, Allen PM, et al. The immunological synapse: A molecular machine controlling T cell activation. Science 1999;285:221–227.

5. Marlin SD, Springer TA. Purified intercellular adhesion molecule-1 (ICAM-1) is a ligand for lymphocyte function-associated antigen 1 (LFA-1). Cell 1987; 51:813–819.

6. Sanders ME, Makgoba MW, Sharrow SO, Stephany D, Springer TA, Young

HA, Shaw S. Human memory T lymphocytes express increased levels of three cell adhesion molecules (LFA-3, CD2, and LFA-1) and three other molecules (UCHL1, CDw29, and Pgp-1) and have enhanced IFN-γ production. J Immunol 1988; 140:1401–1407.

7. Nickoloff BJ, Basham TY, Merigan TC, Morhenn VB. Keratinocyte class II histocompatibility antigen expression. Br J Dermatol 1985; 112:373–374.

8. van Seventer GA, Shimizu Y, Horgan KJ, Luce GE, Webb D, Shaw S. Remote T cell co-stimulation via LFA-1/ICAM-1 and CD2/LFA-3: demonstration with immobilized ligand/mAb and implication in monocyte-mediated co-stimulation. Eur J Immunol 1991; 21:1711–1718.

9. Nickoloff BJ, Griffiths CEM, Barker JNWN. The role of adhesion molecules, chemotactic factors, and cytokines in inflammatory and neoplastic skin disease—1990 update. J Invest Dermatol 1990; 94:151S–157S.

10. Nickoloff BJ, Mitra RS, Green J, Zheng X-G, Shimizu Y, Thompson C, Turka LA. Accessory cell function of keratinocytes for superantigens. J Immunol 1993; 150:2148–2159.

11. Hildreth JE, Gotch FM, Hildreth PD, McMichael AJ. A human lymphocyte-associated antigen involved in cell-mediated lympholysis. Eur J Immunol 1983; 13:202–208.

12. Werther WA, Gonzalez TN, O'Connor SJ, McCabe S, Chan B, Hotaling T, Champe M, Fox JA, Jardieu PM, Berman PW, Presta LG. Humanization of an anti-lymphocyte function-associated antigen (LFA)-1 monoclonal antibody and reengineering of the humanized antibody for binding to rhesus LFA-1. J Immunol 1996; 157:4986–4995.

13. Klingbeil C, Hsu DH. Pharmacology and safety assessment of humanized monoclonal antibodies for therapeutic use. Toxicol Pathol 1999; 27:1–3.

14. Krueger J, Gottlieb A, Miller B, et al. Anti-CD11a treatment for psoriasis concurrently increases circulating T-cells and decreases plaque T-cells, consistent with inhibition of cutaneous T-cell trafficking. *J Invest Dermatol* 2000;115:333.

15. Lowe J, Stefanich E, Rangell L, Pippig S. Efalizumab (anti-CD11a) inhibits transendothelial migration of T cells. Poster Presented at Society of Investigative Dermatology, Los Angeles, California, May 15–18, 2002.

16. Bauer RJ, Dedrick RL, White ML, Murray MJ, Garovoy MR. Population pharmacokinetics and pharmacodynamics of the anti-CD11a antibody hu1124 in human patients with psoriasis. J Pharmacokinet Biopharm 1999; 27:397–420.

17. Gottlieb A, Krueger JG, Bright R, Ling M, Lebwohl M, Kang S, Feldman S, Spellman M, Wittkowski K, Ochs HD, Jardieu P, Bauer R, White M, Dedrick R, Garovoy M. Effects of administration of a single dose of humanized monoclonal antibody to CD11a on the immunobiology and clinical activity of psoriasis. J Am Acad Dermatol 2000; 42:428–435.

18. Papp K, Bissonnette R, Krueger JG, Carey W, Gratton D, Gulliver WP, Lui H, Lynde CW, Magee A, Minier D, Ouellet JP, Patel P, Shapiro J, Shear NH, Kramer S, Walicke P, Bauer R, Dedrick RL, Kim SS, White M, Garovoy M.

The treatment of moderate to severe plaque psoriasis with a new anti-CD11a monoclonal antibody. J Am Acad Dermatol 2001; 45:665–674.

19. Gottlieb AB, Miller B, Chaudhari U, Oh C, Sherr A, Solodkina G, et al. Clinical and histologic effects of subcutaneously administered anti-CD11a (hu1124) in patients with psoriasis. Poster Presented at Society of Investigative Dermatology, Chicago Illinois, May 10, 1999.

20. Dummer W, Joshi A, Beyer J, Garovoy M, Dedrick R, Krueger J, Gottlieb AB, Bauer RJ. Pharmacodynamic effects of subcutaneous (SC) administration of efalizumab (anti-CD11a). 60th Annual Meeting of the American Academy of Dermatology, New Orleans, LA, Feb 22–27, 2002.

21. Leonardi CL, Gottlieb AB, Miller B, Tashjian D, Pariser D, Shapiro W, et al. Efalizumab (anti-CD11a): results of a 12 week trial of subcutaneous administration in patients with moderate to severe plaque psoriasis. Poster Presented at American Association of Dermatology, Washington D.C., March 2–7, 2001.

22. Menter A, Bissonnette R, Gottlieb AB, Goffe B, Beutner KR, Dunlap R, Magee A, Dummer W, Papp KA. Subcutaneous efalizumab (anti-CD11a) provides rapid clinical response in patients with moderate to severe plaque psoriasis. 60th Annual Meeting of the American Academy of Dermatology, New Orleans, LA, Feb 22–27, 2002.

23. Gottlieb AB, Papp KA, Lynde CW, Carey W, Powers J, Rist TE, Rafal E, McCune M, Shear NH, Ouellet JP, Walicke P, Compton P, Tyring S, Garovoy M, Leonardi C. Subcutaneous efalizumab (anti-CD11a) is effective in the treatment of moderate to severe plaque psoriasis: pooled results of 2 phase III clinical trials. 60th Annual Meeting of the American Academy of Dermatology, New Orleans, LA, Feb 22–27, 2002.

24. Finlay AY, Khan GK. Dermatology Life Quality Index (DLQI)—a simple practical measure for routine use. Clin Exp Dermatol 1994;19:210–216.

25. Chren MM, Lasek RJ, Quinn LM, Mostow EN, Zyzanski SJ. Skindex, a quality-of-life measure for patients with skin disease: reliability, validity, and responsiveness. J Invest Dermatol 1996;107:707–713.

26. Gordon KB, Leonardi C, Harvey D, Powers J, Phillips H, Weinstein GD, Compton P, Dummer W, Lowe N. Continuous treatment improves outcomes in patients with moderate to severe plaque psoriasis treated with subcutaneous (SC) efalizumab (anti-CD11a): results from the phase III trial ACD2058g. 60th Annual Meeting of the American Academy of Dermatology, New Orleans, LA, Feb 22–27, 2002.

27. Lebwohl M, Miller JL, Goldman M, Henderson D, Nelson C, Wolf D, Chambers M, Gilbert M, Farber H, Clark S, Edwards L, Stein LF, Wang X, Dummer W, Koo JY. Continued treatment with subcutaneous efalizumab (anti-CD11a) improves outcome in patients with moderate to severe plaque psoriasis. 60th Annual Meeting of the American Academy of Dermatology, New Orleans, LA, Feb 22–27, 2002.

Index